Giandomenico Partipilo

LOGICALLY C

A Rational Introduction To Vitamin C

Hardcover ISBN: 978-1-967828-94-4

Paperback ISBN: 978-1-967828-96-8

Published by:

Pine Book Writing

www.PineBookWriting.com

R-10225 Yonge St Suite #250, Richmond Hill, ON L4C 3B2, Canada.

Printed in the United States of America

This work is dedicated to my guiding light, Vipar, whose vivid wisdom lives on in me, illuminated by his ever-penetrating gaze.

To his brother, my father Raffaele, also known as "The Vitamin C Man", goes my deepest dedication, along with a part of myself. Without him, nothing would have been possible.

Dulcis in fundo, my beloved wife Angelica. To her goes everything I have, including my admiration for having always believed in me.

Special thanks go to the rest of my family, especially my mother Domenica, my brother Gaetano, and my ever-punctual alarm clock, Rio.

Equally heartfelt is my gratitude to the shining Hyakutake, an irreplaceable source of unconditional inspiration.

A huge thank you is also due to all those who support me unceasingly.

And again, my thoughts can only go to the true Hero of our times, the incomparable Dr. Atsuo Yanagisawa. Thank you for the wonderful preface and for believing in me.

Special thanks go to Professor Adolfo Panfili, Linus Pauling's pupil and worthy successor to his work, and to Dr. Paul Marik, the courageous pioneer in the use of vitamin C for the treatment of sepsis.

Adriano Abrusci, Ennio Abrusci, Vito Campanale, Giovanna Gemmato, Vittoriana Laquale, Maria Mitolo, Giovanni Monfreda, Piero Notarnicola with his assistant "Dino Word", Mario Pugliese and Lorenzo Vaiani. Thank you very much for your valuable contribution.

Special thanks also go to those who impeccably structured this new edition, Claudio Lippi and Simona Scarpati. Thanks to Claudio for the professionalism and great adaptability. Thanks to Simona, an extraordinary mind who fully grasped the essence and potential depth of my work.

And thank you too, Foresta Mercadante, for listening with such respectful attention to my daily introspections, gently wiping away those invisible tears imprinted in my heart.

Legal note

The information contained in this monograph is provided for general educational and informational purposes only. It does not constitute medical advice, diagnosis, prevention, or treatment of any disease, and should not be considered a substitute for the doctor–patient relationship or for professional medical consultation.

Before making any decisions regarding your health — including any changes to diet, supplementation, or lifestyle — you should always seek the advice of a qualified healthcare professional. The author of this book is not a medical doctor. While the text cites scientific studies, medical literature, and statements from physicians, these are presented for informational purposes only. The author assumes no responsibility for how individual readers choose to use the information provided.

Technical note

This book is the English translation of the Italian volume 'Logicamente C, un'introduzione razionale alla vitamina C', published in Italy in 2023 by Youcanprint. In addition to the English translation, this edition includes updates with the most recent and relevant studies on the subject. As this is a translated work, some minor grammatical or stylistic imperfections may remain despite careful editing.

Preface

Health is an essential requirement for our well-being and that of our families, friends, and, above all, those who represent the next generation, our children. Food and essential nutrients are fundamental for maintaining a healthy body and fighting disease. Dr. Linus Pauling, a two-time Nobel Prize winner, once stated: "Almost all diseases can be traced to a nutritional deficiency".

As President of the International Society for Orthomolecular Medicine, I have traveled the world and worked with many scientists, doctors, naturopaths, and other experts in nutritional therapy to share the incredible benefits of orthomolecular nutritional therapy.

Orthomolecular Medicine aims to prevent and treat disease by optimizing the use of all substances that are naturally required by the human body. This means we can prevent and cure diseases and maintain ideal health through an appropriate diet, strengthened by the addition of vitamins, minerals, essential fats, and amino acids.

We consider vitamin C a special nutrient in orthomolecular medicine. Historically, vitamin C has protected human health from various bacterial and viral infections, cancer, chronic diseases, and even neuropsychiatric disorders. During the incident at the Fukushima nuclear power plant in Japan in March 2011, vitamin C proved to be the most effective weapon to defend our bodies from radiation. More recently, it has been shown that vitamin C can save the lives of people suffering from sepsis and severe COVID-19 infections.

Giandomenico Partipilo has published a new book on vitamin C titled "Logically C, a rational introduction to vitamin C". Partipilo became interested in vitamin C shortly before his father's serious illness was resolved thanks to a multifaceted therapeutic approach, in which the pharmacological intervention with vitamin C presumably played a crucial role. Since then, vitamin C has become an important part of Partipilo's career as a naturopath and science communicator. Partipilo has dedicated many years to researching vitamin C and has acquired a deep understanding of the subject. His book explores the historical background, the atypical pharmacokinetics, and the multifaceted physiology of vitamin C, as well as the incredible health benefits this molecule can offer, representing the culmination of his knowledge on the topic.

The book captures all the essential knowledge acquired on vitamin C with accuracy and effectiveness. I believe this work should not be limited to the Italian language. It deserves to be translated into English and other languages, making it available to healthcare professionals around the world. We know that some doctors and scholars remain skeptical about this field of medicine. This treatise will spread such an objective scientific truth about vitamin C that it will dispel any possible doubts.

We are living through turbulent times. And in restless times, conventional values change drastically, and familiar ways of thinking no longer function as they should. The COVID-19 pandemic has brought major changes, affecting our health, lifestyles, and even the economy. Many people feel lost, uncertain about the best ways to protect themselves and their families. It is in such moments that a hero often emerges, becoming a guide for many. I am convinced that Partipilo is one of those heroes. His book will serve as a reference key for vitamin C in the years to come.

Atsuo Yanagisawa, M.D., Ph.D.
President,
International Society for Orthomolecular Medicine

Table of contents

Introduction

It was a mild afternoon, wrapped in an ambiguous atmosphere seemingly designed to cause confusion. It was a carefully crafted illusion in which the supposed victim, a calendar about to close October's chapter, appeared to prevail without hesitation. Precisely the kind of absolute certainty that true Science, aware of its own limits, should always avoid.

Let us return to a precise moment that afternoon. As the sun was inexorably relinquishing its strength in favour of a typically October-like display of colours, something unexpected happened. A new sensation pervaded my body, completely trapped in the swirling storms of adolescence. A spark-like sensation, which was the cause of the subsequent fire in which the protagonist longed for nothing more than the advent of such an imposing blaze to regain vigour.

As is often the case, however, looking inside oneself is complicated, and my case was no exception. The lack of introspection, a victim perhaps of a carefree age, was then unexpectedly counteracted by a sudden and unexpected flash of lightning, a flash that illuminated everything inside me. It was thus that a passion for Mathematics was born, which in time turned into a veneration. Yes, veneration, because Mathematics is a subject "in which we never know what we are talking about, nor whether what we are saying is true" (incidentally, do you have a better definition than the one proposed by the mathematician Bertrand Russell?) but which at the same time, according to the mathematician, "possesses not only Truth, but also Supreme Beauty".

A book on vitamin C starting with math? Definitely unusual!

Just think, before I was swept away by the devastating effects of a cyclone so violent that it broke down all resistance, my desire to understand the essence of Mathematics had allowed me to achieve interesting scientific results in a specific branch called "Number theory". Regarding this Number theory, improperly named Higher Arithmetic and surprisingly linked to unusual mathematical areas unrelated to Elementary Arithmetic, C. F. Gauss, also called "Princeps mathematicorum" (Prince of Mathematicians), was one of the most prolific, versatile, and profound mathematicians ever. He also lived an extraordinary childhood. Suffice it to say that at the age of 8, he was among the Greatest: in response to an impossible school assignment, he calculated the sum of the first hundred positive integers in a few seconds using a very original technique. He did this by exploiting the main characteristic of mathematicians, namely imagination, so that he could see the chain of fifty equalities of the type 1+100=2+99=3+98…, astounding the world.

He often liked to say that "Mathematics is the Queen of Sciences and the Theory of Numbers is the Queen of Mathematics". It is a doubly powerful statement that conveys some interesting truths. First of all, it shows the extreme importance Gauss attributed to a branch, Number Theory, that appears "elementary" but is in fact one of the most complicated areas of Mathematics. Although it may seem devoid of practical implications, Number Theory is actually fundamental. The theory of prime numbers, for example, lies at the basis of Cryptography, the scientific field that protects data through special techniques of message representation.

Here we introduce one of the many appearances that deceive, a misleading version that has also polluted the environment that hosts the living being vitamin C, to such an extent as to cause heavy structural modifications reflecting an abstruse paradigm whose simplicity could stage tragicomic spectacles. A simplicity that could then be mistaken for banality, thus obscuring the extraordinary virtues that distance the molecule from an elementary nutrient.

But Gauss' words also make explicit another reality, probably even more interesting and of broader scope, which Galileo Galilei captured in the statement: "Nature is a book written in mathematical characters". To avoid an albeit useful, yet potentially misleading discussion of the countless arguments that support the words of the Pisan scientist, let me give you just one example. Around 200 B.C., Apollonius of Perga studied the properties of certain geometric curves. Eighteen centuries later, those very curves enabled Kepler to mathematically describe the motion of the planets around the Sun. The reference is, of course, to conics, and in particular to the ellipse. In this light, the meaning of Logically C might already appear clearer.

It is therefore no exaggeration to say that mathematical language stands as the only true tool for a full understanding of the laws that govern the entire Universe (a genuine key to accessing knowledge), an understanding that the reality of facts has shown to be characterised by a multi-level scale, the high levels of which necessarily require the help of logic.

It may seem trivial, but even the vitamin C planet is immersed in the Universe and cannot escape the general laws that decree its fate. This necessarily requires the integration of logical criteria in all scientific evaluations that claim to be profound, which is the only way to produce an analysis striving for maximum precision.

The long and troubled history of vitamin C, a molecule that I am as madly in love with as the Number Theory, cannot therefore be correctly interpreted without an adequate logical, almost mathematical view, i.e. a lucid exploration of the immense space that hosts the vast and heterogeneous scientific research on the subject. Despite being uneven, this research is so productive that it requires a laborious interpretative design capable of placing the numerous results obtained in the most appropriate dimension. In short, my work aims to be a harmonious and well-structured project. Initiated a few years ago through the study of holistic and naturopathic disciplines and strengthened by a mathematical spirit, my work can be likened to a probe that seeks to fathom the scientific literature in order to assess human health from the perspective of vitamin C. It is a kind of functional mapping, an attempt to rationalise the enormous amount of data accumulated over almost 100 years of research. The aim of this project is to compact the many fragmentary evaluations that have marked the qualities of vitamin C in the various medical fields, in order to derive general principles to propose for future research. And speaking of principles, one will note the value of Stone's formidable insights, according to which many pathological states are linked to vitamin C deficiency (a rather ambiguous term, around which practically the whole point of the book revolves).

Overall, my project is a complex one, and its realisation was made possible by two elements of great value. Firstly, objectivity: I believe that scientific literature is the only tool that allows an evaluation based on objective, rational and therefore scientific criteria. This is extremely important because, as a professional naturopath and holistic practitioner who has developed a deep passion for the subject, it provides credibility in a field where some may remain sceptical. Just like the algebraic identity $a^2 - b^2 = (a - b)(a + b)$, the Fundamental Theorem of Calculus, or Newton's Third Law of Motion, these are scientific principles accessible to mathematicians, biologists, doctors, engineers, sculptors, and beauticians; in short, they are available to everyone and therefore belong to everyone. Although it may seem risky to compare Medicine to Mathematics, I think the concept is nevertheless functional. In one example we find the equivalence "Pythagoras' theorem is true = It has been preliminarily demonstrated that vitamin C can exert an antitumour action, which is moreover selective and therefore non-toxic". This equivalence is not supported by me, nor by the greengrocer Michele or Dr Emanuele, but by the neutrality of the scientific literature! It is an equivalence that has a dual purpose: to help understand the nature of my book and to propose some relevant considerations that will often sound like a refrain.

In the second place, we find the critical analysis of the literature, which is indispensable in order to avoid any personal opinion, producing a sort of mathematisation of the problem that will make it possible to identify certain elements that can be traced back to the troubled events involving the legendary pioneers of vitamin C, among whom we also mention two Nobel Prize winners. In the perimeter of some contaminated soil, these elements had to counteract a fog created by the eccentric, drug-like nature of vitamin C. A rather atypical nature that is often misunderstood and easily lends itself to dysfunctional interpretations, especially in all those conceptual dives characterised by a lack of logic. Thus, in the course of the book, it will become increasingly clear that a lucid framing of vitamin C issues is conditional on the availability of a sufficient dose of "logical reasoning", indispensable to avoid misinterpretations that could lead to embarrassing misunderstandings.

Here is a significant example: it will be noted that the proposition "Vitamin C does not cure the disease M" is meaningless, whatever the subject M may be. This arises from the great approximation surrounding the therapeutic object when it is unhappily presented in the form "vitamin C", a vagueness that has nothing to do with the scientific approach. And this, obliquely, does not necessarily imply the exact opposite, namely that vitamin C can cure all diseases. A proper logical framing, in fact, suggests that excluding its specific efficacy constitutes one of the most difficult operations in the entire scientific world. And we shall demonstrate this through the immense power of logic.

The systematisation of knowledge on vitamin C, an indispensable ingredient for achieving the book's true objective (we will discover this later), will also grant, almost as a parallel effect, the opportunity to delve deeper into what vitamin C really is, how it works and is absorbed by the body, how it acts in conditions of disease, exactly as any reclassification requires full mastery of the elements to be reordered. All of this would have been impossible without the mediation of that refined probe, the vehicle for a progressive accumulation of information through which the best tools have been prepared to estimate with great precision the true scientific weight of our protagonist. After all, it's all about weight.

All that remains is to fasten your seatbelts (vitamin C, above all, represents safety) and embark on this long journey. Along the way, you will be consistently guided by the wisdom of a map that, while not perfect, reflects the most up-to-date knowledge (the scientific literature), accompanied by a logical commentary framework to which I will devote my full effort.

However, this personal commitment is also something more, perhaps even more ambitious: as with the most meaningful journeys, the kind that leave a lasting mark, my hope is that this one may spark a change within you by the time it concludes. Ideally, the reading will awaken whatever lies dormant or unconsciously neglected. The goal, then, is to catch a series of subtle signals that may prove decisive, just like the flash of lightning on that October afternoon that shaped my own path.

Chapter 1
The Dawn Of Vitamin C

Scurvy and the discovery of vitamin C

There is only one solution, as mathematicians studying the so-called existence and uniqueness theorems would say, that can unite a group of elements such as gingivitis, slow wound healing, edema, anaemia, pneumonia, asthenia, fatigue, haemorrhages, muscle and joint pain and, lastly, some peculiar neurological manifestations, the latter typically appearing at a more advanced stage. The apparently abstruse equation is resolved by a solution called scurvy, a little-known but potentially deadly disorder.

Dubbed "the sailors' disease", scurvy has shown its deadly nature time and again throughout history, with unfortunate sailors serving as ideal victims. Its aggressiveness caused more deaths than shipwrecks or naval battles. One striking example is Magellan's famous circumnavigation (1519-1522), during which an estimated 80% of the crew died of scurvy.

The earliest historical mentions, dating back to 1500 B.C., and the works of Hippocrates show that its existence has been known for a long time, although the issue has only been scientifically addressed since the 1700s, when its great harmfulness was realised. It is, therefore, an ancient disease long misunderstood.

Some attempts to rationalise the problem can be found in the Elizabethan age, when various empirical procedures based on bread, meat and grape juice were used to try to control the increasingly aggressive disease. Despite the disappointing results, these efforts led to the idea, which would become increasingly popular later on, that nutrition was related to scurvy. But why sailors in particular?

While the increasing number of voyages by European explorers, concentrated particularly between 1500 and 1800, made it possible to derive the first useful elements for sketching an aetiological model, this inevitably led to sailors becoming progressively more vulnerable to the deadly consequences of the disease.

The tangled puzzle would only partially settle in 1605, when the enterprising East India Company ventured on a voyage to those very lands. A small breakthrough was achieved. A single act of endurance, in fact, proved capable of preventing scurvy during the long crossing. It was a new strategy devised by Captain Lancaster, namely the supply of lemon juice, a supply that would allow his men, and only his men, to escape danger. This was a crucial strategy, so important that for the first time it steered assumptions about the causes of scurvy in a definite direction, thus integrating a series of ideas that had previously appeared completely unconnected.

John Woodall, the expedition's chief physician, is credited with organising what we might call the first systematic view of the matter, built on the invaluable experiences that would later give rise to his illuminating treatise "The Surgeon's Mate". The use of lemon juice as an anti-scurvy therapy is how one can summarise the main recommendation in the manual, which represented a remarkable step forward in the fight against the disease.

However, the decisive breakthrough would come from another personality, the figure who will always be remembered for providing the first pioneering knowledge on vitamin C.

Here we encounter an interesting first digression. The history of science teaches us that it often takes a genius to effect a change of course in the troubled navigations toward solving the most complex problems, and the case of understanding the aetiological mechanisms of scurvy was no exception. This genius is the extraordinary Dr. James Lind, a name that, with a little more luck, might have been placed alongside scientists such as Archimedes, Einstein, Golgi, Newton, Pauling, Curie, Euler, and Pasteur.

Gauss, as you can see, is not included in this prestigious list because he is regarded as an unparalleled genius, so exceptional that he stands apart from all other great minds. Possible exceptions might include the tormented Ettore Majorana, the brilliant and troubled physicist who disappeared after foreseeing the dire consequences of the research he conducted with the renowned "Boys of Via Panisperna". Their work later contributed to the tragic development of the atomic bomb. Another is the mystical, self-taught Indian mathematician Srinivasa Ramanujan. The story of Srinivasa Ramanujan is one that everyone should know, not only because it is inspiring and moving, but above all because it still highlights a narrative in which Science and Faith appear sinuously intertwined in a powerful union. Ramanujan, discoverer of a multitude of highly original theorems, agreed with Gauss, who famously said that "God does Arithmetic", by repeatedly declaring that "An equation for me has no meaning unless it expresses a thought of God".

Returning to Lind's genius: born in 1716 in Scotland to a wealthy bourgeois family, he was a member of the Royal Navy from 1739 to 1748 and later served as a physician at the Royal Naval Hospital in Haslar from 1758 to 1783, a period in which he mainly worked on preventive medicine.

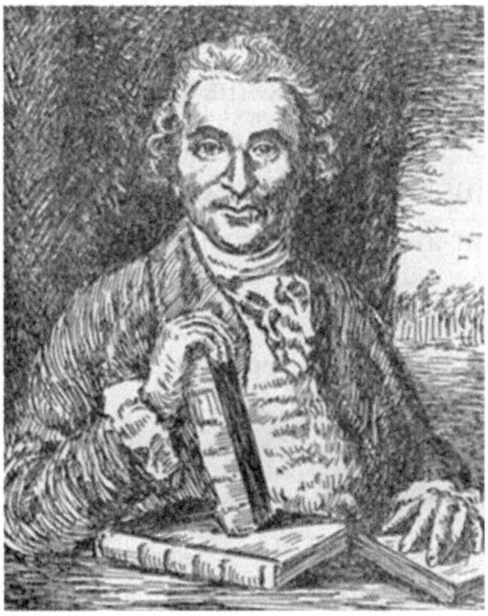

James Lind

Those were the hardest times, when naval expeditions were on the increase and fatally causing growing numbers of deaths because of the disease; this caught the attention of Lind himself and of most physicians, scientists and statisticians. The scurvy epidemic continued unabated due to the substantial lack of scientific evidence supporting the link with lemon juice, despite the promising insights of Lancaster and Woodall. Yet this was precisely the gap that Lind set out to fill, leaving a profound mark on the whole matter. Like his colleagues, he was powerless against the devastating effects of the disease, often exacerbated by the harsh conditions of long sea voyages, such as severe weather, exhausting labor, and malnutrition. He decided to tackle the problem with an original approach that would prove to be crucial.

Lind's work describes a very powerful dynamic that often occurs in scientific research, where solving a complex problem may require the use of unconventional tools, independent and not bound to the gravitational field revolving around the problem. These tools are often so extraordinary that they overshadow the initial problem, revealing new insights that appear secondary only until the problem is solved. One of the most valuable examples can be found in Fermat's renowned Last Theorem: the French mathematician Pierre de Fermat formulated it in 1637, but it took 358 years for Andrew Wiles to provide a complete proof, using highly sophisticated mathematical techniques. What appeared to be a minor arithmetic theorem (the equation $x^n + y^n = z^n$ has no positive integer solutions for $n > 2$) ultimately generated a wealth of profound and innovative mathematical concepts.

Returning to Lind. Before describing his experiment on scurvy, it is worth insisting on the plausibility that the disease, which we shall see later is directly related to vitamin C deficiency, could be aggravated by certain factors capable of rapidly depleting the molecule's residual bodily stores, such as adverse weather conditions or physical stress. It is therefore likely that these factors severely aggravated the effects of scurvy on sailors, making it even more aggressive.

It is important to note that Lind's genius is officially recognised not only for his contribution to the understanding of scurvy, but also for his innovative method of investigation. He validated the results of his experiment using an approach that would later be adopted worldwide to test the efficacy of treatments. Lind's experiment marked a historical moment in Medicine: it clarified, so to speak, the cloudy sky of scurvy and introduced the use of control groups, a principle still central to clinical trials today. This is one of the main reasons why medical science owes so much to vitamin C.

A controlled trial is a scientific study that evaluates whether a treatment works by comparing two groups: one receives the treatment, while the other, the control group, does not. The control group may receive a placebo, standard care, or no treatment. If participants are assigned to these groups at random, the study is called a randomized controlled trial (RCT). Randomization is crucial because it increases the reliability of the results.

Building on Woodall's limited (though essentially correct, as time would prove) evidence, Lind implemented a rigorous investigation to confirm Woodall's insights and provide a more rational view. The results were significant and were carefully recorded in his famous "A Treatise of the Scurvy", one of the most representative works in the history of medical literature. All the data converged on a single conclusion: oranges and lemons contained a yet unidentified compound capable of completely neutralising scurvy.

In May 1747, Lind selected 12 scurvy patients on board the ship Salisbury, ensuring that their general condition and specific symptoms were as similar as possible. This is of paramount importance in this kind of experiment, allowing one to avoid those systematic errors that could distort interpretations.

These are Lind's words, taken from his manual: "On the 20th May, 1747, I took twelve patients in the scurvy on board the Salisbury at sea. Their cases were as similar as I could have them. They all in general had putrid gums, the spots and lassitude, with weakness of their knees. They lay together in one place, being a proper apartment for the sick in the fore-hold; and had one diet in common to all, viz., water gruel sweetened with sugar in the morning; fresh mutton broth often times for dinner; at other times puddings, boiled biscuit with sugar etc.; and for supper barley, raisins, rice and currants, sago and wine, or the like. Two of these were ordered each a quart of cyder a day. Two others took twenty five gtts of elixir vitriol three times a day upon an empty stomach, using a gargle strongly acidulated with it for their mouths. Two others took two spoonfuls of vinegar three times a day upon an empty stomach, having their gruels and their other food well acidulated with it, as also the gargle for the mouth. Two of the worst patients, with the tendons in the ham rigid (a symptom none the rest had) were put under a course of sea water. Of this they drank half a pint every day and sometimes more or less as it operated by way of gentle physic. Two others had each two oranges and one lemon given them every day. These they eat with greediness at different times upon an empty stomach. They continued but six days under this course, having consumed the quantity that could be spared. The two remaining patients took the bigness of a nutmeg three times a day of an electuary recommended by a hospital surgeon made of garlic, mustard seed, rad. raphan., balsam of Peru and gum myrrh, using for common drink barley water well acidulated with tamarinds, by a decoction of which, with the addition of cremor tartar, they were gently purged three or four times during the course. The consequence was that the most sudden and visible good effects were perceived from the use of the oranges and lemons; one of those who had taken them being at the end of six days fit for duty. The spots were not indeed at that time quite off his body, nor his gums sound; but without any other medicine than a gargarism or elixir of vitriol he became quite healthy before we came into Plymouth, which was on the 16th June. The other was the best recovered of any in his condition, and being now deemed pretty well was appointed nurse to the rest of the sick".

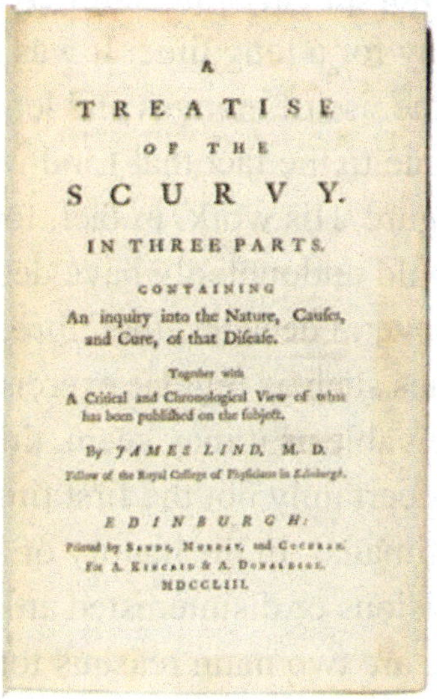
A
TREATISE
OF THE
SCURVY.
IN THREE PARTS.
CONTAINING
An inquiry into the Nature, Cauſes, and Cure, of that Diſeaſe.
Together with
A Critical and Chronological View of what has been publiſhed on the ſubject.
By JAMES LIND, M. D.
Fellow of the Royal College of Phyſicians in Edinburgh.
EDINBURGH:
Printed by Sands, Murray, and Cochran.
For A. Kincaid & A. Donaldson.
MDCCLIII.

The mystery seemed to be solved, consistent with the observation that the effects of scurvy tended to worsen during long sea voyages: the lack of fresh fruit (particularly oranges and lemons), attributable to the short periods of time that greatly affect the biological integrity of vegetables and the absence of adequate preservation techniques, seemed to cause the disease; it was also discovered that the intake of oranges or lemons proved to be a very effective and specific therapy. The innovative aetiological framework will endure steadily in the course of time, consolidating to the point of revealing, as will be noted in detail at various points, a clear congruence with the dual nature marking the magic compound contained in oranges and lemons. Through this dual nature, it will become increasingly evident that vitamin C can help manage a wide range of diseases, expressing a dynamic adhering to the following scheme: low dose-prevention/high dose-therapy.

We return to Lind's ingenious experiment to highlight the new awareness of the fundamental impact that oranges and lemons could have on the health of sailors. Thus, efforts began to focus on strategies for the proper preservation of food, a task that soon proved to be extremely challenging.

Yet, before discussing the importance of food preservation, it should be noted that this awareness was unfortunately not sufficient to extend Lind's fundamental scientific indication worldwide. "How is this possible?" you will rightly ask.

The fascinating story did not immediately have a happy ending as the extraordinary discovery did not quickly find solid ground in which to sow the best prospects, almost fading away for a long time. It was more than forty years before the British Navy mandated the use of oranges and lemons in the diet of sailors, a culpable delay presumably due to the fact that Lind was regarded in scientific circles as an uninfluential figure. His work, in fact, found no place in authoritative medical journals when it would undoubtedly have deserved all the scientific exposure in the world. For several decades, therefore, precautions against scurvy continued to include strategies such as regular exercise, good hygiene and a positive attitude. As inconceivable as it may seem, this fact should not come as much of a surprise, as it was certainly not the first time that an important scientific discovery had been underestimated. In the history of Science, turbulent periods characterised by confused visions or disinterested attitudes have often preceded important discoveries. There are two main reasons for this: social contexts hostile to innovation and rigid ethical and religious opposition. These dynamics found their worst expression in a significant and dramatic triangle formed by Galileo Galilei, Giordano Bruno and heliocentrism.

As for the experiment, one thorny issue was still unresolved: devising effective food preservation techniques in order to safeguard the citrus fruits during the longer journeys and ensure their worldwide export. But why is food preservation crucial?

It is widely demonstrated that the time between harvesting and consumption, cooking, heat, and climate are factors that deeply affect the biological quality of the bioactive nutrients (vitamins, minerals, amino acids) contained in food. Consequently, the integrity of these nutrients (such as the anti-scurvy agent) requires effective preservation, and this meant that, at the time, the global eradication of the disease depended on advances in technology. It is no coincidence that, under specific conditions, scurvy continued to kill.

Two notable examples can be found in Robert Scott's famous polar exploration (Discovery, 1901-1904) and, above all, in the emblematic challenge (1910-1912) launched by the latter to Norwegian explorer Roald Amundsen for the conquest of the South Pole. Perhaps through negligence, or as a result of ill-advised suggestions, this competition saw Scott's team lose out decisively, literally overwhelmed by the cold and above all by the scurvy that did not surprise Amundsen's crew. It was all thanks to his ship's doctor, Frederick Cook, who had gained previous experience during which he realised that Arctic inhabitants, who were particularly accustomed to raw meat, did not fall ill with scurvy. Cook's insight thus ensured the safety of his men, consequently enabling Amundsen to achieve a historically exceptional goal, and at the same time consolidated the association between a diet of fresh Antarctic seal meat (an animal species, as we shall see, capable of producing vitamin C) and the prevention of scurvy. It was a magnificent insight that shifted research into the anti-scurvy molecule to the animal kingdom, forcing the entire research world to radically reorganise its scientific approach to the subject. Amundsen's expedition, in short, had the great merit of shifting investigations towards what would prove to be a veritable mine of information, namely the study of animals.

This is interesting because it contains a description of those methodological transfigurations typically necessary for solving the most refractory problems, through which a different perspective can provide a twofold contribution. Approaching a problem from a different angle, as mathematics teaches, can allow both to test the viability of new paths and to obtain a clearer view of the path previously taken. This is exactly what happened to the research on the anti-scurvy agent. The new perspective, in fact, fuelled a wave of animal investigations with renewed enthusiasm, gradually shaping the belief that the presence of the anti-scurvy agent was a prerogative of the animal kingdom. This theory was consistent with all empirical observations in which animals appeared invulnerable to the terrible disease. Were Cook's insights truly correct?

The issue involved many scientists, including Oslo University Hygiene professor Axel Holst and pediatrician Theodor Frølich, who were firmly convinced of a nutritional defect underlying beriberi and played an almost unwittingly crucial role. Why? And what is beriberi?

The origin of their research was inspired by their investigations into another disease called beriberi. This illness, which can cause serious damage to the nervous system and cardiovascular system, was initially linked to an exclusive diet of polished rice and was later understood to result from vitamin B1 deficiency. This gave strong impetus to consider a previously unimagined scenario, namely the existence of a variety of diseases closely linked to diet and nutritional deficiencies, which would soon lead to the concept of vitamins being formally defined. Holst and Frølich developed a model to search for the anti-beriberi factor, choosing certain animals for their experiments, and focusing in particular on the guinea pig. Here was the turning point!

Whether this was the result of deliberate reasoning or, more likely, a stroke of luck (or GULO, an acronym for gulono-lactone oxidase, and, amusingly, a perfect homophone for the Italian slang word “culo”, meaning both “butt” and “lucky break”), it proved decisive: years later, it was discovered that this species, like humans, is one of the very few unable to synthesise vitamin C. Thus the guinea pig proved to be the best choice to deal with the issue. Going into the specifics of their experiment, Holst and Frølich fed the animals a diet that had previously caused beriberi in pigeons, so essentially a diet of flour and cereals. They observed a surprising fact: the onset of scurvy instead of the expected beriberi. As already mentioned, the choice of animal model based on guinea pigs (pigeons, in the same way as all animals except humans, guinea pigs and other rare species, are able to synthesise vitamin C) momentarily led the two researchers astray, because it was universally accepted that scurvy was a typically human disease.

At this point, Holst and Frølich hypothesised, on the one hand, the concrete possibility of curing scurvy with the use of a fortified diet, thus coming very close to today's general concept of vitamins, and, on the other hand, the existence of animal species vulnerable to scurvy. As for vitamins, it was not long before the concept was finally formalised, elaborated with extreme rigour and announced with great enthusiasm by the Polish biochemist Kazimierz Funk in 1912: “Non-mineral nutrients essential for life, to be taken with the diet”. Thus was born vitamin B1, the anti-beriberi molecule, and vitamin C, the anti-scurvy molecule. It was a historic moment for all of Science, and of course also for all of society, which for too long had been suffering the terrible ravages of the two enigmatic diseases.

Research on the anti-scurvy molecule, driven by continuous technological progress, accelerated in the late 1920s. This led to the formation of two study groups: one led by Albert Szent-Györgyi and the other by Charles Glen King. The Hungarian Szent-Györgyi, whose name is linked not only to vitamin C but also to his famous studies on the Krebs cycle, achieved great fame during his stay at the Mayo Clinic in Rochester in 1928. This was not the last time the Mayo Clinic would be associated with vitamin C, though with alternating fortunes. During that stay, he succeeded in isolating a particular compound from the adrenal glands of an animal model in order to study its anti-scurvy properties. The compound was technically called hexuronic acid. Here too, research into vitamin C may have owed something to luck. It was later discovered that the adrenal glands absorb more vitamin C than most tissues and plasma. Plasma, in turn, is the liquid component of blood, rich in water, nutrients, and hormones, but devoid of cells.

On the other hand, King focused his efforts on investigating the anti-scurvy properties of lemons, going so far as to isolate an acid that he called ascorbic acid. These two important lines of research were only apparently distant. In fact, Joseph Svirbely, through whom King received a sample of hexuronic acid isolated from the competing group, demonstrated how close the two lines of research actually were. A turning point was thus reached. On April 4, 1932, now celebrated worldwide as "Vitamin C Day", King clearly demonstrated that the two acids were in fact the same molecule, thus giving rise to today's definition of vitamin C (or ascorbic acid, to use King's own terminology). This was an immense satisfaction for science, but it was accompanied by rather heated disagreements. Although King had crossed the finish line first in the marathon, it was in fact Szent-Györgyi, who reached the same conclusions a few weeks later, who was awarded the 1937 Nobel Prize for Medicine and Physiology, sparking considerable controversy over the failure to honour his colleague.

Disputes aside, great credit is due to the Hungarian scientist for sending a sample of hexuronic acid (today vitamin C or ascorbic acid) to the British chemist Sir Walter Norman Haworth with the aim of analysing its chemical and physical properties. A fortunate choice, the results of which would enable Sir Walter Norman Haworth to quickly (in 1933) identify the structural formula (the formula indicating the location of chemical bonds between the atoms of a molecule) of vitamin C, thus paving the way for synthetic production. Similarly to Szent-Györgyi for Medicine and Physiology, Sir Walter Norman Haworth also received the Nobel Prize in 1937 (for Chemistry, thanks to the discovery of the structural formula of vitamin C), thus forever tying that lucky year to vitamin C.

These were years of great fervour for the entire scientific spectrum, from the all too effervescent Physics in which Majorana no longer recognised himself, to the Mathematics increasingly studded with extraordinary rising stars such as the Topology of Hausdorff and Kuratowski, and the Analytic Number Theory, masterfully supported by the unforgettable Hardy-Ramanujan partnership. But there were also great advances in the field of Biology. Paul Karrer, the eminent Swiss chemist who shared the Nobel Prize with Haworth in 1937, was achieving extraordinary results in understanding vitamins A, B2 and E. He was able to identify their chemical formulas, enabling the synthetic production that allows us to conveniently use vitamin supplements today.

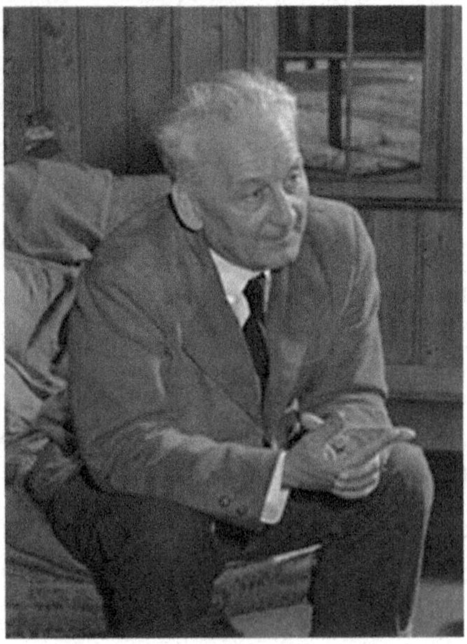

Albert Szent-Györgyi

The endgame?

The complex battle against scurvy sparked much reflection, keeping the issue of ascorbic acid alive, especially in those discerning minds that had already guessed that its scope could go far beyond the sailors' disease. Among these were also Nobel Prize winners, whose prestige, however, was not sufficient to expand research on the topic. It must be noted, in fact, that the space reserved for vitamin

C in academic circles was initially quite limited, as it was confined to the narrow preventive view focused solely on scurvy.

Endgame?

Over the decades, facts would gradually confirm the stereotype that behind every apparent end there may lie a wonderful beginning. In this regard, several scientists, including Nobel laureates Szent-Györgyi and Pauling, have repeatedly pointed out that the main reason for the vitamin C-scurvy association was historical. In other words, had the discovery of vitamin C's anti-scurvy properties been preceded by the discovery that collagen synthesis requires vitamin C, we would most likely have a different name, perhaps "pro-collagen acid" or something similar, a definition that would emphasize the relationship between the two elements. And I insist on asking a question: what would have happened if vitamin C had been discovered through its anti-polio properties, given that its antiviral potential seems to require doses hundreds of times higher than those needed to satisfy the anti-scurvy model?

It seems clear that a different historical sequence of events could have radically redefined the history of vitamin C and, by extension, that of Medicine. Here, then, is a real and logically possible perspective in which the anti-scurvy property is only one of the molecule's many functions, each of which requires specific conditions to be expressed successfully, first and foremost the appropriate dosage. Curiously, vitamin C has historically been predominantly linked to a conceptual model, the prevention of scurvy, which requires only a minimal dose. Although this approach is historically understandable, it has inevitably led to the marginalization of its many essential physiological functions identified later, those that make it a vital component of human health and potentially significant in combating disease.

In line with the remarkable views of Szent-Györgyi and Pauling, I believe that the chronological factor has negatively influenced the scientific understanding of vitamin C, hindering many discoveries that have progressively illuminated the molecule from various biological angles, some of which were unimaginable just a few years ago. Indeed, increasingly original perspectives over the years have allowed for a reevaluation of vitamin C's roles, leading to a structural redefinition of its biological characteristics. This has logically opened up unimaginable scientific horizons, within which vitamin C acts both as a fundamental element in human physiology and as a potentially useful pharmacological agent in the clinical management of numerous diseases.

Szent-Györgyi wrote in the preface to the famous treatise "The Healing Factor" (which will be discussed at length later): "Lack of ascorbic acid caused scurvy, so if there was no scurvy there was no lack of ascorbic acid. Nothing could be clearer than this. The only trouble was that scurvy is not a first symptom of lack but a final collapse, a premortal syndrome, and there is a very wide gap between scurvy and full health. But nobody knows what full health is! If you do not have sufficient vitamins and get a cold, and as a consequence pneumonia, your diagnosis will not be "lack of ascorbic acid" but "pneumonia"".

Thus, Szent-Györgyi's hypothesis suggested that a disguised vitamin C deficiency can impair health without causing scurvy. This enriched the image of the anti-scurvy molecule with an unprecedented range of dimensions, providing evidence of additional biological properties. The Nobel laureate's words allow us to introduce some very interesting topics, through which we will see that correcting some unforgivable inaccuracies and the painstaking search for the optimal daily dosage are essential for understanding the true capabilities of ascorbic acid.

In fact, vitamin C is not the only vitamin to have suffered from this kind of scientific misinterpretation, being considered solely as a remedy for a deficiency disease. Consider, for example, the aforementioned vitamin B1, or thiamine, which is historically associated with beriberi. Advances in scientific research have highlighted its therapeutic potential at high doses, much higher than those used in the anti-beriberi model, which could improve the clinical management of serious diseases such as Parkinson's disease (1) and heart failure (2).

Another perfect example is vitamin D: scientific research is now enthusiastic about new discoveries in its physiology. Eighty years ago, no one could have predicted, not even a fortune teller, that the anti-rachitic molecule would turn out to be an efficient immunomodulator within the complex biochemical network of the immune system (3). Vitamin D was discovered in the 1920s as the only substance capable of preventing and treating rickets, a pediatric disease characterized by severe skeletal deformities. However, research advancements have since revealed new properties unrelated to its classical metabolic role in bone health, now appropriately termed "extra-skeletal". These surprising functions, which require higher doses than those needed for its anti-rickets role, point to a broader conceptual framework that extends far beyond its original anti-rachitic role.

Such ideas form the foundation of what is commonly known as Orthomolecular Medicine, a medical field not yet fully embraced by the mainstream scientific community. This discipline aims to prevent and treat diseases through the use of optimal amounts of bioactive compounds found in food, such as vitamins.

Although this topic will be discussed in greater depth later on, it is important to remember that many doctors, technically known as "orthomolecularists", have successfully used high doses of vitamin C, often exploiting effective synergies with other nutrients. Klenner (who will be discussed shortly), Stone, Pauling, Cameron, Cathcart and Hoffer, leading figures in Orthomolecular Medicine, challenged some of the most insidious diseases, often with impressive results, even in extremely complex areas such as neuropsychiatric disorders. For example, Hoffer specialized in treating mental illnesses using well-known megadoses of vitamin B3, the "antidote" to pellagra, another well-known deficiency disease.

It is precisely vitamin B3 that offers well-established evidence that different intake levels can result in different biological responses. In particular, numerous studies have shown that very high doses of vitamin B3 can modulate cholesterol levels, reducing LDL ("bad" cholesterol) and simultaneously increasing HDL, or high-density lipoprotein ("good" cholesterol) (437).

When it comes to vitamin C, there is considerable confusion regarding the different intake levels: the effectiveness of a minimal dose for preventing scurvy (equivalent to the amount in a quarter of a fresh lemon, just a few milligrams), the effects of the dose recommended by health authorities (the well-known RDA, ranging from 70 to 100 mg per day for vitamin C), the effects of the maximum plasma concentration achievable through oral intake, and finally, its true pharmacological action (typically associated with intravenous administration). As you will see, the maximum plasma concentration achievable through oral administration requires repeated gram-level doses throughout the day, a strategy theorized within the "dynamic flow" conceptual model.

The scientific lesson of vitamin B3 should have established that different intake levels can trigger markedly different reactions; yet over time, the confusion surrounding vitamin C has never been fully resolved and has, in fact, seriously damaged its biological image. Clarifying this state of confusion, a dense haze that seems to confuse part of the scientific community, is the ambitious goal of this book, the success of which necessarily depends on a functional systematization of knowledge around vitamin C. As a result, several important ramifications will emerge. Some will aim to raise awareness within the medical research world regarding Stone's new/old unconventional perspective, first inspired by Szent-Györgyi's words. Others will seek to shed light on aspects still shrouded in unreasonable ambiguity, from physiological dosage to the excessive fear of "serious side effects".

As mentioned in the introduction, extensive reference will be made to the scientific literature, thereby avoiding unsupported scientific claims, the only appropriate choice for the sake of objectivity, and to substantiate my role as mediator between Science and the reader. Nonetheless, my responsibility will also be to develop hypothetical-deductive reasoning. And so, through this intermediation, we will make room to formulate some potentially useful proposals for improving various aspects, thus opening a reasoned critique of the sometimes unconvincing methodological approaches that have shaped vitamin C research.

In essence, this work aims to guide the reader along a clear and structured path, maintaining a neutral and objective stance. As previously mentioned, this approach is enriched by a network of secondary branches that trace parallel paths and recurring connections, above all, an objective critique of the scientific literature, supported by a comprehensive and detailed exploration of the physiology and pharmacology of vitamin C. Building on this, the goal is to identify a potential optimal dosage through pharmacokinetic analysis and consistent hypothetical-deductive reasoning. These two main axes, critical review and theoretical modelling, intersect in ways that may inform clinical practice and contribute to a broader shift in perspective. The hope is to provide the tools necessary to develop a new awareness of the topic, guided by logic and an increasingly refined understanding of the multifaceted nature of vitamin C, which is now beginning to be the focus of intense and systematic research. Indeed, a "new" conception of vitamin C is not only possible but perhaps necessary, even essential, to restore scientific credibility to a field long met with skepticism.

This work is, in essence, a careful effort to fuel such innovation, or what I prefer to call an "advanced renaissance". Borrowing the expression used by several scientists in a leading intensive care journal, this could be described as a case of "Vitamin C revisited". This is, in fact, the title chosen by a group of authors for a landmark article published in 2014 in the prestigious journal "Critical Care" (165), which highlighted a bimodal model of ascorbic acid, with evidence pointing to its dual role in both the prevention and treatment of disease. Treatment? Yes, treatment, because the pharmacological version of vitamin C is increasingly being recognized as a multifunctional, versatile, inexpensive, readily available and non-toxic therapeutic agent. It is a very promising drug, indicated by a growing body of research as a valuable resource in managing numerous conditions, including severe and even critical ones. These conditions often have a common feature: a rapid and massive depletion of the body's vitamin C reserves, with potentially dramatic health consequences.

Anyone who still considers the idea of vitamin C as an emergency drug to be unscientific should carefully reflect on the conclusions drawn by the scientists in reference (165): "High-dose vitamin C provides a cheap, strong and multifaceted antioxidant, especially robust for resuscitation of the circulation. Vitamin C given as early as possible after the injurious event, or before if feasible, seems most effective. The latter could be considered at the start of cardiac surgery, organ transplant or major gastrointestinal surgery. In critically ill patients, future research should focus on the use of short-term high-dose intravenous vitamin C as a resuscitation drug, to intervene as early as possible in the oxidant cascade in order to optimize macrocirculation and microcirculation and limit cellular injury" (165).

Jungeblut, Klenner and polio

The first scientific initiative that sparked renewed interest in vitamin C was undertaken by a pivotal figure in the history of medicine: Professor Claus Washington Jungeblut, initially affiliated with Stanford University and later a full professor of bacteriology for over thirty years at the prestigious Columbia University. It was largely due to his pioneering research that a significant breakthrough was achieved, one that paved the way for a radically innovative interpretation of the anti-scurvy agent, marking the early phase of a new scientific era.

On September 18, 1939, the renowned "Time" magazine reported on a series of discoveries presented at the esteemed Manhattan International Congress for Microbiology. Among the findings, one in particular attracted both scientific and public attention: the potential role of vitamin C in combating poliomyelitis (4). The article described Jungeblut's experimental research from previous years, which had uncovered an unexpected correlation between vitamin C deficiency and the progression of polio. "Under certain restricted experimental conditions, vitamin C is capable of influencing favorably the course of the infection in monkeys", the article reported. This was the first time that vitamin C was attributed a pharmacological effect, thus introducing a concept entirely unrelated to its historical role in preventing scurvy.

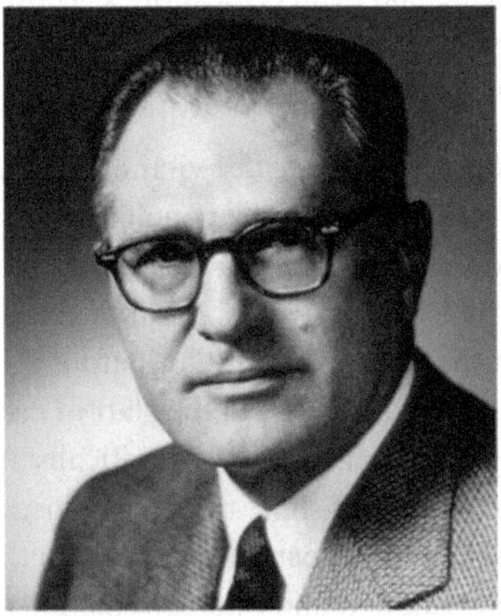

Claus Washington Jungeblut

Jungeblut's claims regarding the possible antiviral properties of vitamin C date back to 1935, when he began publishing a series of in vitro studies (6) suggesting the molecule's potential efficacy against the poliovirus. As he reported: "Multiple doses of the polio virus become non-infectious when mixed with very small amounts of crystalline vitamin C (ascorbic acid)". By 1937, his hypothesis gained further credibility through an intriguing in vivo experiment (5) conducted on groups of monkeys deliberately infected and subsequently treated with vitamin C. This study opened new perspectives, particularly on the critical issue of dosing, while also providing encouraging evidence of the molecule's anti-polio potential.

Having alluded to the crucial matter of dosage, it is useful to undertake a brief historical detour before delving into the extended debate on this topic, in which the role of Dr. Klenner will prove pivotal. The scientific investigations of that time unfolded against the dramatic backdrop of the polio epidemic, which provided an ideal scenario for exploring the possible antiviral properties of vitamin C.

During the first half of the 20th century, poliomyelitis outbreaks grew to pandemic proportions across Europe, North America, Australia and New Zealand. Around 1950, the epidemiological peak shifted notably toward pediatric age groups, leading to the establishment of the first hospital intensive care units (ICUs) specifically designed to manage respiratory complications from polio (7). The severity of the epidemic spurred global research initiatives aimed at developing an effective vaccine, engaging some of the greatest scientific minds of the time, including Albert Sabin and Jonas Salk. It was the latter who provided the world with a long-awaited breakthrough, announcing on April 12, 1955, the development of a viable vaccine against poliomyelitis (8).

This historical context, characterised by a complex network of challenges later addressed by Sabin through the development of a second vaccine, highlights a key consideration: these important scientific advances came more than a decade after Jungeblut's pioneering observations and, as we shall see shortly, several years after the emergence of data favourable to the therapeutic model used by Dr. Frederick Klenner, which involved the administration of doses of vitamin C never used before. It is now essential to clarify a preliminary point: between 1937 and 1955, and, regrettably, even in the years that followed, the potential anti-polio properties of vitamin C were never seriously pursued by the scientific establishment, despite the remarkable empirical evidence gathered by Klenner. Why was this the case?

The widespread lack of interest can be traced back to the outcome of a specific experiment conducted in 1939 by Albert Sabin, the very scientist who would later develop the second polio vaccine. Sabin sought to replicate Jungeblut's promising results using appropriately infected monkey models (9). Unfortunately, the conclusions were discouraging: "In the experiments reported in the present communication it was found that vitamin C, both natural and synthetic preparations, had no effect on the course of experimental poliomyelitis induced by nasal instillation of the virus".

It is reasonable to infer that this outcome dealt a significant blow to the credibility of Jungeblut's research, especially since the challenge came from a figure of considerable scientific influence on the international stage.

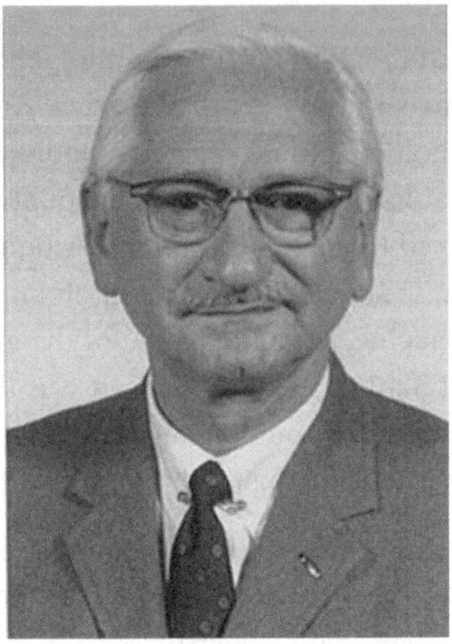

Albert Bruce Sabin

One recommendation may provide a valuable perspective for interpreting the turbulent history of vitamin C: the reader is invited to take note of the methodological asymmetries between the studies conducted by Jungeblut and Sabin. These discrepancies would reemerge, in a substantially similar manner, some forty years later, when Linus Pauling first provided clinical evidence of the potential anti-tumour role of vitamin C.

The figure who most vehemently contested Sabin's conclusions was the brilliant Dr. Frederick Klenner, a pulmonologist from North Carolina, considered the first great pioneer in the therapeutic use of vitamin C. Regarding the apparent failure of Sabin to replicate Jungeblut's promising results in poliomyelitis research, Klenner, affectionately referred to by his patients as "The Country Doctor", published a critical article in the "Journal of Applied Nutrition" in 1953, titled "The Use of Vitamin C as an Antibiotic" (10). There, he wrote: "One of the most unfortunate mistakes in all of the research on poliomyelitis was Sabin's

UNSCIENTIFIC attempt to confirm Jungeblut's work with vitamin C against the Polio virus in monkeys. Jungeblut in infecting his Rhesus monkeys used the mild 'droplet method' and then administered vitamin C by needle in varying amounts up to 400 mg/day. Even this method did not give him absolute control over the degree of infection that would result. However, his antibiotic (vitamin C) remained relatively constant. With almost infinitesimal amounts, as we at present recognize, he was able to demonstrate in one series that the non-paralytic survivors were six times as great as in the controls. On the other hand, Sabin, in infecting his monkeys did not follow the procedure given by Jungeblut whose experiments he was attempting to repeat, but instead employed a more forceful method of inoculation which obviously resulted in sickness of maximum severity. Sabin further refused to follow Jungeblut's suggestion as to the dose of vitamin C to be used. By Sabin's actual report the amount given was rarely more than 35 per cent of that used by his associate. Sabin makes this significant statement (1939), 'One monkey was given 400 mg of vitamin C for one day at the suggestion of Jungeblut who felt that large doses were necessary to effect a change in the course of the disease.' Yet on the basis of Sabin's work the negative value of vitamin C in the treatment of virus diseases has been for years accepted as final".

"Final" is an adjective as rigid as it is definitive, perhaps suitable for the realm of mathematics, but decidedly less appropriate in medicine, a discipline inherently linked to the probabilistic and statistical dimensions of knowledge, domains often far from offering absolute certainty.

With this brief epistemological parenthesis concluded, we can now shift focus to Klenner himself. His critique centred on the pronounced methodological discrepancies between the studies of Jungeblut and Sabin, most notably, the fact that Sabin employed both a higher viral load and a lower dose of vitamin C. In essence, as Klenner argued, Sabin executed a methodological inversion.

This brings to the fore one of the most enduring challenges in the therapeutic use of ascorbic acid: dosage adequacy. According to Klenner's incisive reconstruction, Sabin's methodological error, namely, the use of insufficient ascorbic acid, amounted to a misrepresentation of Jungeblut's work. Consequently, the absence of therapeutic results may not have been due to a lack of antiviral efficacy, but rather to the inadequate dosage used. Even today, Sabin's experimental decisions remain difficult to interpret. Do you share this view?

Beyond interpretations, there is a highly questionable aspect: the decisiveness with which Sabin's study labeled the antiviral potential of vitamin C as negative.

In addition to the asymmetries highlighted, Klenner's skepticism also stemmed from his work between the late 1940s and early 1950s, during which he produced notable theoretical insights and described numerous clinical cases that were extraordinarily resolved thanks to the "massive" use (as he himself liked to call it) of vitamin C. This was an absolute novelty in the scientific world, through which vitamin C quickly transitioned from being a mere anti-scurvy micronutrient to a sophisticated broad-spectrum therapeutic weapon, theoretically effective against various viruses. From low dosage to massive dosage, then. A transition with far-reaching clinical consequences, but one that required an essential paradigm shift, a new vision of the anti-scurvy molecule: using doses vastly higher, even up to 2500 times the survival-level dose for scurvy. A coefficient of 2500 is so excessive that it is unimaginable to apply it to any traditional pharmacological model, since the resulting drug would be so toxic that any attempt to enhance its therapeutic effects would be nullified. This, in summary, is the first atypical feature of vitamin C as a pharmacological agent.

Among the various articles written by Dr. Klenner, the one published in the "Journal of Southern Medicine and Surgery" in July 1949, titled "The Treatment of Poliomyelitis and Other Virus Diseases with Vitamin C", is particularly significant. The article presented the effectiveness of so-called "megadoses of vitamin C", an approach based on the daily administration of many thousands of milligrams of vitamin C, therefore, doses much higher than those used in Sabin's experiments. Particularly interesting is the therapy implemented during the poliomyelitis outbreak that ravaged North Carolina in 1948, during which dozens of recoveries were achieved using continuous vitamin C administration. This means that the molecule was administered at short intervals, using both oral and intramuscular routes, reaching total daily dosages that usually exceeded 30000 mg.

Beyond the practical implications, which were nonetheless remarkable (the reference is obviously to the many people saved), Klenner's work still appears extraordinary today as it enabled some important pharmacokinetic and pharmacological concepts to be grasped for the first time, which time would largely confirm. First of all, Klenner described the molecule as a "powerful reducing agent" and "an integral part of the oxidation-reduction system of the body", thus highlighting its notable antioxidant ability to neutralise the damaging action of free radicals, a fact historically relevant because it separated vitamin C from its exclusive association with scurvy (11). Furthermore, in (11) it is possible to intercept some pharmacokinetic concepts: "Hawley and others have shown that vitamin C taken by mouth will show its peak of excretion in the urine in from four to six hours. Intravenous administration produces this peak in from one to three hours. By this route, however, the concentration in the blood is raised so suddenly that a transitory overflow into the urine results before the tissues are saturated".

But it is above all through the disquisitions around the "Fluid dose schedule", a modality based on those continuous administrations that are essential to maintain a robust and constant presence of the molecule in the plasma and also in the tissues, that we can perceive the immensity of Klenner's talent. In fact, thanks to the meticulous description of this innovative approach, it is possible to illustrate another crucial aspect for the effectiveness of vitamin C therapy, concerning the importance of maintaining high levels. I repeat, therapy. Not a dietary factor or, worse still, an antiscorbutic agent.

There are indeed many therapeutic schemes through which Klenner has succeeded in coping with a wide range of challenging clinical situations, in which he has often achieved favourable outcomes, being well aware of how best to use a drug that appeared increasingly surprising in terms of potency and versatility. Not just an anti-polio solution, then, but much more. A valid testimony can be found in the treatment of shingles: "In herpes zoster 2000 to 3000 mg of vitamin C was given every 12 hours, this supplemented by 1000 mg in fruit juice by mouth every two hours. Eight cases were treated in this series, all of adults. Seven experienced cessation of pain within two hours of the first injection and remained so without the use of any other analgesic medication. Seven of these cases showed drying of the vesicles within 24 hours and were clear of lesions within 72 hours. They received from five to seven injections" (11).

These statements cannot leave us indifferent, as they are surprising when compared to standard nutritional concepts and suggest two points of great historical importance. First, the pulmonologist referred to uncommon routes for administering vitamin C: intramuscularly and intravenously. These are very unusual methods for assimilating a nutrient into the body, but even then they were considered much more efficient than the traditional oral route, as they were able to produce plasma levels that were impossible to achieve with classic oral intake (remember Hawley's discoveries).

The second point concerns the broad versatility of vitamin C, a peculiarity that extended its range of action beyond polio treatment. "The response of virus encephalitis to ascorbic acid therapy was dramatic. Six cases of virus encephalitis were treated and cured with vitamin C injections. Two cases were associated with virus pneumonia; one followed chickenpox, one mumps, one measles and one a combination of measles and mumps. In the case that followed the measles-mumps complex, definite evidence was found to confirm the belief that massive, frequent injections are necessary in treating virus infections with vitamin C", Klenner continues in the article (11) concluding with another fundamental consideration: "In using vitamin C as an antibiotic no factor of toxicity need be considered. To confirm this observation 200 consecutive hospital patients were given ascorbic acid, 500 to 1000 mg every four to six hours, for five to ten days. One volunteer received 100000 mg in a 12-day period. It must be remembered that 90 per cent of these patients did not have a virus infection to assist in destroying the vitamin. In no instance did examination of the blood or urine indicate any toxic reaction, and at no time were there any clinical manifestations of a reaction to the drug".

With these words, Klenner was revealing something extraordinary that makes vitamin C unique, thanks to the fact that it is essentially non-toxic in all its forms of use, ranging from dietary to massive oral doses, ultimately to the injection route. These were scientific suppositions that time would turn into an increasingly established reality, and which seemed truly significant, considering that the pharmacological use of vitamin C (not nutritional!) seemed capable of exerting an antiviral action desperately required at a time in history when there was a dramatic shortage of anti-polio treatments.

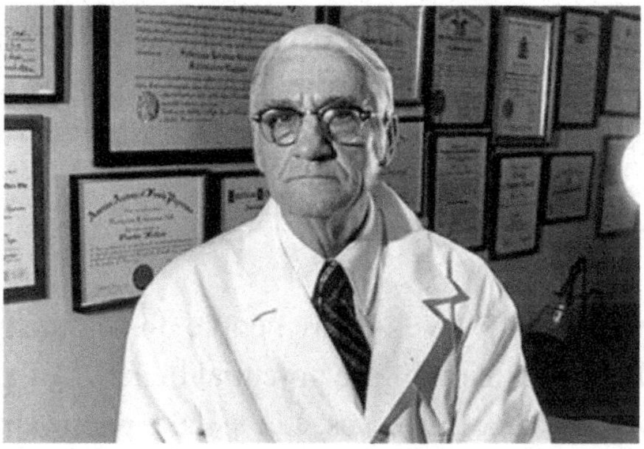

Frederick Robert Klenner

Some logical introspection deserves to be shared. Although Klenner's remarkable results did not entirely meet the standards of scientific rigour, and moreover were based on a few patients and an unclear rationale (the pulmonologist was essentially referring to the antioxidant effect of ascorbic acid, without knowing, unfortunately, about the immunomodulatory action, "pro-interferon", anti-inflammatory, analgesic, anti-stress and epigenetic action), in my opinion the negligent attitude expressed by health institutions remains enigmatic, especially since it occurred during a violent health emergency in which specific therapies were lacking and anti-polio vaccine research was in its early stages.

In practice, there seemed to be no good reason why the scientific community would reject an accurate assessment of the anti-polio potential of vitamin C that emerged from Klenner's work. Although his studies had obvious limitations, the results were very encouraging, especially considering the very low toxicity of vitamin C therapy. After clarifying the causes of Sabin's failed experiment, categorically ruling out this therapy seems irrational and incompatible with the drama of historical events.

"When you got nothing, you got nothing to lose" suggested Jack Dawson in the cult movie Titanic. And during Klenner's hot years, apart from vitamin C, it seemed that nothing could curb the uncontrollable advance of the devastating polio. Nonetheless, in spite of the resulting "nothing to lose" and although the ship was sinking, vitamin C was dismissed.

This will not be the last time that vitamin C is enigmatically sidelined.

Vitamin C as a broad-spectrum anti-infective agent

'The patient should get large doses of vitamin C in all pathological conditions, while the physician ponders the diagnosis'

Frederick Klenner

Klenner's genius not only saved many people during the polio epidemic, but also provided an advanced vision of the potential benefits of ascorbic acid in the management of a wide range of diseases. Let us take pneumonia as a model. In 1948, he published a twofold study (12), in which he provided, on the one hand, empirical evidence of therapeutic efficacy (through the indispensable massive and frequent doses) against a possible manifestation of scurvy, and, on the other hand, a biological rationale to support treatment with ascorbic acid.

As was often the case, Klenner had seen this clearly. The idea of treating pneumonia with vitamin C would, indeed, receive partial scientific confirmation many decades later in several significant studies (13). Some of these studies also provide evidence supporting a key conclusion: the "partial" results may be attributed to the insufficient use of vitamin C.

In this regard, the authors of an interesting systematic review (a systematic review is a method of critically summarising the results of individual studies concerning a particular health intervention) published in 2007 in the "Journal of the Royal Society of Medicine" (13) stated: "We carried out a systematic review, published in the Cochrane Library, in which we examined the role of vitamin C supplementation on preventing and treating pneumonia. We identified three controlled trials reporting on the preventive effect and two on the therapeutic effect of vitamin C against pneumonia. Each of the trials found a statistically significant benefit of vitamin C supplementation on at least one clinically relevant outcome". The authors therefore focused on the efficacy of vitamin C "supplementation", as opposed to Klenner's vigorous "therapies" based on massive and frequent dosing.

It should now be clearer to the reader what I meant by "insufficient use of vitamin C", having clearly distinguished the term "supplementation" (which, in any case, was associated with positive results in the review) from the more potent concept of "therapy", referring to multiple oral and intravenous administrations.

Although it will be observed throughout the course of the book that the fate of vitamin C as a drug depends on the supplementation-versus-therapy dualism, what we have just explored represents a first element that aims to clarify all those obscure dynamics that have often altered interpretations of vitamin C research.

We have thus encountered a crucial question. The issue, which will be addressed repeatedly in the book, is absolutely central within a context where misunderstandings, mystifications, prejudices, and ambiguities, fueled by a logic in which semantics has sometimes been misused, have circulated too freely.

We continue with an article by Klenner entitled "Massive doses of vitamin C and the virus diseases" (14), which contains an interesting analytical description of the organism-acute infections-vitamin C triangle. What mechanism could cause its structural alteration?

This refers to Klenner's extraordinary intuition that any acute infection tends to rapidly deplete vitamin C concentrations, both in the plasma and in the tissues. This assumption, which was to be widely confirmed over the years, on the one hand justified the intensity of the therapies adopted by Klenner (the prospect of replenishing the vitamin C depleted by the disease), and, on the other hand, it highlighted for the first time the biological importance of the molecule for the functioning of the immune system. Klenner, in fact, identified many infectious diseases theoretically susceptible to vitamin C, including viral encephalitis, measles, parotitis, shingles, pneumonia and tetanus. Although these were essentially speculative hypotheses, Klenner reinforced them with clinical evidence, illustrating a number of very complex clinical cases in which the vigorous use of ascorbic acid proved decisive (14).

In today's view, we can compare Klenner's scientific work to a monumental structure, originated on a solid theoretical foundation and strengthened by the incredible clinical results and influence he was able to bring to bear on subsequent scientific research into ascorbic acid.

Among the many researchers who were fascinated by Klenner was Berzin, a talented scientist who in the mid-1950s examined diphtheria and hypothesised an immune involvement of vitamin C in both the pathogenesis (the biological process through which a disease develops) and the course of the disease (15), (16), (17). For the second time, therefore, vitamin C was associated with new biological functions, broadening the antioxidant vision and fading the naive anti-scurvy perspective even further. Similarly to diphtheria, tetanus has also been related to vitamin C, as evidenced by some authoritative studies by Jungeblut (18), (19).

The time has come to use a very efficient time machine, one that will truly serve our purposes. With it, we will take a few brief dives into modern literature, showing the dimensional heterogeneity that has characterised, and to some extent still characterises, scientific research on vitamin C. At the same time, we will discover just how profound the vision of the vitamin C pioneers was, a vision that even today is not easy to refute.

As far as tetanus is concerned, a clinical trial involving 117 patients in Bangladesh in the early 1980s (20) yielded noteworthy results despite the fact that vitamin C was used in much lower dosages than Klenner's therapies, an example of dimensional heterogeneity. The study explored the potential of vitamin C by dividing tetanus patients into two treatment groups: conventional therapy, conventional therapy combined with a single daily intravenous administration of 1 g of vitamin C. We are about to learn an unexpected fact, at least for some. The combined treatment with vitamin C, in fact, produced a remarkable reduction in mortality compared to standard therapy, a reduction that in the subgroup of patients under 12 years of age was as much as 100% (20).

It is time to ask a couple of questions, starting from a fundamental assumption, already briefly mentioned and to be explored in greater depth both in the following pages and in the chapter on pharmacokinetics: a single dose (oral or intravenous) of non-dietary vitamin C (i.e., not accessible through food) tends to remain in the body for only a few hours. Therefore, based on a reality that will be amply demonstrated throughout the book, it is reasonable to ask: would "continuous" use, repeated frequently throughout the day (in the "Klenner manner," so to speak), of the intravenous dose of 1 g have been even more effective?

And again: why was a therapy used whose effectiveness is evidently limited to only a few hours (i.e., a single administration in 24 hours)?

Would a single meal be enough to sustain you throughout an entire day? And above all, in anticipation of an event that sharply increases the body's metabolic demand for ascorbate (such as tetanus or intense physical exertion), would the energy derived from just one meal, such as breakfast, be adequate?

Although the rationale behind the tetanus study (20) raises some doubts, one meaningful conclusion can still be drawn: it provides valuable evidence of the broad-spectrum anti-infective properties of ascorbic acid, even when used in a manner that is not entirely appropriate, or at least insufficient.

A valuable synthesis of modern evidence supporting the pathogen-neutralising potential of vitamin C was provided by the specialist Hemilä in a 2017 review (21). This paper is significant for several reasons, and it allows us to revisit and analyse some of the key points introduced earlier. Through this analysis, it becomes possible to properly contextualise certain partial or total failures in vitamin C research.

For instance, while the review (21) highlights its efficacy against many infections caused by bacteria, viruses and protozoa ("A total of 148 animal studies indicated that vitamin C can alleviate or prevent infections caused by bacteria, viruses and protozoa"), the results reported appear limited, perhaps due to another heterogeneity. Regarding the most investigated infectious disease, the common cold, the author writes: "The role of vitamin C in common cold treatment is unclear. Two controlled trials found a statistically significant dose-response, for the duration of common cold symptoms, with up to 6-8 g/day of vitamin C. Thus, the negative findings of some therapeutic common cold studies might be explained by the low doses of 3-4 g/day of vitamin C". This statement seems to contradict other research in which the efficacy of vitamin C appeared minimal. What might explain this discrepancy?

Hemilä formulates a very plausible hypothesis: "The negative findings of some therapeutic common cold studies might be explained by the low doses of 3-4 g/day of vitamin C".

In essence, the dose-dependent response principle is firmly affirmed, a logical tool capable of rationally explaining some of the vitamin C failures, largely attributable to the use of low dosages (the reference to Sabin's unfortunate polio studies cannot be missed!). The hypothesis that the inappropriate use of vitamin C as a pharmacological agent may have caused many unsatisfactory clinical results, not only in the treatment of infections, thus gains considerable weight.

Recalling that the topic of the common cold will be revisited later when discussing the work of Nobel Prize winner Pauling, and that Hemilä himself still calls for more in-depth studies ("The effects of vitamin C against infections should be studied further"), we continue by highlighting a point that underscores the wide asymmetry in the literature on ascorbic acid. Much of it is in fact characterised by considerable methodological heterogeneity in terms of therapeutic approaches, and not only in terms of dosage. We must not overlook either the method of administration (oral, intramuscular or intravenous) or the frequency with which vitamin C was administered over a 24-hour period during clinical investigations. In the following chapters, we will find a therapeutic arsenal that is as vast as it is heterogeneous: 200 mg orally every 8 hours, 500 mg orally twice a day, 1 g orally once a day, 1 g intravenously once a day, 1.5 g every 6 hours intravenously, 50 mg/kg every 6 hours intravenously, 100 g intravenously. This arsenal is so heterogeneous that it suggests wide divergences in terms of results, something we will fully understand when highlighting the profound variability of vitamin C pharmacokinetics, whose capacity to accumulate in the body is extremely sensitive to the route of administration (22).

But it is not only the dosage that has an impact: stating a dosage of 3-4 g or even 6-8 g without specifying the timing of intake (single dose? multiple fractions?) could lead to vague or misleading interpretations, since we will show that different fractionation schemes produce different plasma levels and thus, ultimately, potentially different clinical results. For example, it is easy to show that 8 g of vitamin C taken as a single oral dose results in lower average 24-hour concentrations than a regimen of 2 g every 6 hours. In summary, identical 24-hour dosing but possibly different outcomes.

We have gathered, therefore, several elements in favour of the following thesis: regardless of the dosage, the application of an inadequate frequency could lead to inconsistent interpretations, underestimating the true abilities of ascorbic acid. All this only serves to reinforce Klenner's talent: despite his extremely limited theoretical knowledge, he had probably grasped the essence of vitamin C treatment during acute illness, setting up highly fractionated treatment regimens, even going as far as those hourly administrations that would be proposed again by Linus Pauling.

This method, as will be demonstrated later, is particularly suited to the pharmacokinetics of high doses and is inspired by a fundamental insight: the neutralisation of acute diseases requires a constantly high level of vitamin C. It is a preliminary version of the modern concept of "Dynamic Flow" (which Klenner himself referred to as "Fluid Dosing Scheme"), a model that will never be rigorously formalised in the book. This stems from the lack of pharmacokinetic knowledge on high oral doses of vitamin C and also from the broad category of factors influencing absorption and metabolism of the molecule. In the course of the book, however, it will be possible to gather data useful in formulating an ideal model of dynamic flow, towards which, in fact, some authors have gone as far as a possible definition. These are Cathcart (of whom we shall speak at length), Hickey and Roberts.

In conclusion, the principle of dynamic flow embraces a more conceptual and qualitative form, and in essence aims at imitating that natural process of biosynthesis that ceased too early in the long human, and I stress almost uniquely human, evolutionary history.

The work of Hickey and Roberts, the essence of which will be better grasped in the last chapters of the book, may help to clarify the mentioned misgivings about studies on oral vitamin C. An article of theirs from 2005, entitled "Misleading Information on the Properties of Vitamin C" (23), contains evidence supporting the theory that some failures of oral vitamin C therapy (for example, in the treatment of colds) are due to its being taken too discontinuously. Inappropriate use, in essence, through which the restoration of ascorbic concentrations depleted by the disease would be incomplete and fleeting because it would be limited to a few hours, and therefore inadequate for a lasting and effective therapeutic action.

What has been presented allows us to return to the general principle mentioned earlier in connection with the tetanus study (20), the principle that, irrespective of the route of administration, any dose exceeding dietary intake persists in the body for only a few hours. And this, as you might guess, is exactly why the mistaken idea persists that non-dietary doses are useless because they are poorly absorbed. In truth, what is really useless is the unnecessary confusion surrounding this topic.

Hickey and Roberts are of the same opinion when they criticise Douglas and Hemilä, two respected researchers in the field: "Douglas and Hemilä give a misleading impression by not making it clear that the doses they consider are not pharmacological. They claim that the results of one study, giving an 8-g dose at the start of symptoms, are tantalising and deserve further assessment. However, once this single dose has been excreted, the protective effects will be lost. During illness, ascorbate is depleted rapidly and higher oral intakes are tolerated—up to 200 g per day. It would be surprising if this 8-g dose had a large effect" (23).

Hickey and Roberts, in essence, confirmed Klenner's brilliant ideas by reiterating the importance of keeping vitamin C concentrations constantly high, a practice only achievable through repeated administration. This would be the only way, and I stress the only way, to counteract the rapid and severe vitamin C depletion typical of acute illness.

But let us return to Hemilä's review (21), in which it is suggested that 6-8 g might offer greater benefits than 3-4 g (consistent with the concept of dose-dependent response) but still limited, not fully satisfactory. It is logical that this should be the case, it could not be otherwise! Nor is it too difficult to prove. Hickey and Roberts readily did so by reaffirming that such a large oral dose, when taken in one go, produces limited benefits because the body has a reduced capacity to retain a high dose. In fact, we will notice that massive doses cannot be fully retained for more than 3-4 hours, basically due to increased renal elimination.

To put it more clearly, do you think you could drive for 10000 km without stopping to refuel? Imagine that the 10000 km distance stands for the whole day, the fuel is vitamin C, the tank is the body, and the typical dwell time of a high concentration corresponds to the time needed to cover enough distance to empty the tank. At this point, nothing should seem strange anymore.

However, this clear theoretical notion oddly clashes with clinical practice, where almost all oral trials have systematically administered vitamin C in just one daily dose, or at most two, and almost never with amounts exceeding 1 g. In practice, the molecule was treated as a dietary ingredient or, at best, as a food supplement, rather than as a full-fledged pharmacological weapon. Supplementation versus pharmacological use, that is.

Hickey and Roberts's rational thought fits perfectly in this context; they bluntly attacked the vitamin C studies: "Studies on ascorbate require appropriate doses. Douglas and Hemilä have only confirmed that 60 years of vitamin C research has largely been wasted because of confusion between nutritional and pharmacological intakes, and because of a misunderstanding of the pharmacokinetics. It is essential that high-dose studies take into account ascorbate's dual-phase pharmacokinetics. The dosing regime should allow sustained high plasma levels to be achieved. The claim that vitamin C cannot prevent or cure the common cold is both premature and unwarranted" (23).

In conclusion: a single daily dose, however high, may not be sufficient to achieve the maximum therapeutic response because it cannot cover the entire 24-hour period. Does the confusion now appear more evident?

The authors of an interesting prospective controlled study (24) added further perplexity, at least with regard to the common cold and influenza: hundreds of students were divided into a test group (treated with hourly doses of 1 g of vitamin C in the first six hours after the onset of symptoms and then 1 g three times a day) and a control group (treated with analgesics and decongestants). The results were clear: "Overall, flu and cold symptoms reported in the test group decreased by 85% compared to the control group after administration of megadoses of vitamin C. Megadoses of vitamin C administered before or after the onset of flu and cold symptoms alleviated and prevented symptoms in the test population compared to the control group", said Gorton and Jarvis (24). This study seems "extravagant" compared to the available literature on oral vitamin C, to the point of raising some questions.

One such reflection deserves to be shared: why have the dosages used in studies on oral vitamin C been progressively reduced over the years? The lack of an answer anticipates the careful analysis that will be organised in the final part of the book, through which a strong association between the various disappointing results and the use of insufficient dosages will be identified.

The ideas of Hickey and Roberts, which Klenner had put into practice over fifty years earlier with remarkable insight, find further theoretical support, as we shall see, in Stone's work begun in the 1960s. This theory focuses on the profound difference between humans and the vast majority of animals with regard to the biosynthesis of vitamin C. This is another key point that will be analysed in detail.

It should be pointed out that the need to resort to the dynamic flow theory relates mainly to oral administration. It will be noted, in fact, that strict intestinal control, which dynamically modulates the absorption of vitamin C taken in oral form, can be circumvented, albeit only partially, by the artifices of dynamic flow. This is in contrast to intravenous administration, whose pharmacokinetic laws, while preserving the law of short-stay, allow for markedly higher plasma concentrations than oral administration.

This chapter concludes with a tribute to the pioneer who first identified vitamin C as a pharmacological agent capable of optimally combining efficacy, versatility and safety. The reference is clearly to Dr Klenner, the hero of North Carolina, the genius who helped save lives by using an original but effective therapeutic approach, the result of an explosive mixture of intuition, courage, and self-sacrifice. To be honest, Klenner went much further, as he was the first to highlight key mechanisms of action of vitamin C, a hallmark of brilliant minds. He rightly criticised all those who stubbornly rejected the view of vitamin C as a pharmacological agent, thereby confining it, as Irwin Stone later pointed out, to the limited concept of a dietary element.

"No one would expect to relieve kidney colic with a five-grain aspirin tablet; by the same logic we cannot hope to destroy the virus organism with doses of vitamin C of 10 to 400 mg. The results which we have reported in virus diseases using vitamin C as the antibiotic may seem fantastic. These results, however, are not different from the results we see when administering the sulfa, or the mold-derived drugs against many other kinds of infections. In these latter instances we expect and usually get 48- to 72-hour cures; it is laying no claim to miracle-working then, when we say that many virus infections can be cleared within a similar time limit" (11).

A passage of extraordinary symbolic power and great communicative expressiveness, theoretically suitable to sweep away those clouds that continue enigmatically to cover the vitamin C sky. In theory, yes, but even today, unfortunately, a striking lack of practical implementation still persists.

Thank you, Dr. Klenner, for all you have done.

Chapter 2
The Genetic Disorder
And The Other Pioneers Of Vitamin C

'One might imagine animals exchanging knowing glances whenever a nutritionist talks about vitamin C'

Irwin Stone and the genetic disorder

Why is scurvy almost non-existent in the animal world? How do animals react when they encounter hostile conditions such as attacks by dangerous pathogens, poor nutrition, physical trauma, unfavourable climatic events, or predators?

There are some indisputable facts in this regard: stray animals cannot benefit from adequate nutrition or medical care.

Finally, is a piece of fresh lemon, capable of preventing scurvy for several days, really enough to ensure the proper functioning of our body?

These are questions of considerable scientific interest that can serve as a starting point for an advanced discussion on vitamin C. It was another brilliant mind, that of Irwin Stone, the proponent of a unique theory long marginalised and underestimated, that provided many of the answers. Over time, evidence has confirmed what was once dismissed or underestimated: thanks to Stone's bold insights, we now have a perspective that extends Jungeblut's and Klenner's pioneering insights through a solid scientific foundation. It was his revolutionary ideas that paved the way for a new era in ascorbic acid research, ultimately inspiring the man who would become its greatest advocate, Linus Pauling.

Irwin Stone (1907-1984, who, remarkably, was born and died in the same years as Klenner) was a prominent American biochemist, chemical engineer and author who spent many years studying vitamin C. Although his scientific output was not extensive, his works in the 1960s exerted such an overwhelming influence that they shaped all subsequent scientific research on ascorbic acid.

Only today are we fully aware of this, recognising in his literary masterpiece "The Healing Factor" a majestic scientific work in which the essence of vitamin C is enshrined. This is not an exaggeration. On the contrary, I take this opportunity to recommend reading this wonderful text, and not only for the fact that the preface boasts the seal of Nobel Prize winners Albert Szent-Györgyi and Linus Pauling.

Impressive, isn't it? How many books can boast such a gem?

Pauling wrote in the preface: "Irwin Stone deserves much credit for having marshalled the arguments that indicate that most human beings have been receiving amounts of ascorbic acid less than those required to put them in the best of health. It is his contention, and it is supported by much evidence, that most people in the world have a disease involving a deficient intake of ascorbic acid, a disease that he has named hypoascorbemia. This disease seems to be present because of an evolutionary accident that occurred many millions of years ago".

What disease was Pauling referring to?

It is a disease, more precisely an enzymatic disorder of the liver called "hypoascorbemia" by Stone, which denotes an inadequate level of vitamin C (ascorbate or ascorbic acid) in the blood and tissues. Literally, the term hypoascorbemia means ascorbate deficiency, i.e. a deficiency of ascorbic acid in the blood.

Why are we affected by this disorder?

We owe the answer to Stone's extraordinary insights: humans suffer from a genetic alteration (the evolutionary accident referred to by Pauling) that has irreversibly impaired the biosynthesis (spontaneous synthesis from within the body) of vitamin C, which is diametrically opposed to what occurs in the vast majority of the animal kingdom.

The whole affair revolves around the bizarre behaviour of a particular enzyme, namely the enzyme L-gulonolactone oxidase (GULO or GLO), the same enzyme that is directly involved in what Stone unhesitatingly described as "The greatest catastrophe ever to befall mankind in the course of its evolution". The GULO (forgive the preference over GLO, full of spirit in associating the acronym with an anatomical element traditionally associated with a lucky component) represents the last of a series of enzymes in the biochemical pathway used by the mammalian liver to synthesise ascorbic acid. Technically, GULO catalyzes the final step of ascorbic acid biosynthesis, in which glucose is the starting molecule.

Vitamin C, therefore, originates from glucose, a clear subordination in which one will notice that the two protagonists prefigure a sort of "biochemical competition" resulting from their strong chemical affinity.

What are the causes of this genetic disorder?

The problem stems from an unfortunate combination of events that occurred during the long course of evolution, leading a primate ancestor of humans to undergo a series of mutations in the gene encoding the GULO enzyme, progressively degrading and ultimately nullifying its activity, thereby eliminating the natural ability to complete vitamin C synthesis. Due to this build-up of mutations, the animal, that is, the primate ancestor of humans, and all its descendants, forever marked by the genetic disorder, lost their inborn ability to synthesize ascorbic acid; this inevitably established total dependence on external sources rich in vitamin C.

In summary, the human liver is unable to complete the natural conversion of glucose into vitamin C.

There are various views on this genetic disorder, one of the most credible being that the phenomenon was the result of a change in dietary style: at the point in history when primates began to feed on fresh vegetables, which at the time were very rich in vitamin C, its biosynthesis, due to some form of energy-saving principle linked to natural selection, was interrupted because it was deemed no longer energetically convenient. A conceptual extension towards Physics, in this sense, supports the energy optimisation hypothesis, considering the existence of an analogue known as the "Variational Principle of Least Action", according to which the nature of physical actions always tends to be minimal.

Whatever the cause, we must admit that the effect has been tragic. At present, there is no way to restore GULO activity through genetic intervention.

Despite the wide variability in the degree of preservation of GULO in the animal kingdom, there is no doubt that vitamin C biosynthesis is still preserved in all animal species, with the exception of a few "unfortunate" ones including guinea pigs, certain types of monkeys, an Indian fruit bat and rare fish specimens.

And humans, of course. This process, therefore, although not totally intact in some "lucky animals" (some scientists hypothesise that it is not totally efficient in dogs, for example), still manages to guarantee them, unlike humans and the very few other species that share the same misfortune, a continuous internal production of vitamin C.

To conclude on the subject of animals, some researchers have hypothesised that there is a direct correlation between the amount of vitamin C synthesised and the structural integrity of the GULO enzyme. These are technical subtleties that must not, however, obscure the core, i.e. the significant difference that separates humans from animals, a difference as decisive as it is unfortunately underestimated. This discrepancy has been constantly emphasised by Stone: the total inability of the human liver to synthesise vitamin C, the biochemist emphasised, placed humans at a great metabolic disadvantage compared to other mammals, outlining an anomalous condition of absolute dependence on external supply.

What is the problem, since the shortage of fresh citrus fruits typical of the scurvy era no longer exists?

Clearly, there is something else, something that science has overlooked. In fact, "lucky animals" (i.e. almost the entire animal kingdom) are equipped with an extraordinary mechanism that maintains the homeostasis of ascorbic acid in the blood and tissues (175). It may sound far-fetched, but it is true. This mechanism, dubbed the "feedback mechanism" by Stone, tends to regulate vitamin C levels in all circumstances by modulating its biosynthesis. This is analogous to the functioning of those fundamental chemical messengers called hormones.

To understand this mechanism, consider glucagon, a key hormone secreted by the pancreas that regulates blood glucose levels. As a hyperglycaemic agent, it responds to any fall in blood glucose by promptly increasing its secretion. In animals, vitamin C biosynthesis behaves in a similar way under stress. The modulation of this biosynthesis occurs in response to threats that may arise during life, just as a hormone responds appropriately to metabolic imbalances regarded as dangerous.

In other words, vitamin C biosynthesis is dynamically regulated to respond appropriately to all endogenous and exogenous stresses that threaten the body.

The implications of this phenomenon are remarkable: during any kind of stress (prolonged fasting, contact with an insidious pathogen, an attack by a predator, a disease, physical, chemical or thermal trauma, exposure to adverse climatic conditions), the mammalian liver reacts swiftly by releasing a supraphysiological, i.e. above-ordinary amount of vitamin C. The significance of the rapid increase in biosynthesis is twofold: to immediately replenish the ascorbic acid reserves depleted by the threat (outlining a compensatory mechanism) and to counteract the disturbing event. Such dynamization, therefore, provides the organism with a new equilibrium through the realisation of an effective response against the stressful event (175).

Stone provided an illustrative example that has become well-known among vitamin C advocates: a 70 kg goat, under normal conditions, produces approximately 13 grams of ascorbic acid per day. Under stress, such as a predator attack, this production can rapidly rise to peaks of 30 grams or more.

Simply put, stress places a heavy demand on vitamin C, which acts as an essential fuel to counteract the stressful event, leading to a rapid depletion of the body's stores. This, in turn, activates a feedback mechanism designed to restore normal ascorbic acid levels as quickly as possible.

Although the American biochemist's hypothesis of hypoascorbemia has been unparalleled in both scientific and media impact, it's important not to overlook the independent studies published since the 1960s (444), (445), (415). These works reconfirm the biochemical differences between humans and animals in vitamin C metabolism. Particularly noteworthy is the animal research by Lahiri and Lloyd (415), which provides compelling evidence for the existence of sophisticated adaptive mechanisms that enhance ascorbic acid synthesis under stress. Equally significant were the histamine experiments conducted by the Japanese duo Suzuki and Nakano, who were especially active in the 1980s (444), (445).

Consistent with previous findings, a 2009 study on hospitalized cats showed that severe stress, such as serious illness, can markedly increase vitamin C concentrations, resulting in plasma levels that appeared to be three times higher than those observed in healthy animals (574).

However, stress is not the only factor that sets humans apart from animals. Even in the absence of stress, animals generally maintain proportionally higher levels of vitamin C than humans. For example, the adrenal glands of rats naturally contain at least twice as much vitamin C as those of humans (67). This finding is significant because, as we will soon discuss, it highlights the fundamental role of vitamin C in responding to stressful events.

At this point, a deep breath may help to process these important concepts, and to prepare for the fascinating discussion ahead. I am confident that one striking observation has not escaped your attention: why do institutional guidelines recommend a daily intake of just 70-100 mg of vitamin C, when a goat typically produces about 150 times more?

This is a critical question, one we will return to and attempt to answer in the final part of the book.

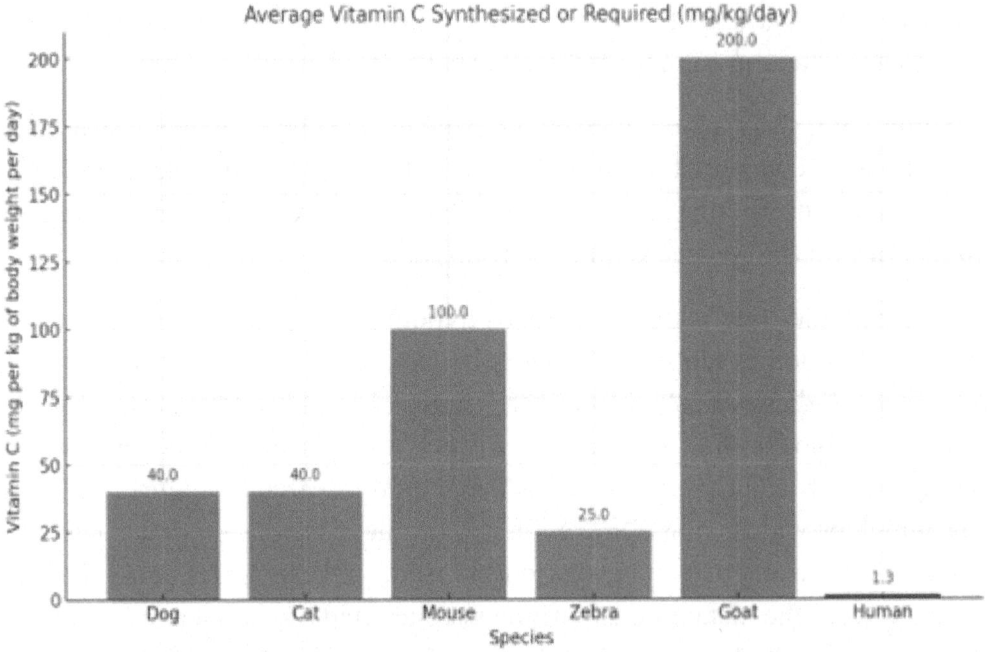

Let's now return to the biosynthesis of vitamin C, particularly during the manifestations of that overwhelming metabolic storm called stress. We will exploit the effectiveness of the time machine we have already inaugurated, discovering how pioneering the ideas of past specialists were and how fortunate animals are to possess this biosynthetic capacity.

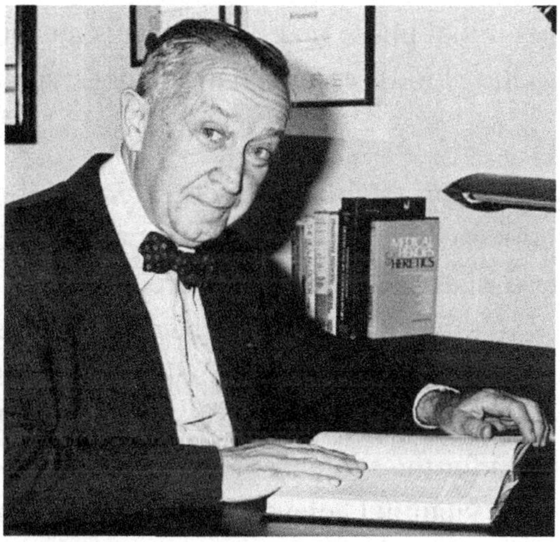

Irwin Stone

Vitamin C: the true anti-stress agent

What is stress and why is vitamin C essential in this condition?

Stress is a physiological response triggered when an individual perceives a significant imbalance between external demands (stressors) and their available resources to cope. This reaction, often referred to as the "General Adaptation Syndrome", aims to quickly restore internal balance (homeostasis) disrupted by stressors.

The physical response to stressful exposure requires the intervention of the nervous and endocrine systems, and is divided into two phases: an immediate and a delayed response. The former, evoking Stone's goat that promptly releases enormous amounts of vitamin C following a predator's attack, involves the release of specific hormonal compounds known as catecholamines, particularly adrenaline and noradrenaline, into the bloodstream. These hormones increase muscle tone and heart rate, enhance attention, and activate other processes essential for survival. This is the well-known "fight or flight" response, typically triggered by a perceived threat, such as a violent predator attack. Within moments, crucial biochemical reactions are set into motion: the liver releases glucose to provide immediate energy; the heart rate increases to optimize blood flow to vital organs; and the pupils dilate (a phenomenon known as mydriasis) to improve vision, among other vital adaptations.

As anticipated, this initial phase involves mainly catecholamines, released by the adrenal glands into the bloodstream. What role does vitamin C play in this biochemical vortex?

Let us now consider a few established facts. First of all, the adrenal glands represent an area with a very high concentration of vitamin C, far higher than plasma and most other tissues. Therefore, the adrenal glands constitute a privileged, "favourite" site for vitamin C. Furthermore, as we will see in detail in the chapter on physiological functions, vitamin C acts as an enzymatic cofactor (for now, suffice it to say that it is an element necessary for the proper functioning of biochemical reactions) for the synthesis of catecholamines, particularly noradrenaline. Therefore, vitamin C plays an active role in the construction of these very important anti-stress compounds.

These data provide a "heuristic" demonstration of the great value of vitamin C in the immediate response to stress, in line with the increase in its biosynthesis that occurs whenever animals with preserved GULO undergo stressful events.

Can you now understand, at least to a partial extent, the human disadvantage due to the genetic defect that Stone called hypoascorbemia? Indeed, it seems that a little GULO wouldn't hurt!

The role of vitamin C does not stop there: in the second response phase (slow or delayed response phase), the body attempts to counteract the negative effects of prolonged fatigue by providing specific hormonal responses via various endocrine glands. In particular, the hypothalamus secretes release factors for another vitamin C-rich site, the pituitary gland, initiating the production of ADH (vasopressin, a molecule dependent on vitamin C) and ACTH (adrenocorticotropic hormone). This activates the famous hypothalamic-pituitary-adrenal axis, a very important system in which ACTH, acting at the level of the adrenal cortex, causes the release of certain corticosteroids including aldosterone and cortisol. While the former is concerned with maintaining a regular fluid level by balancing sodium and potassium concentrations, cortisol, which is much more involved in reaction mechanisms (it is called, not surprisingly, the stress hormone), operates in a completely different and more specific manner. In fact, it stimulates gluconeogenesis (the process aimed at converting compounds other than carbohydrates, such as proteins, into glucose) and reduces the action of insulin (the hormone that facilitates the passage of glucose from the blood to the cells).

These actions are intended to increase blood glucose levels to effectively support the delayed response phase.

It should be emphasised, however, that a prolonged excess of cortisol can cause very negative effects on the organism, not only related to a disproportionate increase in blood glucose. The weakening of the immune response and the decrease in collagen and bone matrix synthesis, paradoxically three effects opposite to those that vitamin C can produce, provide sufficiently strong reasons to fear elevated cortisol levels.

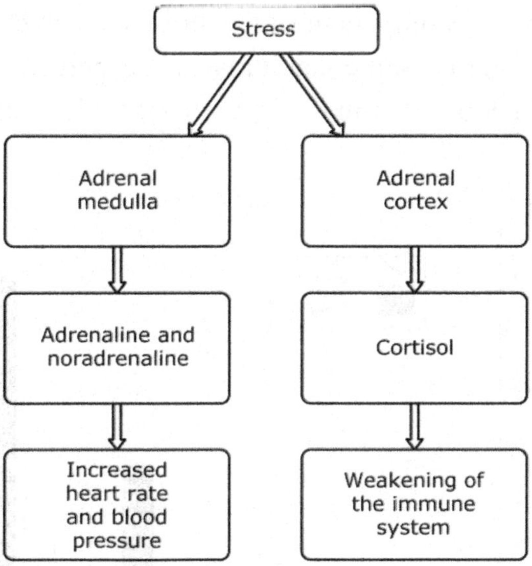

This theoretical premise is the ideal spark to warm up the engines of our time machine and set a very recent date, taking us on a particularly exciting journey.

In 2020, Paul Marik (his name, profoundly linked to research on pharmacological vitamin C in the treatment of sepsis, will be taken up several times) produced a paper (25) in which he refined Stone's original view that vitamin C plays the role of a "stress hormone" in the animal world.

Marik, an internationally renowned American scientist and author of more than 450 peer-reviewed articles, states that the rapid release of adrenal ascorbic concentration (very abundant there, as already mentioned) in response to ACTH during stressful events provides compelling evidence of the fundamental role of vitamin C in stress-response processes. This role, for obvious reasons, is more intense in the animal world.

If these arguments are an extension of Stone's insights, what we are about to illustrate now requires the utmost attention because it is, in a sense, quite surprising. In the same paper (25), in fact, there is evidence to support an inverse correlation between an animal's ability to produce vitamin C endogenously (an ability directly related to the relative degree of GULO preservation) and the amount of cortisol secreted in response to stress (see figure). This suggests two extremely significant corollaries: the ability to increase vitamin C production and secretion is a fundamental component of the stress response. Fundamental. Moreover, it is plausible to assume that humans "desperately" try to compensate, under stress, for the lack of vitamin C biosynthesis by increasing cortisol production (25).

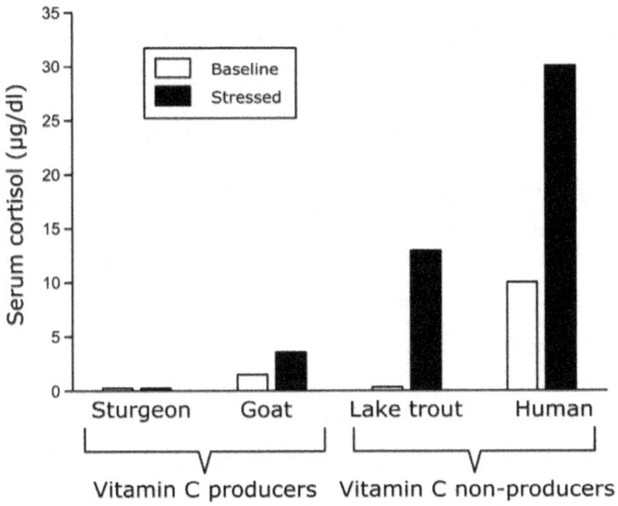

graph adapted from (25)

An abnormal response to stress, probably less efficient than in animals, altered by nature. This is how humans react to stress, implementing a forced substitution that would not have made sense in the absence of the genetic accident that compromised biosynthesis.

It is therefore reasonable to say that the inability to produce vitamin C exposes humans under stress (any type of stress, including psychological, physical and pathological) to the risk of developing more complications than mammals normally equipped with biosynthesis. "Due to an unfortunate evolutionary mutation, humans have lost the ability to synthesize vitamin C (Homo Sapiens Ascorbicus) and consequently have an impaired stress response. The inability to produce vitamin C during stress increases the vulnerability of humans to infectious disorders. Therapeutic doses of vitamin C in combination with other biologically active agents likely improves the outcomes of humans with serious infections", Marik wrote at the conclusion of his paper published in the "Journal of Thoracic Disease" and focused on the deadly sepsis (25).

It is therefore clear that, at least on a theoretical level, the concepts appear to be well defined. But have they actually been confirmed in practice?

In a randomized, double-blind, placebo-controlled study (26), researchers found that oral administration of vitamin C at a dose of 1000 mg three times daily for two weeks reduced blood pressure, cortisol synthesis, and subjective responses to acute psychological stress. Although the intervention was structurally different from Klenner's therapeutic approaches, the study suggests a strong anti-stress effect of vitamin C, consistent with the findings of Stone and Marik. Furthermore, the fact that vitamin C supplementation reduced cortisol levels confirms its significant influence on the mechanisms regulating cortisol release under stress (26).

To conclude for now with Marik, it may be of interest to preview the potential contributions of vitamin C in the treatment of sepsis. As the scientist himself notes in (25): "The inability of humans to produce vitamin C is likely highly deleterious during sepsis due to the rapid metabolic consumption of this stress hormone". This is one of the reasons why adequate ascorbic acid therapy could be beneficial against this insidious disease, given that sepsis rapidly depletes vitamin C levels, potentially pushing the body toward scurvy. From the prevention of scurvy to the treatment of one of the most challenging diseases, sepsis, this represents an acrobatic leap that nevertheless calls for a fundamental paradigm shift.

Returning to the anti-stress reactivity of cortisol, it is useful to note that its intimate relationship with vitamin C under stressful conditions has been extensively analysed (27), (28). While the ascorbic modulation of cortisol has been detected since the early 1980s ("Adrenal ascorbic acid concentration falls as cortisol secretion into the plasma increases", Odumosu wrote in 1982 at the end of an animal experiment (27)), we must nevertheless note that it was not until 2007 that knowledge received sufficient clarification. In this year, researchers were able to describe for the first time the dynamics regulating the release of vitamin C under the stimulus of ACTH (28). The study involved 26 patients who received an intravenous ACTH infusion, designed to stimulate the release of cortisol and vitamin C. The aim was to compare both locally, i.e. in the adrenal veins, and globally, i.e. in the peripheral veins, the amounts of ascorbic acid and cortisol released in response to the ACTH stimulation. In a nutshell, a vitamin C-cortisol competition was staged in the setting of a highly stressful field (the ACTH stimulation).

The results of the study, published in the renowned journal "The American Journal of Clinical Nutrition", supported the findings of Stone, Odumosu and Marik: in the adrenal veins, ACTH induced an immediate increase in vitamin C, which peaked at about four times the baseline level approximately two minutes after adrenocorticotropic stimulation. The release of adrenal ascorbate was therefore rapid, robust, although rather transient (it took less than 20 minutes for adrenal values to return to baseline levels). More importantly, the release of adrenal ascorbate clearly preceded the peak in cortisol levels (28).

The above paints a remarkable picture in which vitamin C appears to play the dual authoritative role of "cortisol-sparing anticipator" under stress. This saving, a clear consequence of the ability to precede the release of cortisol, seems to have very important biological impacts, because it is plausible that a pre-existing and adequate amount of ascorbic acid can limit the release of cortisol during stress, supporting the theory of constantly elevated concentrations.

The study went further. It was observed, in fact, that the ACTH stimulus did not induce an increase in vitamin C concentration in the peripheral veins. According to the authors, this finding indicates that vitamin C reacts to stress through a paracrine secretion, meaning a local action on surrounding cells rather than a systemic one. It should be noted that these dynamics were observed on a human model, clearly deprived of that feedback mechanism that allows lucky animals to develop a much more rounded, and therefore not only local, reaction to stress.

Ultimately, the study suggested that adrenal vitamin C secretion is an essential part of the mechanisms regulating the stress response in humans (28).

This highlights an often underestimated quality of vitamin C: its role as a powerful anti-stress compound. Its involvement in all phases of the stress response, primarily through the modulation of cortisol and support for catecholamine synthesis, forms the basis of a compelling theory: adequate vitamin C intake is essential, truly essential, for effectively supporting the body's response to stress. This view is further supported by the fact that, in the animal kingdom, such intake occurs automatically, wisely ensured by Mother Nature.

At this point, it is worth considering: the harsh fate that Mother Nature has reserved for us seems to dictate the need for a substantial intake of vitamin C as soon as a harmful event occurs, thus making an attempt to mimic the animal model. Or perhaps, as we'll soon explore, a more strategic approach might be possible: a form of preventive action.

In any case, the surprises about vitamin C never end. Another crucial contribution is its powerful antioxidant defence, which protects the body from the overwhelming action of free radicals unleashed by intense stress. This represents a real threat to cellular integrity: oxidative stress, which we will describe in detail later. Under such conditions, another damaging factor also comes into play, inflammation, against which vitamin C proves to be a declared enemy. We will review several studies on this, including one focusing on a group of marathon runners.

I am convinced that a question is forming in your mind: from a practical point of view, how much vitamin C is needed to neutralise the negative effects of stress?

The hectic pace of daily life, environmental and electromagnetic pollution, poor nutrition, psychological discomfort, work-related stress, smoking, alcohol abuse, intense physical activity and the use of drug therapies are some of the main stress factors. I answer this question with another question: is a daily intake of 70-100 mg (RDA) sufficient to effectively counteract the numerous stressful stimuli?

It is not difficult to see that a standard intake (50-150 mg per day), easily obtained through diet, is characterised by a static nature that reflects an "insensitivity" to the external conditions that increasingly permeate our lives. This static nature is the opposite of the dynamism that characterises the animal organism, which, under stress, is able to respond to any danger through effective modulation of biosynthesis. It could therefore be useful to work in advance, implementing a sort of anti-stress prophylaxis. How?

A few more questions. Could it be beneficial to supply our bodies with high and repeated amounts of ascorbic acid?

Despite the lack of certainty (Medicine is a long way from Mathematics, and not only in terms of the soundness of statements), logic suggests that such a regimen may provide the best conditions (i.e. a consistently high ascorbic content, as occurs in animals that synthesize vitamin C endogenously) to cope with the consequences of a stressful episode, which, as is well known, tends to deplete vitamin C and induce the release of large amounts of cortisol and free radicals.

It is reasonable to state, therefore, that consistent supplementation would grant maximum preparation for the inevitable encounter with stress. It is not irrelevant to note that the numerous authors of the previous study (28) expressed themselves in similar terms in their conclusions: "If adrenal vitamin C secretion has physiologic consequences, consideration should be given to vitamin C intake above that possible from foods alone".

And in the case of an overt pathology, would the recommended 70-100 mg daily be sufficient, considering that the pathological state may intrinsically represent a form of stress?

These very interesting questions raise a logical perspective that will be developed further in the overall assessment at the end of the book. In any case, among the various hypotheses and questions, there is one fact that remains indisputable: stress increases the metabolic requirement for vitamin C, distancing us from animals.

This paragraph concludes with a unique source of stress already mentioned, which is interdependent with pathological conditions: the use of drugs, whose necessity, in the case of chronic diseases, can be prolonged. As logic suggests, the administration of any pharmacological agent tends to reduce vitamin C levels, in some cases quite markedly. Numerous animal studies (29), (30), (31), in fact, have shown significant increases in vitamin C in response to pharmacological administrations, indicating a vigorous response of the animal organism under pharmacological stimulus, evidently indispensable for rapidly restoring weakened concentrations due to the stress caused by exposure to drugs.

Overall, what has been examined supports the need for appropriate vitamin C supplementation during illness. In the case of certain drugs (sedatives, analgesics, muscle relaxants), in fact, the increase in biosynthesis observed in animal experiments was so high (up to eightfold the baseline production) that it raised significant questions (29), (30), (31). We will examine one in particular, developed using a model that may help to clarify the issue. A diabetic patient undergoing drug therapy has at least three compelling reasons to consider supplementation with adequate amounts of vitamin C:

1- The disease itself – Diabetes can significantly deplete vitamin C levels, leading to low concentrations both in plasma and within cells, particularly red blood cells;

2- Chronic exposure to antidiabetic medications – These drugs introduce an additional source of stress and oxidative stress, which can further lower vitamin C levels;

3- The anti-stress prophylactic model.

A fourth and more direct reason will be examined later, when the potential hypoglycaemic properties of ascorbic acid are discussed in detail.

Together, these factors support the rationale for vitamin C supplementation during the course of diabetes. In this context, ascorbate depletion caused by the disease itself may be further exacerbated by drug therapies. The result is a concerning scenario in which persistent vitamin C deficiency seems a likely outcome in many chronic illnesses requiring ongoing pharmacological intervention. What is particularly surprising is how rarely these arguments are reflected in clinical practice or scientific discourse. It is therefore reasonable to assume that the marginalisation of the importance of vitamin C supplementation, both in the context of maintaining general health and during illness, is a highly questionable approach. Admittedly, this is a personal interpretation, but it is reinforced by a critical point: vitamin C therapy is characterised by few side effects, even when administered in high oral doses or via intravenous routes.

Chronic subclinical scurvy

The long parenthesis on stress serves as the ideal preamble for a new journey through time, one that will take us back to the 1960s, where something truly exciting awaits us: Stone's prolific and groundbreaking work.

We thus encounter one of the American biochemist's key contributions: he hypothesised a compensatory mechanism that would allow human physiology to adapt to low levels of vitamin C, thereby staving off (or perhaps cunningly disguising?) the symptoms of scurvy. Beware of false illusions, however: such an adaptation, being a form of forced "metabolic reprogramming", may not guarantee the optimal efficiency of the countless biochemical processes linked to ascorbic acid. The idea that low levels of ascorbic acid may weaken the biochemical processes related to it, causing implicit suffering in the body, is increasingly supported by scientific evidence. This insidious suffering, referred to by Stone as "chronic subclinical scurvy", seems to involve several manifestations, including reduced stress tolerance, clearly compatible with the weak anti-stress reactivity extensively described above. But that is not all: there would be other outcomes, about which I ask you to be patient for a moment.

Stone was so original as to theorise the existence of three categories of physiological-pathological states, thus framing human health in an unusual three-dimensional vision. These are frank scurvy, chronic subclinical scurvy and full health. It is a list in which there is a third part that falls between scurvy and health, a third part that tends to largely separate the state of optimal health from the state of apparent good health, highlighting that masked scurvy, despite the typical tendency not to express striking symptoms, is far from full health. More explicitly: not having an empty tank does not necessarily imply full health.

In this regard, the biochemist associated the disease state with chronic subclinical scurvy, hypothesising for the first time that ascorbic acid deficiency could be involved in the pathogenesis of many diseases. This insight has been confirmed over time by numerous specific epidemiological studies: chronically low vitamin C levels increase the overall risk of disease, as suggested by the numerous inverse correlations between plasma concentrations and the risk of contracting a wide range of diseases, from cancer to vascular events, metabolic diseases and neurodegenerative diseases. These would be the other important "symptoms" of chronic subclinical scurvy. These symptoms are different from those we are used to, more subtle and less immediate, but they could nevertheless act by progressively weakening our defences until the numerous concomitant causes trigger the pathological state.

It is therefore plausible to formulate a pragmatic thesis that the greatest benefits of vitamin C are paradoxically invisible, especially when the tank is not completely empty. Benefits tied to the slow but relentless passage of time, arguably the only judge of vitamin C's true weight. A judge, however, who may need time, a lot of time, to gather evidence of efficacy. After all, Voltaire was probably not wrong when he claimed that "Time is a gentleman".

Stone's vision introduced a remarkably original perspective, whereby analytical observation of many diseases produces images that identify them as symptoms of chronic vitamin C deficiency. This, and this is not a marginal fact, is in complete agreement with Szent-Györgyi's thinking, also expressed in the preface of "The Healing Factor".

Although Stone's conception may appear simplistic, I believe that a judicious interpretation may instead lay the groundwork for formulating a sort of Grand Unification Theory, the theory constructed by physicists to achieve the unification of the three fundamental interactions of physics; this analogy suggests that any pathological state is correlated with inadequate levels of vitamin C. I repeat: inadequate, and therefore not necessarily close to zero. What does this mean, practically speaking?

An example might clarify the concept: as we will discuss in more detail in the specific chapter, various studies (32), (33) have indicated that cancer patients exhibit much lower ascorbic levels than the general population, with a significant portion approaching levels typical of scurvy. This raises a curious question: do cancer patients die from the disease itself, or from the profound vitamin C deficiency it often induces?

Perhaps Stone was not entirely off the mark when he argued that serious disease states such as cancer, being potential causes of scurvy (which, for those who may have forgotten, is a fatal disease), can lead to death directly from vitamin C deficiency. A supporting argument for this conjecture is found in the concluding chapters of his book, where he refers to an interesting study by

Hawley. This study found that white blood cells contain at least 30 times more vitamin C than plasma. Hawley's discovery, of great historical significance, introduced two central concepts: the compartmentalisation of vitamin C within the body and its primary role in immune functions. Building on Hawley's findings, Stone hypothesised that the residual vitamin C reserves in leukaemia patients must be concentrated almost exclusively in white blood cells. This, in turn, would prevent tissues from utilising vitamin C for various metabolic functions, including its potential anti-haemorrhagic action. From this, he outlined a potential association between leukaemia and scurvy, supported by the similarities in symptoms that the two diseases can manifest, particularly haemorrhaging.

In other words, according to the biochemist, leukaemia would be able to consume vitamin C so voraciously (consistent with the already reported association between cancer and vitamin C deficiency and with what we will document later (507)) as to project a scenario whereby death could be blamed on its deficiency, essentially therefore on scurvy. A vision undoubtedly fascinating and perhaps not so far from reality.

In any case, Stone's discoveries provide an effective insight into his profound scientific thinking, based on the concept of hypoascorbemia (which he later redefined as a "congenital error of carbohydrate metabolism") and its important interdependence, i.e. the invisible but robust link between vitamin C deficiency and the pathogenesis of a wide range of diseases. No less important is the sagacity with which he hypothesised the progressive depletion of ascorbic levels that characterises the various stages of a serious disease. This depletion, already observed by Klenner in the context of infectious diseases, can be so severe that it quickly leads to scurvy.

A very interesting question is the following: regardless of specific therapies, would it be reasonable to consider vitamin C treatment for serious diseases?

A potential answer will be provided later, when we will also observe how the combination of logic and science allows us to add another piece to the puzzle, namely, the synergy that typically characterises combination therapy involving vitamin C. It is no coincidence that Klenner used to recommend to his colleagues in emergency medicine the immediate use of intravenous vitamin C in any critical condition. But is this really sound advice?

There is a rationale behind this suggestion. At its core lies a fact that will be thoroughly discussed and documented throughout this book: critically ill patients very often exhibit drastically reduced vitamin C levels (34). Consistent with the typically inadequate levels observed in cancer patients, this finding seems to support Klenner's pioneering proposal. It is reasonable to assume that restoring normal plasma concentrations may help limit the progression of a critical condition, while also supporting specific therapeutic interventions. This suggests the importance of rebalancing ascorbic acid levels depleted by severe illness, a need that holds intrinsic value, even independently of any potential direct therapeutic effect. You may already have anticipated the reason: the negative impact of low vitamin C levels in critically ill patients is well documented, and this deficiency can exacerbate pre-existing dysfunctions as well as trigger further serious complications (34).

Let us return to Stone's scientific output. Once the concept of chronic subclinical scurvy had been clarified, all that remained was to define a recovery manoeuvre that could heal the wounds of hypoascorbemia. This led to the strategy known as "correction of hypoascorbemia", which consists of administering ascorbic acid in doses equal to those that the human liver would have produced if it had not been affected by the genetic disorder. Stone essentially had in mind a form of imitation of animal behaviour, a sort of symptomatic therapy for the genetic defect. It was purely symptomatic, considering the impracticality of the interventionist approach on the defective gene, which is also impractical for modern genetic engineering techniques.

Let us consider the comparison with a rare disease known as "primary coenzyme Q10 deficiency", a genetic disorder caused by a mutation in one of the genes involved in the biosynthesis of this molecule. This is a serious metabolic disorder, underlying the deficiency of a compound that is strongly involved in human physiology. Coenzyme Q10 is abundant in the myocardium and supports energy metabolism by promoting the proper functioning of mitochondria, the intracellular organelles that act as the powerhouses of cells. It also provides protection against oxidants, as it is one of the antioxidants belonging to the very important class of endogenous antioxidants. Therefore, a deficiency due to this genetic disorder would represent a serious danger against which, since we cannot intervene genetically, we have only one effective weapon, perhaps inconvenient but of vital importance: the normalisation of physiological concentrations. The treatment of primary coenzyme Q10 deficiency therefore involves the administration of coenzyme Q10 supplements in order to keep the body free from deficiency.

Using similar logic, albeit on a different scale (vitamin C, in addition to having a much higher requirement than all essential micronutrients, including coenzyme Q10, is subject to depletion with extensive etiological roots), Stone proposed correcting the damage caused by the genetic defect. However, he pointed out that this was impossible through dietary sources due to the low amounts of ascorbate present in food and the physical limits on the volume of food that can be consumed. This was a commendable project, but it was systematically rejected by the scientific community, which continued to view vitamin C as the "orange of health", a restriction that unfortunately still applies today.

He persistently challenged the narrow view of vitamin C as just a micronutrient, going so far as to call it "the most obtuse concept in nutrition", dominant in the medical profession of yesterday and, unfortunately, at least in part, still today. He also emphasised another crucial fact: vitamin C does not meet all the criteria of a vitamin, i.e. it does not universally meet the criteria required by the formal definition of a vitamin (organic chemical compounds essential for survival and not synthesised by the body). It is in fact an atypical vitamin compound, ruined by time and the vagaries of fate, and therefore not fully compliant with other vitamins. This clearly stems from animal biosynthesis and the unfortunate genetic accident suffered by humans, without which we would have no doubt about the non-vitamin nature of ascorbic acid. I emphasise: the non-vitamin nature of ascorbic acid.

The non-vitamin essence of ascorbic acid introduces the long list of reasons that make this substance unique: in fact, there is no other vitamin compound in nature whose "vitamin" status disappears when confined to the animal world, or that has lost its original non-vitamin status during evolution.

Stone's work sparked a significant trend that gradually intrigued many scientists, some of whom, notably Linus Pauling, became so fascinated that they devoted their best energies to the courageous project of debunking the mythology that restricted vitamin C to the realm of nutrition. Stone's preference for the term "ascorbate" (equivalent to ascorbic acid or vitamin C), with which he constantly highlighted the "psychological difference" between vitamin C produced in the liver of animals and that introduced by humans through diet, is effectively complemented by the following comparison: musicians teach us that F sharp and G flat, though acoustically identical, are not considered the same note at all.

Stone also presented some arguments in support of the very low toxicity of vitamin C. The reason given by the biochemist is evolutionary: if it had been in any way toxic, given its extremely wide distribution in all forms of life, it would have been eliminated by a series of evolutionary processes. Although the real underlying reasons are still partially unknown, the water-soluble nature and the existence of rigorous homeostatic mechanisms constitute evidence for the substantial non-toxicity of vitamin C, which has been confirmed in practice by numerous clinical evaluations.

The masterpiece "The Healing Factor" concludes with an astounding list of contributions that vitamin C could make in the treatment of many diseases, including cardiovascular disorders, asthma, glaucoma and mental illness. Stone also raised an issue that is still relevant today. The protagonist is the lack of pharmacological preparations, both for infusion and oral administration, containing high doses, which are clearly essential to ensure the pharmacological action that could be useful in clinical practice.

So here we are again: supplementation versus pharmacological agent. This issue continues to hinder any high-dose pharmacological approach involving ascorbic acid, which is particularly relevant in contexts such as adjuvant cancer therapy. In such cases, the need for massive intravenous administrations (70-80 grams or more), likely required to achieve clinically significant antitumour effects, underscores the inadequacy of standard pharmaceutical formulations, which are generally limited to modest 500-1000 mg injectable solutions. This represents a significant technical barrier within the framework of vitamin C drug therapy, while also drawing attention to one of the most emblematic issues in the field: the dualism between the concept of nutritional intake (a notion extensively criticised by Stone) and the more advanced concepts of correction of hypoascorbemia and, above all, pharmacological use. This dualism, already widely heralded, has given rise to an embarrassing state of confusion in the scientific community, which is still so widespread today as to direct specialists towards the urgent need for a radical change of mindset, now indispensable in order to identify the exact nature of vitamin C, or even better, ascorbate.

Linus Pauling

"I think that mankind owes a serious thanks to Irwin Stone for having kept the problem alive and having called Linus Pauling's attention to it", Szent-Györgyi wrote in a notable passage of the preface to "The Healing Factor". This is a very important quote, highlighting another fundamental contribution made by Stone: that of informing Linus Pauling of the surprising advances made in the field of ascorbic acid.

Endowed with a profound sense of peace, the American chemist Linus Pauling is considered one of the greatest scientists of the last century, the only person in the world to have won two Nobel Prizes without sharing them with anyone else. The first, for Chemistry, was awarded in 1954 for his sophisticated description of the nature of chemical bonds, while the other, dating back to 1962, embraced what he had always fought so hard for: Peace. A career of infinite value, therefore, which would see further merits in the early 1970s, when he began a remarkable love affair with vitamin C. His passion for vitamin C was such that it prompted him to inaugurate, with the collaboration of Cathcart and Hoffer, a new field of science, namely Orthomolecular Medicine. This is based on a fundamental principle: full health requires optimal levels of essential nutrients such as vitamins, amino acids, and minerals. According to this logic, any imbalance would therefore require adequate replenishment, and the correction of hypoascorbemia is the central example around which further indications can be built.

The birth of Orthomolecular Medicine did not go unnoticed in the scientific community, which did not take long to pour out fierce criticism on the founders, justifying it by the lack of solid scientific evidence. What was probably missing at the time of the events, I report this as a personal impression, was a logical vision that would allow orthomolecular theories to be linked to the rigorous criteria of Science. Nothing more!

Pauling, in fact, emphasised the importance of replenishing vitamin levels (remember that these are essential substances for life) depleted due to any aetiological factor, while also pointing out that the dosages considered ideal by health institutions are probably underestimated compared to the body's actual physiological requirements. The example of vitamin C is illuminating in this regard: the recommended dosages are probably insufficient to ensure full and lasting health.

The Nobel Prize winner's ideas, which were not limited to vitamin C, make it possible to identify certain typicalities of orthomolecular philosophy, one of which can be easily understood through a rather pertinent comparison. Pauling offered the example of type 1 diabetes therapy as a model for the orthomolecular approach, a disease in which the replenishment of the hormone insulin, which is in short supply due to the autoimmune-based destruction of the beta cells of the pancreas, is indispensable to ensure the body's proper metabolism. There's nothing strange about that, is there?

With a similar logic, Pauling proposed to monitor and eventually replenish all those nutrients essential for human biology. Essentials, I repeat, whose deficiency can therefore lead to dysfunctions of varying severity up to and including serious diseases such as scurvy, beriberi and pellagra, just as insulin deficiency correlates with potentially dramatic metabolic consequences.

As anticipated, many of the arguments of the orthomolecular planet were also harshly attacked because of the thickness of the main promoter: it seemed totally unacceptable, in the eyes of the medical establishment, that a Nobel Prize winner acted apparently without scientific evidence.

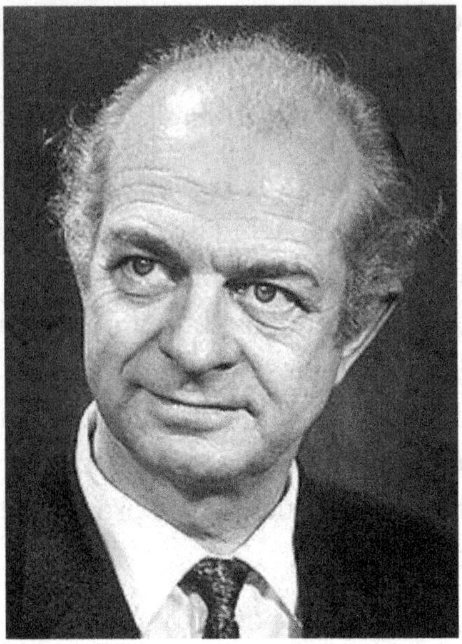

Linus Pauling

Pauling's position plummeted to a worrying low point, an event that will be illustrated in the chapter on cancer through a detailed historical reconstruction, when he and the talented Scottish surgeon Ewan Cameron published data from a courageous clinical study on terminal cancer patients. The results, which astonished the world, suggested a noteworthy anticancer effect of vitamin C. The leap from scurvy to cancer was so dramatic that it inevitably ignited an electrifying battle, both social and scientific, in which the first major "academic confrontation" saw vitamin C fall under a storm of skepticism and controversy. However, over time, there has been a progressive reevaluation through which their controversial studies have come to be regarded as increasingly plausible.

Driven by Stone's formidable structuralist vision, the double Nobel Prize winner oriented his interests in multiple directions and came to highlight a variety of points of tangency between vitamin C and medical science. One of these inevitably brings us back to the subject of the common cold, a condition that, for better or worse, has historically elevated media interest through the promotion of its "immunostimulant" properties. It should be noted that the term immunostimulant lends itself to ambiguous, potentially misleading interpretations. Indeed, even today, there is a tendency to associate certain pharmacological capacities of vitamin C, such as its immunostimulant properties, with what is mistakenly considered by many to be a remedy against the common cold, i.e. the biological effect of a simple glass of orange juice. Vitamin C, which is not a mere remedy but a vital substance, and not an immunostimulant, but an immunomodulatory agent, reminds us how easily we fall into the ever-persistent trap of mistaking a fruit vendor for a pharmacist.

The first research on the common cold concerned the dual preventive-therapeutic role. We are in the early 1970s, a time when the literature was already smiling at vitamin C: “A statistical analysis of these four studies leads to rejection of the null hypothesis that ascorbic acid has no more protective power than the placebo”, reads a review by Pauling in 1971 (35).

The studies on the common cold, initially included in the book inspired by constructive conversations with his friend Stone, entitled “Vitamin C and the Common Cold”, were updated many years later in his famous book “How to Live Longer and Feel Better”. A broader and deeper book, in which the description of the treatment of the common cold is just one of many concerning the benefits of vitamin C and orthomolecular medicine.

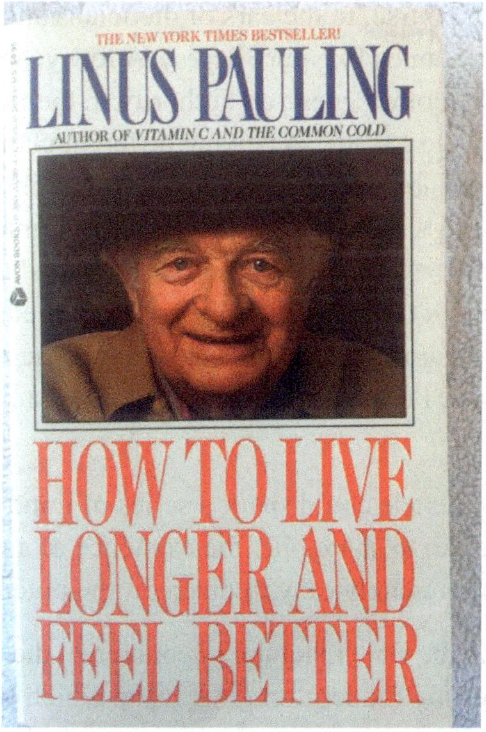

Regarding the common cold, Pauling noted that taking large hourly doses, a strategy similar to Klenner's therapeutic regimen, could alleviate symptoms and shorten its duration. He reported in his book: "When you feel the first symptoms of a cold, you should immediately increase your intake of the vitamin to a therapeutic level. In my experience, this means taking 1 g or more per hour, throughout the day. In this way, cold symptoms would be suppressed immediately and would not reappear should the therapeutic dose be maintained as such throughout its predictable duration. The only discomfort caused by this regimen might manifest itself, in the first few days, with some discomfort in the bowels (soft stools)". While this statement tends to reiterate how essential it is to properly set up a vitamin C treatment (a timely, repeated, and high-intensity treatment), it also describes the only potential discomfort, which Cathcart had associated with "bowel tolerance".

Before organizing a time travel with 2016 as a destination, it might be useful to remark that the Nobel laureate's ideas had little "appeal" in the scientific community. An anecdote illustrated in his book perfectly captures the stormy climate at the time: "Of course, to the ears of dieticians and orthodox physicians, my simple prescription sounds like pure heresy. A few years ago I was invited to a TV show together with another guest, an authority in the field of nutrition, Dr. Fredrick J. Stare. Stare and I made somewhat different claims about vitamin C and its efficacy. The hour-long program was almost coming to an end when Stare said: «'I know Dr. Pauling's method of preventing the common cold is useless; I tried it and it didn't work'». I made to ask him how he had tried it, but the host interrupted us by saying: «'Gentlemen, I'm sorry, but time is up; thank you for participating in our program'». So, as we were leaving the room, Stare turned to me and said: «'Of course, I did not use the astronomical amounts you recommend'»".

I believe that this episode could spark a series of important reflections. Among these, I would like to share one: the existence of an ambiguous position through which it is unfortunately easy to discredit the potential of vitamin C.

Let us now resume the time machine to concretize the booked trip, in which we encounter an interesting modern review (36) in which Bucher and White pointed out the remarkable anti-stress role of vitamin C during the common cold. From the body of research examined, a greater effectiveness has in fact emerged in subjects exposed to high physical stress. This finding reaffirmed the fundamental role of vitamin C in stressful conditions, evoking the hormonal effect of stress, which is entirely natural for animals capable of biosynthesis.

Bucher and White (36), demonstrating that therapeutic efficacy requires vigorous (8 g per day) and timely (essentially at the first onset of common cold symptoms) treatment, joined Hemilä (21) in reiterating the importance of properly characterising vitamin C therapy, indirectly providing valid justifications for the disappointing clinical results. A note: the thesis that the time factor may indeed be decisive will be demonstrated on several occasions.

What has been described reveals how marginalized the work of orthomolecularists has been throughout history, beginning with Klenner's work. The use of hourly doses, for example, has rarely been considered in scientific research. While the rationale for excluding modern, and I emphasize modern, studies from making use of such a treatment is scarce, we are still forced to wonder what its actual clinical weight might be. The specification "modern" comes from the fact that several decades ago hourly doses were more common. Some traces can be found in Pauling's book: "The best study of the therapeutic effect of vitamin C was carried out by Asfora (1977), who distributed 30 g as an alternative to a placebo to 133 subjects (medical students, physicians or patients hospitalized in Pernambuco) who had reported the onset of a cold. The vitamin C was distributed in 1000 mg effervescent tablets, along with instructions recommending taking six a day (two at a time, three times a day) for five days; the placebo consisted of similar effervescent tablets. Some patients began treatment on the first day of the cold, some on the second, and some on the third, as is shown in the table below. The percentage of subjects for whom the treatment could be said to have totally failed, as they developed secondary bacterial infections and were sick for an average of fifteen days, was 13% for those who took vitamin C on the first day, 20% for those who took it on the second day, and 41% for those who took it on the third day (and 39% for the placebo group). For the remaining subjects in each group, whose colds were uncomplicated, the mean number of sick days was 1.82, 2.71 and 5.10 at the said days on which intake had occurred, respectively. We therefore observe that 6 g of vitamin C, taken on the first or second day of a cold, stopped the disorder in most of the subjects in the survey".

In addition to their intrinsic value, these studies (Pauling cited several in his book) reinforce the importance of a crucial aspect of effective acute treatment with vitamin C: the timeliness of intervention, which is probably no less important than dosage or frequency. It should be noted that optimal timing is essential to maximize the therapeutic potential of vitamin C, especially in complex clinical settings such as septic shock or severe burns.

Let us now turn to one of Pauling's most intriguing contributions. It consists of a set of hypotheses linking the pathogenesis of certain cardiovascular diseases to vitamin C, a theory that will be explored in greater depth in the following chapters. At the origin of this theory is the so-called lipoprotein-a, a lipoprotein structurally similar to the famous LDL (but metabolically different) which numerous epidemiological studies have identified as a risk factor for atherosclerotic diseases (473). It all began with a 1990 study (37) that laid the foundations for the theory thanks to a surprising link between lipoprotein-a and ascorbic acid. This study reported evidence supporting an inverse association between the two components, some of which came from the observation that lipoprotein-a is abundant in animals deprived of biosynthesis. As we will see, this represents a starting point from which some scientists will develop a theory that the aetiology of many cardiovascular disorders has different answers than those accepted by most of the scientific community.

Let us turn the page, because the repertoire of the two-time Nobel laureate is truly vast. Encouraged by Klenner's work and the subsequent developments in which the antiviral capabilities of vitamin C seemed increasingly real, he decided to test its pharmacological abilities against a very insidious virus, HIV, the agent responsible for AIDS. Vitamin C was able to pass even this preliminary test. In a 1990 in-vitro experiment published in the prestigious journal "Proceedings of the National Academy of Sciences of the United States of America" (38), Pauling, Harakeh and Jariwalla provided preclinical evidence of a significant anti-HIV effect mediated by vitamin C. This result was unexpected, as it was obtained with merely physiological levels of the vitamin. The finding gave rise to a hypothesis, consistent with Stone's ideas and still debated today, suggesting that the normalization of plasma concentrations may be sufficient to offer antiviral benefits in infected patients, who are clearly vulnerable to viral depletion. This hypothesis will be discussed later through a personal perspective.

We have reached the final years of the double Nobel Prize winner's life (early 1990s), almost ten years after the oncological controversy that damaged his prestige, which had already been undermined by his orthomolecular leadership, which he never abandoned. But these were also the years when decisive efforts were made to understand the pharmacokinetics of vitamin C, highlighting the profound differences between oral and intravenous administration, a fact that would provide the arguments for "rehabilitating" the criticised anticancer studies.

The great relationship with vitamin C offers numerous points of reflection about Pauling's scientific work, two of which appear particularly relevant: his intuition regarding its anticancer properties, explored for the first time in a clinical context, and his unparalleled scientific determination. These two elements would earn him the permanent role of the world's greatest promoter of vitamin C in history.

We close by quoting a review by the Kodama brothers (39) entitled "Is Linus Pauling, a Vitamin C advocate, just making much ado about nothing?".

The review focuses on an aspect repeatedly emphasised by the Nobel Prize winner himself. The reference is to the "paradigm shift" of vitamin C, an ideological transposition that becomes the leitmotif of the book. The Kodama brothers joined other specialists in believing that a radical ideological change in clinical research on vitamin C was necessary, thanks to which misunderstandings and confusion could finally be avoided. "We also refer to a series of scientific debates to show that a paradigm shift is indispensable to achieve a full understanding of the benefits of vitamin C, including the control of diabetes mellitus and the autoimmune disease/allergy complex", they stated encouraged by their research in which high-dose vitamin C appeared effective against diabetes and allergies (39).

And it is precisely the topic of allergies that provides an interesting conclusion. We are, in fact, examining a condition in which adequate treatment with vitamin C seems to align perfectly with those dynamics that only a genius like Stone could have foreseen so early on: it is well known that animals respond to sudden increases in histamine with a rapid surge in biosynthesis, thus identifying allergic reactions as significant sources of stress.

Pauling's death on 19 August 1994 marked the close of a unique chapter in the history of vitamin C, a symbol of perfection in which Irwin's contribution, namely introducing Linus to the magic of ascorbic acid, could not have received greater recognition, both in prestige and emotional intensity. It was an unprecedented exchange, made even more remarkable by the dedication with which both scientists risked their credibility and placed their distinguished careers in jeopardy. All in the name of vitamin C.

'Measures to improve one's health and prolong life should not be so burdensome and unpleasant as to seriously interfere with the quality of life or make it difficult to maintain the regimen day after day, year after year. Willingness to comply is very important'

Linus Pauling

Cathcart and Hoffer

'The number-one side effect of vitamins is failure to take enough of them'

Abram Hoffer

At the other two corners of the orthomolecular triangle are Robert Cathcart and Abram Hoffer, two great scientists thanks to whom vitamin C will continue to be the subject of profound scientific interpretation, controversy included.

Originally from California, Dr Robert Fulton Cathcart acquired extensive clinical experience with vitamin C, gained after devoting the early part of his career to his specialty, orthopaedic surgery, a branch in which he produced significant innovations (467). Fascinated by Pauling's work, Cathcart shifted his interests to vitamin C and came to conceive the treatment of infectious diseases through what would later go down in history as ascorbic acid megadoses. He followed numerous clinical cases, producing an iconic report in 1981 containing the main clinical observations of his long career, in which thousands of patients are said to have benefited from an original therapy using massive doses of vitamin C, based on reaching the so-called bowel tolerance.

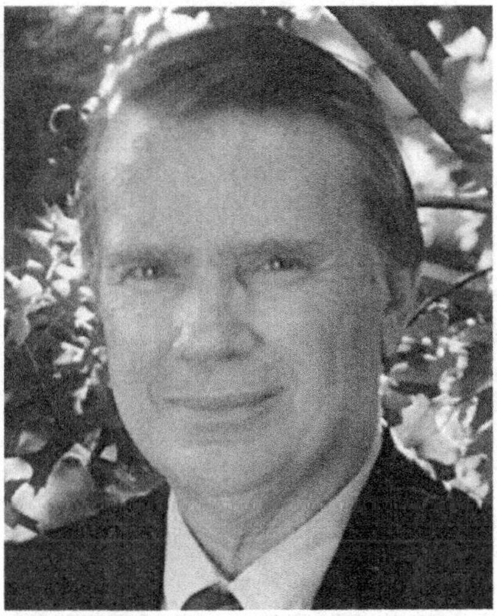

Robert Cathcart

This term refers to the maximum dose of vitamin C that the intestine can tolerate, i.e. that it is able to absorb without developing intestinal symptoms. The practice aims to seek out the smallest intake that can cause an intestinal reaction, usually a mild laxative effect, achieved through progressively increasing doses. Reaching this "intestinal limit", which is rather variable as it is influenced by multiple factors, would correspond to the maximum effectiveness of oral (I stress, oral) ascorbic therapy. Basically, Cathcart's method aims to prepare the human body to counteract adverse events, mimicking the spontaneous dynamics through which the livers of animals capable of synthesizing vitamin C naturally operate.

There are numerous publications on bowel tolerance, some of which include other innovations such as Cathcart's famous "empirical therapeutic tables" and the notion of "anascorbemia" (40).

Usual doses based on intestinal tolerance		
Disease	Grams in 24 h	Number of doses in 24 h
Normality	4-15	4
Mild cold	30-60	6-10
Severe cold	60-100	8-15
Flu	100-150	8-20
ECHO	100-150	8-20
Mononucleosis	150-200 and more	12-25
Viral pneumonia	100-200 and more	12-25
Hay fever, asthma	15-50	4-8
Environmental and food allergies	0.5-50	4-8
Burns, wounds, surgical procedures	25-150	6-20
Anxiety, athletic perf., and other minor stresses	15-25	4-6
Cancer	15-100	4-15
Ankylosing spondylitis	15-100	4-15
Reiter's syndrome	15-60	4-10
Acute anterior uveitis	30-100	4-15
Rheumatoid arthritis	15-100	4-15
Bacterial infections	30-200 and more	10-25
infectious hepatitis	30-100	6-15
Candida infection	15-200 and more	6-25

"The amount of oral ascorbic acid tolerated by a patient without producing diarrhea increases somewhat proportionately to the stress or toxicity of his disease. Bowel tolerance doses of ascorbic acid ameliorate the acute symptoms of many diseases. Lesser doses often have little effect on acute symptoms but assist the body in handling the stress of disease and may reduce the morbidity of the disease. However, if doses of ascorbate are not provided to satisfy this potential draw on the nutrient, first local tissues involved in the disease, then the blood, and then the body in general become depleted of ascorbate (anascorbemia and acute induced scurvy). The patient is thereby put at risk for complications of metabolic processes known to be dependent upon ascorbate", he stated with great conviction in the article "Vitamin C, titrating to bowel tolerance, anascorbemia, and acute induced scurvy" (40).

To modern eyes, these statements appear interesting not only because they contain the concept of anascorbemia, i.e. the form of scurvy triggered not by a dietary deficiency but by an induced erosion (acute induced scurvy) from stressful or pathological factors. Cathcart went a step further by providing his interpretation of a dynamic that is still unclarified and unfortunately marginalised today: what are the first areas to suffer a depletion, an actual erosion, of ascorbate during the acute phase of a disease?

Although it is now beyond dispute that there are many pathologies that tend to deplete vitamin C, and this will be amply documented, the anatomical mapping of depletion mechanics seems unclear. Moreover, what is meant by "depletion of ascorbic acid", given that it is distributed with great variability in plasma and tissues?

Let's start with a conventional fact: when referring to deficiency, hypovitaminosis, or more generally vitamin C levels, the reference is usually to plasma concentrations, which are much lower than the amounts distributed in the various tissues of the body.

Cathcart added an important piece to the understanding of the anatomical mapping of depletion mechanisms by identifying the "chronologically most sensitive" target to acute disease-induced depletion, namely anascorbemia: the area directly involved in the disease, where vitamin C deficiency precedes plasma deficiency and then spreads throughout the body.

In detail (personal hypothesis), it could happen that the area affected by the disease becomes so depleted that it requires immediate replenishment, to which the plasma would respond in the first instance (this would explain the subsequent plasma depletion). However, the issue seems to be much more complex in reality, due to some fundamental exceptions that should make research on ascorbic acid even more interesting and which could have clinical implications. Why?

An example might make it easier to understand the answer, diagonally flanking a modern confirmation of vitamin C's antiviral qualities. Suppose we wanted to analyse the depletion mechanics by which vitamin C is depleted in the various tissues during the acute phase of viral myocarditis, a dangerous inflammation of the myocardium caused by the activity of a virus. To avoid misunderstandings, it should be noted that the idea of combining vitamin C supplementation with antiviral therapy is supported by some studies, including a recent review and meta-analysis focusing on children (41).

Let's put ourselves in the shoes of a doctor who wants to set up a combination therapy with pharmacological ascorbate. A number of conceptual obstacles may arise, one of which concerns the preliminary measurement of the concentration of ascorbic acid in plasma (or blood, it makes no difference). This strategy, which appears to be functional for efficient pharmacological correction, could actually prove misleading. For what reason?

If we accept the local depletion hypothesis, we must anticipate the fact that a momentary regularity of plasma levels may mask very low local (cardiac in this case) concentrations. In short, plasma levels might be misleading, and the most appropriate choice would fall to measuring concentrations at the site where the very first depletion of ascorbic acid is presumed to have occurred, in this case the myocardium. This would have difficulties, both because there are no studies that have estimated the time interval between local and plasma deficit, and because of the complexity of the procedure, associated with complex laboratory techniques. Better therefore to give up and rely only on traditional therapies?

Here too, logic could help formulate the answer: considering the low toxicity of vitamin C therapy, starting such therapy quickly could be reasonable regardless of plasma or intracellular levels. Without neglecting an essential requirement for effective treatment, the already introduced "rapidity of intervention", which is so crucial that it is potentially preferable to the "measure and correct" approach. This perspective recalls the valuable suggestion that Klenner did not fail to give to his colleagues in Emergency Medicine, now finally re-evaluated and made the subject of interesting study by the scientific community, which is beginning to frame vitamin C as a valuable resource to add to specific therapies in the management of the most dangerous acute conditions, from sepsis to the very delicate phase following cardiac arrest. In conclusion, the myocarditis model offers a conceptually robust example, indicating that adjuvant therapy with pharmacological ascorbic acid may not require any initial assessment of vitamin C status. After all, what disadvantages could there be to a treatment that is readily available, inexpensive and non-toxic?

This is also confirmed by the numerous authors of the review (41): "Vitamin C is widely available and inexpensive and has few adverse effects, making it worth promoting".

There were also other dynamics that caught Cathcart's attention, with particular interest in oxidative stress and disease-associated depletions. "In most pathologic processes, the rate at which free radicals and highly reactive oxidants are produced, exceeds the rate at which the ordinary rate-limited antioxidant free radical scavenging mechanisms can quench those free radicals and oxidants", he wrote in 1985 in the article "Vitamin C: the nontoxic, nonrate-limited, antioxidant free radical scavenger" (42).

Further evidence for his acumen can be found in a 1984 paper entitled "Vitamin C in the treatment of acquired immune deficiency syndrome (AIDS)"

(43), a genuine source of reflection. First of all, the date reference shows that Pauling's investigations into HIV (38) were anticipated by Cathcart, whose clinical experience led him to hold the following view: "My previous experience with the utilization of ascorbic acid in the treatment of viral diseases led me to hypothesize that ascorbate would be of value in the treatment of AIDS (acquired immune deficiency syndrome). Preliminary clinical evidence is that massive doses of ascorbate (50-200 grams per 24 hours) can suppress the symptoms of the disease and can markedly reduce the tendency for secondary infections. In combination with usual treatments for the secondary infections, large doses of ascorbate will often produce a clinical remission which shows every evidence of being prolonged if treatment is continued".

It is worth pausing on the excerpt "In combination with usual treatments for the secondary infections", which is useful in reiterating the view that orthomolecularists had of vitamin C, namely that of a pharmacological agent to be included in the broad class of pharmacological solutions. An agent that is as intelligent as it is harmless, to be used in synergy with all the targeted therapies that various clinical cases may require.

Despite this view, which in some circumstances reflected an excessive humility stemming from the fact that vitamin C had already delivered several solos worthy of the best jazz musicians, the hostilities against the orthomolecularists were so relentless as to create portrayals of scientific persecution.

Let us return to the Cathcartian statements in (43) to emphasise the quantities described, quantities of extraordinary magnitude. Indeed, 200 grams taken orally may seem like an astronomical and excessive amount. Although this is debatable, it is a figure that highlights the enormous ascorbic metabolic effort required by an organism during a major acute illness, presumably useful to avoid a collapse into scurvy or its many "disguises". Megadoses that are reminiscent of Klenner's empirical strategies, defining a notion whose formalisation would have been impossible without the observations gathered throughout Cathcart's relentless clinical practice. Megadoses that would be essential, at least according to him, to neutralise the avalanche of free radicals released by critical illnesses (44).

It is also worth mentioning a reference to allergy, a disorder which, as previously mentioned and further discussed below, appears to be highly sensitive to the action of vitamin C. In an article (45) published in the journal "Medical Hypotheses" in 1986, Cathcart highlighted what he considered to be the main dynamics behind the anti-allergic action, placing free radical control at the forefront.

We will return to Cathcart in the final stages of the book when describing the concept of dynamic flow, which is also closely linked to the notions of intestinal tolerance and megadoses. This seems the ideal preamble for a brief historical digression, as his fascinating therapeutic strategies have been scaled back over time. Although the method of intestinal tolerance may have a role to play in conditions of full health, we must admit that its use during acute illness appears less advisable today than in the past, unless intravenous administration is impossible. In short, oral megadoses would be a fallback solution. Why?

As anticipated, the bowel tolerance-dynamic flow-megadoses triangle (the reference is exclusively to oral intake) is an artificial strategy to circumvent rigid intestinal control mechanisms. A noble but elaborate attempt, and above all of limited effectiveness. This cumbersome approach contrasts with the efficiency of intravenous administration, which instead allows plasma concentrations inaccessible to the oral route to be rapidly achieved by bypassing intestinal absorption. However, as mentioned, pharmacokinetic theories will be clarified after most of Cathcart's scientific output, thus relieving him of any irrationality. In short, there is a truly rational basis for his doctrines, a mark of absolute genius.

Equally remarkable was the genius of the third vertex of the orthomolecular triangle, the one who continued the tradition of vitamin megadoses by confirming that vitamin C is only one of the arrows, and perhaps the sharpest, in the broad arsenal of Orthomolecular Medicine.

Abram Hoffer, who died in 2009, was a Canadian psychiatrist who dedicated his life to the treatment of psychiatric and oncological diseases.

Pauling wrote (46): "In 1967, I happened to read a number of papers published by two psychiatrists in Saskatchewan, Canada. Dr. Abram Hoffer and Dr. Humphry Osmond. (T)here was something extraordinary about their work. They were giving very large amounts of niacin to the schizophrenic patients, as much as 17000 milligrams per day, which is 1000 times the RDA. I was astonished that niacin and ascorbate, with the striking physiological property, when given in very small amounts, of preventing death from pellagra and scurvy, should be so lacking in toxicity that 1000 times the effective daily intake could be taken by a person without harm. This meant that these substances were quite different from drugs, which are usually given to patients in amounts not much smaller than the lethal dosages".

Pauling was fascinated by the magnitude of the so-called therapeutic window (the interval between the minimum concentration below which a compound is clinically ineffective and the maximum concentration above which very toxic effects appear) of vitamins, which is considerably wider than that of most drugs. This gap, which is now irrefutable, puts the drugs at a disadvantage compared to vitamins understood as pharmacological agents, arousing scientific curiosity about the non-toxicity that some vitamins retain even when taken in astronomical doses. Might there be a reason why Mother Nature has made such high amounts tolerable, up to 1000 times higher than the amount needed to prevent scurvy or pellagra?

If "God does not play dice", as Einstein resolutely stated in relation to quantum theories, we might have a reasonable answer since it is permissible to imagine that vitamins, or at least some vitamins, go far beyond prophylaxis of deficiency diseases.

From Pauling's aforementioned statements (46) it is easy to deduce that Hoffer devised a cure for schizophrenia based on the cooperation between high doses of niacin (or vitamin B3) and vitamin C. This original therapy enabled him to achieve remarkable results, which have led to numerous books and a series of highly influential scientific articles.

Let us begin with a curious epidemiological observation resulting from his relentless clinical practice, through which he conjectured a statistical link between the main diseases studied, schizophrenia and cancer. "I have treated 4000 schizophrenics since 1952. Only four of these patients have developed cancer. Since low cancer incidence has been recorded amongst patients treated by both conventional physicians using pharmaceuticals and by orthomolecular doctors who emphasize vitamins and minerals, it follows that this depressed cancer incidence must be related to the biochemistry of the disorder itself. Taken as a whole, therefore, the evidence seems to suggest that schizophrenics, their siblings and parents are less susceptible to cancer than the general population" (47).

Underlying the supposed protection offered by schizophrenia would be a compound derived from the oxidation of adrenaline, adrenochrome, a molecule with hypothesised neurotoxic properties, whose levels, in addition to being high in many schizophrenics, might therefore correlate inversely with the likelihood of developing certain types of cancer. This supposition, epidemiologically very intriguing though mechanistically rather enigmatic, never however caught Hoffer's attention as much as the inseparable tool with which he built his greatest successes: niacin.

Also known as nicotinic acid or vitamin B3, niacin is a water-soluble vitamin essential for numerous metabolic processes, including those involving carbohydrates, fatty acids, and amino acids. A deficiency of niacin causes pellagra, a disease whose main manifestations include neurological symptoms such as depression, anxiety and fatigue, which may progress to hallucinations, delirium and confusion. Niacin is particularly important for the nervous system and, in high doses, also acts as a powerful cholesterol-lowering agent (437). It was precisely this symptomatology that led Hoffer to explore the therapeutic potential of high-dose vitamin B3 in the treatment of mental disorders. The idea turned out to be successful: over the years, it produced positive results in various psychiatric conditions. Not only schizophrenia, although the reduction in anxiety and stabilisation of mood that he often achieved in treating this disorder were considered remarkable.

The literature is rich with his contributions (48), (49), (50), (51), (52), (53), (54), including two notable reviews co-authored with fellow orthomolecular pioneer Humphry Osmond, published in leading journals such as “The Lancet” (53) and “Nature” (51). Therefore, Hoffer was an authoritative scientist, although understandably prone to irritation at times. When a patient expressed concern about the potential side effects of niacin therapy, his response was famously blunt: “You're going to live a lot longer. Is that a problem for you?”

A stinging remark, which in truth was intended to challenge the exaggerated fears about the toxicity of vitamin-based therapies.

“Won’t it be too much? Won’t it hurt? I decided to add vitamin C to the prescribed antibiotic therapy, noticing after a few days a slight abdominal discomfort. It was definitely due to vitamin C, so I stopped it immediately...”

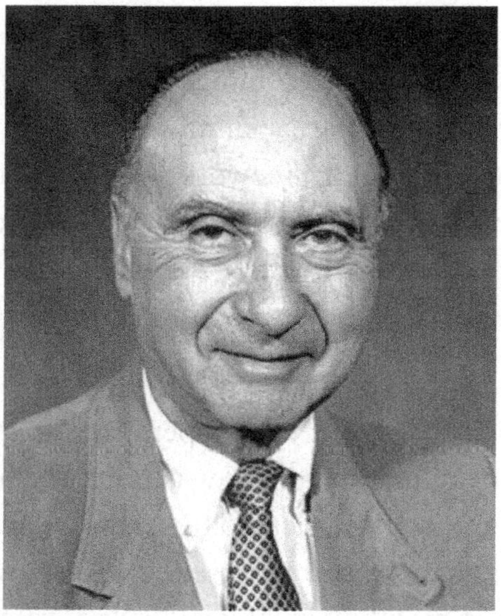

Abram Hoffer

Let us continue with a jump into the recent literature through which it is possible to identify some research that highlights the great scientific soundness of Hoffer's ideas, despite the heavy attacks he endured from the scientific community, which might suggest otherwise. In a paper published in 2015 in the journal "European Review for Medical and Pharmacological Sciences" (55), for example, scientists analysed the involvement of vitamin B3 in the pathogenesis of schizophrenia, outlining three main mechanisms. In summary, it appears that inadequate levels of niacin can trigger neurodegeneration, reduce the presence of so-called membrane phospholipids (substances involved in the structure of cell membranes) and dangerously increase adrenochrome levels. "We, thus, propose that niacin deficiency is a contributory factor in schizophrenia development in some patients and symptom alleviation in these patients will benefit from niacin augmentation, especially in some particular psychotic features", the scientists concluded, supporting Hoffer's hypothesis that high doses of niacin improve schizophrenia by lowering adrenochrome levels (55).

As mentioned, mental disorders were not Hoffer's only interest. He also devoted himself to cancer therapy (56), co-writing with Pauling a book entitled "Healing Cancer".

Paradoxically, one of the most valuable aspects of his scientific output appears to go beyond clinical practice and remains highly relevant today. It lies in his ideological effort to place vitamins on the same level as traditional pharmacological agents. This effort led him to generalize the vitamin C phenomenon, demonstrating that the "vitamin C as a drug" paradigm was not an isolated case, but part of a broader framework with significant therapeutic potential. It helped stimulate further research into so-called megavitamin therapy, grounded in the recognition that, while this regimen is characterized by low toxicity, it often requires very high dosages to be clinically effective.

All efforts to promote the concept of megavitamin therapy were met with unwavering resistance. For example, the cooperative model advocated by Pauling and Hoffer, in which megavitamin therapy was proposed as a supportive adjunct to standard treatments, as also documented by Cathcart, was dismissed outright. The scientific community consistently refused to engage with these ideas, maintaining its opposition by citing an alleged lack of robust scientific evidence.

Explicit confirmation of the stormy climate comes from the book written jointly with Pauling: "In 1971 he had set up the Linus Pauling Institute of Science and Medicine to study Orthomolecular Medicine, in particular the relationship between vitamin B3, vitamin C and schizophrenia. Dr Pauling's efforts filled those practising megadose therapy of these two vitamins (as well as others) with satisfaction, but provoked a wave of hostility and criticism from psychiatric specialists. The American Psychiatric Association (APA) tried to prevent the publication of any information on the efficacy of high doses of vitamins in the treatment of schizophrenia. Eventually, in 1971, they invited me and Dr Osmond to appear before their ethics committee because a Californian psychiatrist had complained about an article I had written describing the recovery of a patient whose father had been indirectly introduced to our ideas by Dr Pauling". Why so much furore, one might ask?

Needless to say, hostilities escalated towards the end of the 1970s, when vitamin C began to be considered by Pauling and Cameron as an anticancer agent, a fact that pushed to its highest level the uncomfortable paradigm of "vitamins as drugs" so strongly opposed by the medical establishment. Not only an anti-infective, antihistamine and anti-schizophrenia agent (some modern clinical studies support the use of vitamin C for the treatment of schizophrenia (515)), but also an innovative anticancer strategy. It was probably too much. A thesis that was perhaps untenable for the science of the time, accustomed to looking at reality with eyes so enchanted that they failed to grasp the great potential of vitamin C.

The efforts of Abram's son, Leonard John Hoffer, professor of medicine at McGill University, who is actively engaged in scientific research on vitamin C (57), (58), could be described as a sign of destiny. Personally, I see Leonard John's work as an attempt to lucidly re-evaluate the ideas that have characterised the troubled history of vitamin C and orthomolecular medicine. Often underestimated, these ideas still retain such freshness that they constitute an original reservoir from which doctors could draw "new" therapeutic resources at a modest cost in terms of both economics and toxicity.

But there's more: in addition to low toxicity, there are valid arguments in favour of very high demand (i.e. megadoses) of vitamins, mainly related to the negative metabolic impacts that serious illnesses and highly stressful events can cause. These pitfalls, at the top of the list of what I personally call "vitamin devourers", therefore have the insidious ability to devour micronutrients, with a preference for vitamin C. Yes, vitamin C, which is often at the top of the list of "strategic targets" for diseases, perhaps because it is considered the most insidious "threat". A note: although this continues to be underestimated, it is a crucial point that will be analysed in detail during the discussion. Vitamin depletion, in fact, entails several insidious consequences, through which stress and disease could progressively and significantly weaken the human body, potentially leading to the most extreme outcomes such as scurvy, beriberi or pellagra.

This may sound like an exaggeration, but scientific evidence shows that it is not: a hint extracted from the section on surgery shows that a very stressful event such as surgery can hold great nutritional risks for the body. "Studies have revealed a potentially severe depletion in plasma/serum concentrations of numerous vitamins following these surgeries acutely. Vitamins C, D and B1 appear particularly vulnerable to significant depletions, with vitamin C and D depletions consistently transpiring into inadequate and deficient concentrations, respectively" (383). Travica and colleagues were unequivocal in their review focusing on the depleting effect that surgery can have on vitamins (383). There is no doubt that deficiency diseases such as scurvy, beriberi and rickets, or even "simple" subclinical forms, still represent real threats today, ready to re-emerge opportunistically when certain conditions arise that can profoundly alter the balance of our bodies.

Adolfo Panfili and Atsuo Yanagisawa: two worthy heirs of Orthomolecular Medicine

Anyone who believes that the star of Orthomolecular Medicine faded with the passing of Cathcart and Hoffer is seriously mistaken. Alongside the important work of Hoffer's son, two genuine cornerstones of the modern orthomolecular landscape stand out: Professor Adolfo Panfili and Dr. Atsuo Yanagisawa.

Adolfo Panfili, a specialist in Orthopaedics and Traumatology, is a pioneer in endoscopic, radio-guided robotic, and minimally invasive surgery of the spine and both small and large joints. He boasts a prestigious international curriculum, with scientific interests ranging from Homeopathy to Phytotherapy, expanding into Orthomolecular Medicine. At the explicit request of his mentor, Linus Pauling, Panfili founded the International Association of Orthomolecular Medicine (AIMO) in 1988, aiming to integrate orthomolecular principles with other specialized disciplines, including Regenerative Medicine.

In 2015, he was honored with the "Leonardo Da Vinci Award for his humanitarian scientific effort in the world to protect children with cerebral neurological damage", and, the following year, he received another prestigious award from the World Organisation for the Achievement of Human Potential for his contribution to improving global quality of life. Panfili is the author of several significant books, including "Orthomolecular Medicine" (582), a true milestone filled with in-depth cross-disciplinary insights into Orthomolecular Medicine and related fields such as Kinesiology and Phytotherapy.

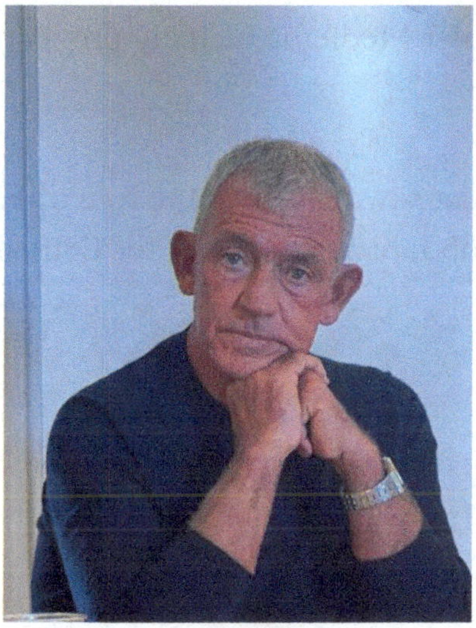

Adolfo Panfili

On the other hand, Japanese physician Atsuo Yanagisawa, a cardiologist and professor at Kyorin University, distinguished himself particularly through his books on Chelation Therapy (581), Nutrition, and the General Theory of Intravenous Vitamin C Therapy (580), in which he is one of the world's leading proponents and experts. It is precisely this role that earned him the presidency of the International Society for Orthomolecular Medicine (ISOM), an organization established to promote the advancement of Orthomolecular Medicine worldwide.

What stands out most about Yanagisawa goes beyond his vast scientific output, which includes over one hundred in-depth articles. His greatest contribution lies in his consistent efforts to educate the public and healthcare professionals alike on the importance of proper nutrition as a defense against disease. In this regard, the Riordan Clinic (a U.S.-based center of excellence in intravenous vitamin C therapy and complementary cancer care) recognized his outstanding commitment to advancing global health by awarding him the prestigious Pearl Maker Award.

Panfili and Yanagisawa thus serve as solid bridges between past and future: on one hand, they keep alive the legacy of the legendary pioneers of vitamin C; on the other, they look ahead by integrating orthomolecular theories with the latest scientific discoveries and educating future generations on the fundamental principles of Orthomolecular Medicine, namely prevention and the promotion of health.

Note: since 2023 Yanagisawa has held the role of Past President of ISOM and is currently President of the Japanese Society for Orthomolecular Medicine.

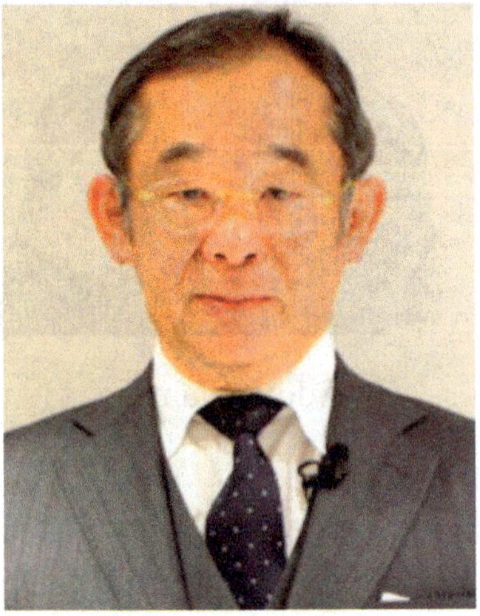

Atsuo Yanagisawa

Chapter 3
The Pharmacokinetics Of Vitamin C

Introduction

After discussing the historical aspects, it is time to delve into the technical details. Although this may seem challenging, the exploration will be gradual and will clarify many of the questions raised, while at the same time offering a critical reinterpretation of the exciting events that have shaped the history of the molecule and its pioneers. We will come to understand that some supposed scientific errors were inevitable, as they were based on knowledge that was still evolving. Consider, for example, Cathcart's astronomical megadoses of 200 grams.

This is a truly fundamental chapter, focused on a comprehensive description of a series of technical aspects such as dietary sources, absorption, transporter activity, bioavailability, tissue distribution, in other words, everything concerning the so-called pharmacokinetics of vitamin C.

Chemical characteristics and food sources

Ascorbic acid, or L-ascorbic acid, is essential for humans owing to the lack of endogenous biosynthesis, making a continuous dietary intake necessary. Moreover, severe deficiency results in scurvy, a debilitating and potentially fatal disease.

Ascorbic acid is a white solid (or yellowish when oxidized), mildly acidic, water-soluble, and appears as odorless crystals. Due to its strong reducing power, it is widely used in the food industry as an additive, a role that introduces its multifunctionality. For example, it is commonly used as a preservative to prevent food browning (browning is a chemical reaction that results in the formation of dark-colored substances, think of a freshly cut apple turning brown) and also as an antinitrosating agent.

Beyond its uses, we must not overlook the fundamental role of vitamin C: donating electrons, a function made possible by its pronounced antioxidant nature, which we will discuss in more detail later. This activity occurs through the donation of two electrons. Upon losing its first electron, ascorbic acid is converted into a relatively inactive free radical known as semidehydroascorbic acid. Semidehydroascorbic acid can then follow two pathways: it can either return to its original form (technically, it is reduced back to ascorbic acid) or, upon losing another electron, be converted into what is known as dehydroascorbic acid, also referred to as DHA. This latter form, the oxidized version of vitamin C, has some characteristics that differentiate it from ascorbic acid, including its low stability.

DHA is involved in a reversible process that allows it to regain its original antioxidant nature. This is a reduction mechanism that leads to the regeneration of vitamin C, which is particularly important for the physiology of red blood cells. This reduction mechanism is ensured by an intracellular recycling system capable of converting DHA back into ascorbic acid.

What is the chemical and physical structure of vitamin C?

The two forms of vitamin C, ascorbic acid and DHA, have the molecular formulas $C_6H_8O_6$ and $C_6H_6O_6$, respectively. This indicates 6 carbon atoms, 8 (or 6) hydrogen atoms, and 6 oxygen atoms, revealing two structures similar to that of glucose ($C_6H_{12}O_6$), offering a chemical analogy that may also be clinically significant, particularly in therapies for cancer and diabetes.

The molecular mass of vitamin C is 176.12 g/mol; this means that 1 micromole of vitamin C equals 0.17612 mg, and 1 millimole of vitamin C equals 176.12 mg. It is useful to specify that the mole, micromole (1/1000000 of a mole), and millimole (1/1000 of a mole) are units used to measure the quantity of a substance. Conventionally, 1 mole is defined as the amount of a given substance that contains exactly $6.02214076 \times 10^{23}$ elementary entities, where $6.02214076 \times 10^{23}$ is the value of the famous Avogadro's constant.

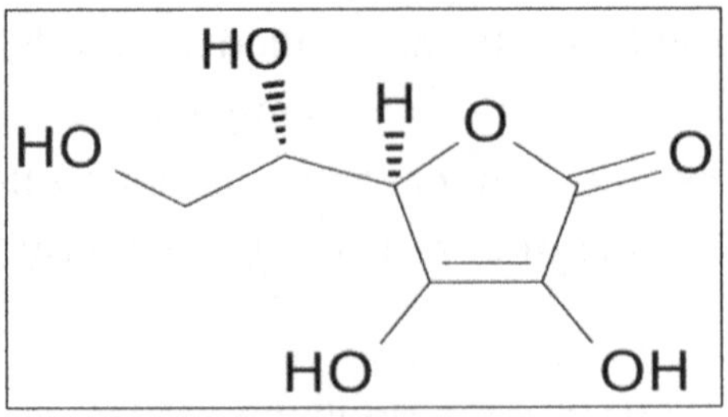

Structure Of Ascorbic Acid

Vitamin C is chemically quite delicate: it is extremely sensitive to certain transition metals and a range of factors such as heat, including cooking, and especially light and oxygen. This requires careful handling of both synthetic formulations and natural plant sources, as exposure to these factors can deteriorate its biological value. Being a water-soluble molecule, that is, soluble in water, vitamin C is easily absorbed by the body, though only in limited quantities. This is a crucial point, as the ease of absorption is counterbalanced by a short retention time. On one hand, this necessitates a constant intake; on the other, it prevents excessive accumulation, thereby eliminating the risk of hypervitaminosis. In fact, the high water solubility of vitamin C, as we will see shortly, ensures very low toxicity, thanks to the mechanisms of intestinal absorption, renal reabsorption, and especially renal excretion.

It is virtually harmless and fully integrated into Nature. In the plant kingdom, for instance, vitamin C is the most widespread antioxidant. This is due to its involvement in growth processes and, above all, to the remarkable protection it provides plants against solar radiation. This defence is regulated by light stimuli and is effectively mediated by biosynthesis, analogous to the way animals respond to environmental, traumatic or infectious stress factors.

Vitamin C is abundantly present in vegetables, and its levels vary depending on ripeness, storage conditions, and processing methods. Its highest concentrations are found in chili peppers, parsley, blackcurrants, bell peppers, arugula, and kiwi. What about the famous orange-lime duo?

It does not appear among the foods richest in vitamin C, a typical example of common misconceptions regarding the vitamin.

There are also three plants with extraordinarily high concentrations: rose hips, camu camu and acerola. From these, vitamin C can be extracted to produce synthetic formulations, and also consumed directly from the fruit.

Food	Vitamin C (mg/100g)
Hot peppers	229
Currants	200
Peppers	166
Parsley	162
Rocket	110
Kiwi	85
Brussels sprouts	81
Turnips	81
Broccoli	77
Cauliflower	59

Transport systems

The inability to synthesise vitamin C did not go unnoticed by Nature. This favoured the establishment, probably as a compensatory element, of certain balancing mechanisms designed primarily to avoid a deficiency state. Thus, intestinal absorption, tissue distribution, intracellular recycling, renal reabsorption, and renal excretion are fundamental processes primarily mediated by an essential family of sodium-dependent proteins known as sodium vitamin C transporters (SVCTs), which occur in two forms: SVCT1 and SVCT2.

Although both essential transport proteins are selectively specialised in transporting ascorbic acid and therefore do not transport the oxidised form DHA, they act differently and in a complementary manner (62), (67). SVCT1 (encoded by the SLC23A1 gene, discovered about 20 years ago (78)) is responsible for transporting (with low affinity) ascorbic acid to the area where it is first absorbed, the small intestine, and then to the liver, lungs and, above all, the kidneys. Among these tissues, the expression of SVCT1 in the renal tubule, the portion of the nephron (the functional unit of the kidney) responsible for the reabsorption of water and nutrients, is particularly crucial. This reabsorption also modulates vitamin C homeostasis by seeking to ensure an adequate balance (62).

Why are they called "essential transport proteins"?

It may be of interest to note that in studies in which mice were subjected to a knockout of the SLC23A1 gene (gene knockout, or gene inactivation, is a genetic technique in which the expression of a given gene is suppressed for research purposes), huge urinary losses of ascorbic acid were found, a finding attributable to inefficient renal reabsorption. This is a significant finding: low plasma and tissue levels due to an SLC23A1 knockout are in fact associated with increased mortality (59). This association suggests potentially serious implications in humans, considering that even a limited loss of SVCT1 expression would logically be more harmful in humans than in animals regularly endowed with the ability to synthesize vitamin C.

However, there are other potential issues. Encoded by the SLC23A2 gene, the SVCT2 protein is responsible for transporting ascorbic acid into nearly all tissues, cells, and extracellular fluids in the body. Its high affinity enables remarkably high accumulation in many tissues, with the brain and adrenal glands showing unmatched concentrations. It is therefore not surprising that mouse models in which SLC23A2 was genetically modified showed even more alarming results, often dying from cerebral hemorrhage or respiratory failure (59), (60). This is an extremely significant discovery, demonstrating beyond any doubt that SVCT2 expression is vital.

Having established the essentiality of transporters in vitamin C homeostasis, it may be interesting to ask whether there are any alterations that may compromise their activity and thus systemic balance. Unfortunately, over time, multiple factors have been identified that can alter the functioning of transporters. Some of them, such as so-called genetic polymorphisms, can markedly impair vitamin C accumulation in plasma or tissues. What are genetic polymorphisms?

Let's start with the concept of genetic mutation, which is closely related to that of polymorphism. A genetic mutation is an alteration in an organism's genetic material, the well-known genome. Although the concepts of mutation (in simple terms: a permanent change affecting the sequence of that fundamental "genetic blueprint" called DNA) and polymorphism are not sharply distinguishable, the latter refers to genetic variations that are more frequent than typical mutations (i.e., with a prevalence of over 1% in the population). These variations, which are often insidious, can obviously also involve the SLC23A1 and SLC23A2 genes, and therefore the SVCT1 and SVCT2 proteins.

Indeed, various pharmacokinetic models have identified numerous polymorphisms in SVCTs, some of which are of particular concern as they can cause plasma and/or tissue reductions severe enough to alter vitamin C homeostasis, thereby increasing the risk of vitamin C hypovitaminosis or even outright deficiency (59). By a vitamin C hypovitaminosis state, most authors mean a plasma level < 23 micromoles/L. A minority, on the other hand, are more cautious as they have broadened the reference to a plasma level < 28 micromoles/L (62).

Vitamin C deficiency is less debated: scientists fully agree on defining it as a plasma level < 11 micromoles/L (62).

Returning to polymorphisms, what do we know about them?

In the scientific literature, unfortunately, there are a limited number of clinical evaluations that have investigated polymorphisms of the SLC23A1-SLC23A2 genes and their biological and clinical implications. Most of these evaluations are included in an emblematic review published in the highly regarded journal "Annual Review of Nutrition" (60). In this review, there is sufficient evidence to confirm that genetic variations in SLC23A1 can actually subvert vitamin C homeostasis in the human body by decreasing both plasma concentrations and intracellular stores.

Even more explicit are the studies on genetic variations affecting the gene encoding SVCT2. Their results have suggested a relevant role for vitamin C in the prevention of a wide range of diseases including certain types of cancer and glaucoma. More generally, several studies have suggested that SVCT2 polymorphisms may increase the risk of a wide range of diseases, thus contributing to a broadening of the problem (60). One consideration, in this regard, deserves to be shared: the presence of such polymorphisms (we do not currently have solid data on their incidence in the world population) could lead to a hypovitaminosis or even a deficiency of ascorbic acid, regardless of dietary intake. These alterations are difficult to detect because they require highly complex laboratory procedures. If present, such polymorphisms would add to the permanent inefficiency of the GULO enzyme, creating a "double genetic dysfunction" that is subtle but potentially very dangerous.

This leads to a logical question: given the difficulties of carrying out the appropriate genetic investigations and monitoring plasma and intracellular concentrations, can the undefined risk of genetic polymorphism be an additional reason to consider the possible use of dynamic flow?

Let us return to the two forms of vitamin C, ascorbic acid (i.e. the reduced form) and its oxidised form, DHA. It is necessary to specify that DHA circulates in the body in a very small ratio compared to ascorbic acid: it ranges from 1-3% during physiological states to slightly higher percentages under pathological conditions (62); even more important is to specify the differences in transport: while ascorbic acid is transported exclusively by SVCTs, the transport of DHA instead relies solely on a family of transporters known as glucose transporters (GLUTs) (67). As one might expect, we are introducing a group of proteins whose primary role is to transport glucose across the boundary that defines the cell and regulates the exchange of chemical substances with the external environment, the plasma membrane (also known as the cell membrane).

"Primary role", however, does not mean exclusive. As previously mentioned, the large GLUT family is also involved in the absorption of vitamin C, specifically in its oxidized form, DHA. This means that any area accessible to glucose is likewise accessible to vitamin C. This important implication is due to a specific subset made up of the GLUT1-GLUT2-GLUT3-GLUT4-GLUT8 group, which plays a central role in an adaptive mechanism where glucose, due to its structural similarity to DHA, is forced to share its transport pathways with the "opportunist" DHA (62), (67).

However, DHA is an unstable and, more importantly, oxidized molecule, making it metabolically unfavorable. Fortunately, a mechanism exists to convert (technically: reduce) DHA back into ascorbic acid immediately after it enters the cell. This crucial process is known as ascorbate recycling, and it relies on certain intracellular enzymes that depend on a key reducing agent known as glutathione. Given the universal importance of glucose, it should come as no surprise that this mechanism allows vitamin C to be delivered virtually everywhere in the body.

What contribution can the oxidised form make to systemic vitamin C levels?

A preliminary observation might generate an interesting ambiguity: surprisingly, some GLUTs appear to have a higher affinity with DHA (67), a finding which does not rule out the possibility that a subset of GLUTs actually has vitamin C transport as a priority.

In short, the issue appears entangled and full of uncertainty. What we do know for certain, however, is the predictable turbulence that characterises the DHA-glucose relationship, the cause of a competition that, in some circumstances, takes the form of a true metabolic conflict.

In line with these observations and the dual functionality of GLUTs, several cell culture studies have suggested that the GLUTs-DHA transport system may be as efficient as SVCTs in supporting vitamin C accumulation (61), (67). However, in scientific research, in vitro results do not always translate to in vivo models, given the complexity of whole-organism physiology. One example is the ascorbic contribution of GLUTs: the aforementioned study (59) clearly showed that SVCT2 knockout in mice was lethal, despite normal GLUT function. This provides clear evidence that has led to a reassessment of the role of GLUTs in vitamin C transport, with one notable exception: red blood cells.

What is so special about erythrocytes?

Red blood cells (or erythrocytes) are an exception, as they are one of the very few cell populations that do not express any SVCTs. This forces GLUTs, essentially GLUT1, to mediate the transport of vitamin C within them, exclusively in the form of DHA (67). Since cells cannot be deprived of vitamin C, this transport is clearly indispensable for the survival of red blood cells, even though it is not completely efficient. In fact, the amount of ascorbic acid that the GLUT-DHA system can supply to erythrocytes is much lower than in other parts of the body, which, unlike erythrocytes, can benefit from the much more substantial contribution of SVCTs.

Let us conclude the discussion on GLUTs by examining their potential role in cancer therapy. Several studies have demonstrated a key function of GLUTs in transporting vitamin C into cancer cells, which are known to exhibit high glucose uptake. This naturally creates a strong competitive dynamic between DHA and glucose. As we will see, many researchers are seeking to exploit this competition to develop therapies capable of selectively targeting certain types of cancer.

Oral pharmacokinetics

The term pharmacokinetics has been used without offering a clear definition. What is it? And why specify the adjective oral?

Pharmacokinetics is concerned with describing the absorption, distribution, metabolism and excretion of drugs or any biologically active substance. Using mathematical models, pharmacokinetics thus seeks to analytically elucidate the processes that govern the achievement of an adequate concentration of a given compound in the various compartments of the body.

Compared to most orally administered drugs, vitamin C differs in several pharmacokinetic aspects, highlighting one of its many distinctions from conventional drugs.

As the title of this section suggests, our attention will focus momentarily on oral intake, which can clearly be via food or supplements. This is the main route of administration of vitamin C, given also the presence of relatively large quantities in Nature.

It is important to specify that, as far as healthy individuals are concerned (by the way, what does "healthy" or "in good health" really mean?), many experts believe it is possible to obtain sufficient amounts of ascorbic acid through diet, an idea that this book will nonetheless challenge. Criticisms aside, there is an objective fact regarding people who are not in "good health." A highly significant point (already mentioned) concerns individuals exposed to adverse conditions such as acute stress, illness, or ascorbic acid deficiency, situations in which dietary intake tends to become insufficient to meet the body's vitamin C requirements. This conclusion is now supported by compelling scientific evidence, is of utmost relevance, and will be revisited several times throughout the book.

How does absorption of vitamin C occur?

Ascorbic acid (hereafter, for the sake of brevity, sometimes referred to by the acronym AA) and DHA are absorbed by enterocytes in the intestinal lumen, a process that occurs throughout all segments of the small intestine, followed by their release into the plasma and kidneys. It is worth emphasizing that the mechanisms regulating these movements are still under investigation, reflecting the sea of uncertainties in which vitamin C specialists still navigate.

After absorption into the intestinal-plasma-renal compartment, where the kidneys help maintain vitamin C homeostasis thanks in part to their valuable reabsorption activity, AA and DHA are ultimately released into the bloodstream (plasma) and subsequently distributed to all the cells of the body.

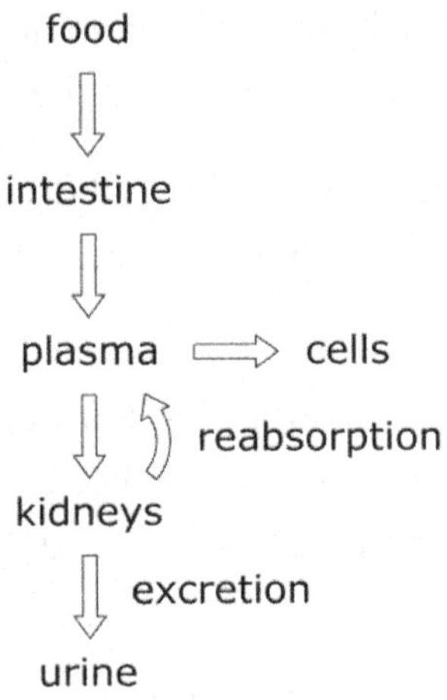

As previously mentioned, the transport systems, composed of SVCTs and GLUTs, can experience dysfunction due to genetic polymorphisms and are also vulnerable to other, perhaps more tangible, insults. This refers to the aging process and pathological states, both of which can impair the transporters to such an extent that a vitamin C deficiency may occur despite an adequate intake (62), (63). It is therefore reasonable to hypothesize that the triad of polymorphism-aging-disease can degrade these transporters to the point where a normal diet becomes insufficient, much like a household budget where expenses exceed income. This would begin as a minor deficit (chronic subclinical scurvy), but could escalate into a dangerous one (scurvy) if not properly addressed.

The sharing nature of GLUTs also contributes to a similar dynamic: an excess of glucose can inhibit DHA absorption, so it's not surprising that maximum absorption of AA and DHA occurs when glucose levels are low (62). Incidentally, we will analyze in detail how the competition between glucose and DHA becomes particularly intense during a condition typically associated with elevated glucose levels, diabetes, of course, to the point of affecting its progression.

As schematic as the last part of the discussion may appear, it is useful to emphasise that these are preparatory notions for subsequent understanding.

Is it true that a large amount of vitamin C is not effectively absorbed by the body?

It has been widely known since the 1970s that the bioavailability (a term describing the fraction and speed with which any compound reaches the systemic circulation without undergoing chemical changes) of vitamin C is inversely proportional to the dose (62). This means that an increase in dosage (oral, mind you!) corresponds to a reduction of intestinal absorption, as if vitamin C transporters had a limited capacity. This fact has made it possible to accumulate more and more evidence in favour of the existence of a precise transport mechanism, which has been shown to be both saturable and active ("active transport" means a transport of molecules across the plasma membrane that requires the mediation of a transport protein and, unlike so-called passive transport, involves an expenditure of energy) (64).

The saturation of transporters (in particular SVCT1, which is directly responsible for intestinal absorption) tends to limit plasma concentrations, setting a limit beyond which certain control mechanisms are activated, including renal excretion. More specifically, massive dietary intakes (in the order of 200-300 mg of vitamin C, obtainable from a diet rich in fresh vegetables) usually correspond to plasma concentrations of 60-70 micromoles/L. 60-70 micromoles/L (equivalent to 10.57 mg/L-12.33 mg/L) is considered an optimal plasma level and one that is difficult to exceed, mainly due to the strict intestinal control (resulting from transporter saturation) that manages ascorbic traffic in the intestine. Therefore, a diet rich in fresh vegetables, typically associated with an intake of 200-300 mg of ascorbic acid, can stabilise a plasma level of 60-70 micromoles/L for a period of approximately 24 hours (in conditions of full health and in the absence of AA deficiency and intense stress) (62). But is this really an insurmountable level?

Absolutely not! The 60-70 micromoles/L plasma level hurdle is indeed surmountable, albeit with some "sacrifice". There is, however, an inherent difficulty, consistent with the fact that quantities of vitamin C in excess of 200-

300 mg (defined as "non-dietary" because they cannot be achieved by diet) cause a very temporary increase in plasma concentration. This is clearly the well-known law of short stay, the reality of which speaks in favour of the great pioneers (remember Cathcart's megadoses?), the first practitioners of an unwritten but abundantly intuited law that frequent and high dosing is indispensable for appreciating the full potential of the oral pharmacological version of vitamin C.

To recapitulate: the higher the dose taken, the shorter its residence time in the body, a theorem that indicates the need to subdivide a high dose to avoid it being largely dispersed.

How long can a high dose remain in the body?

The frequency useful for "fooling" strict intestinal-renal control is suggested by the so-called plasma peak time, i.e. the time required for a dose of a compound to reach maximum plasma concentration; with regard to oral ascorbic acid intake, several studies have estimated that the plasma peak time varies between 120 and 180 minutes (62).

Given the importance of the issue, it is useful to highlight a study that was approved by the Institutional Review Board of the National Institute of Diabetes and Digestive and Kidney Diseases and published in the prestigious journal "Annals of Internal Medicine" (22). The study involved 17 healthy young volunteers, 7 men and 10 women, who participated in a "depletion-repletion" experimental design. They first followed a prolonged diet extremely low in vitamin C (5 mg per day), which was then followed by repletion through various oral doses of AA. The aim was to analyze the absorption rates and plasma concentrations associated with the different doses. The results, which were highly insightful, brought significant clarity, partly destabilizing traditional thinking on the matter. Specifically, it was observed that single doses of 3 grams of vitamin C (a dosage that necessarily requires supplementation) can produce transient plasma concentration peaks that are 3-4 times higher (approximately 220 micromoles/L) than the levels achievable through a vitamin C-rich diet. To reiterate: a diet rich in vitamin C-containing foods typically provides a maximum of 200-300 mg per day, which, in healthy individuals, results in stabilized plasma concentrations of around 60-70 micromoles/L.

Moreover, it was found that two markedly different single-dose regimens (3 grams once daily versus 200 mg once daily) surprisingly produced identical long-term outcomes. In both cases, plasma concentrations returned to baseline levels, those observed prior to supplementation, within approximately 24 hours. This indicates that either dosing pattern reestablishes the previous steady state within a day. The term steady state refers to the equilibrium point at which the plasma concentration of a compound tends to stabilize over time.

We have thus reached a turning point. This study clearly demonstrated that, in healthy individuals, high oral doses can considerably elevate plasma concentrations beyond those achievable through even a diet rich in fruits and vegetables. Specifically, a single 3-gram dose can, albeit temporarily, triple or quadruple the peak plasma values attained through robust dietary intake.

It is essential to emphasize that this transience can be overcome with appropriate dose repetition. Supporting this, the authors, based on their pharmacokinetic models, reached a valuable conclusion: fractionating a total daily intake of 18 grams (specifically, administering 3 grams every 4 hours) is associated with a constant plasma concentration of approximately 220 micromoles/L (22). This regimen would thus ensure effective 24-hour stability (i.e., a “high” steady state), in contrast to the transient nature typical of single daily doses (see figure).

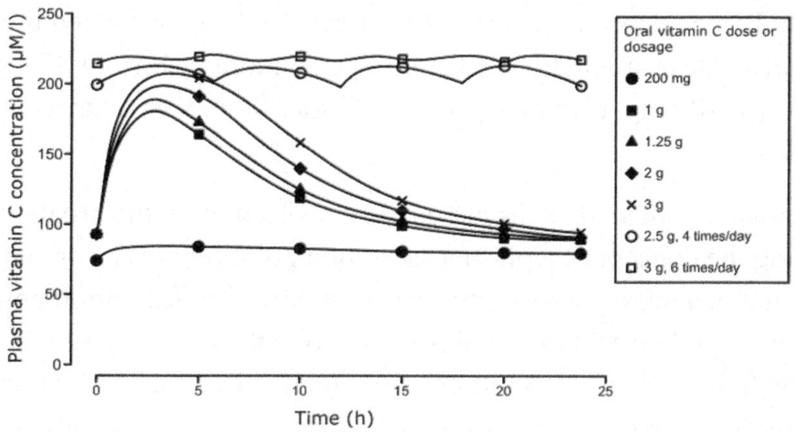

graph adapted from (22)

Other studies have identified similar dynamics. For example, a study published in the journal "Advances in Nutrition" (65) confirmed that, in healthy and non-stressed individuals (a repetitive but necessary clarification, as these considerations primarily apply under conditions of good health and absence of significant stress), oral intake of 200-300 mg of vitamin C can stabilize plasma levels at 60-70 micromoles/L (or simply micromoles, for brevity) without triggering an "impulsive," i.e., rapid, renal excretion. Renal excretion, on the other hand, would be triggered quickly, but only after the plasma peak is reached (i.e., around 120-180 minutes), if a higher dose were administered. This is consistent with the dynamics governing the intestinal-plasma-renal control system. As we've seen, bypassing this control is a demanding procedure, as it requires a "point-to-point" delivery system, that is, one capable of promptly compensating for renal losses caused by previous doses.

In a nutshell, dosages in excess of 200-300 mg (i.e. "non-dietary" dosages) stimulate the "renal taps" to open immediately after the plasma peak is reached: I repeat, after the plasma peak is reached and therefore not immediately after ingestion. This can be seen visually from the line parallel to the time axis that describes the plasma concentration trend relative to a 200 mg intake (22). This parallelism, a clear indication of temporal stability, can only be replicated by using a dosing schedule aligned with plasma peak times, such as the "3 g every 4 hours" regimen described above (22).

The study models from the previous article (65) also calculated the bioavailability rate as a function of the dose taken: it ranged from 87.3% for 30 mg, to 80% for 100 mg, then dropped to 63% for 500 mg, and ended at 46% for a 1250 mg dose.

In summary, both studies discussed are consistent with the broader literature in supporting the concept of a plasma saturation point (emphasis on plasma saturation, not general or tissue-specific saturation). This saturation point, estimated at around 70-80 micromoles/L, supports the existence of a threshold beyond which the intestine and kidneys coordinate to activate strict homeostatic mechanisms aimed at preventing plasma concentrations from stabilizing at higher levels. These mechanisms involve a reduction in intestinal absorption and an increase in renal excretion.

As already mentioned, this "check-up" mechanism, arising from a saturation point that is perhaps too easily reached, is so strict that breaking through it orally becomes almost a challenge. Almost, I emphasize. Various attempts, mainly referring to Cathcart's proposals and the more modern findings of the previous study (3 grams every 4 hours, i.e., 18 grams per day), have yielded limited results, since quadrupling the plasma levels typical of a strong diet required a considerable effort. However, "limited" does not mean null; rather, it implies a contribution that could, as we'll soon demonstrate, add something to the benefits of vitamin C obtained purely through diet. After all, increasing one's ordinary salary by three or four times, however demanding, could bring such satisfaction as to make one forget the effort involved.

It is important to reiterate: anyone claiming that the excess portion of a single oral dose greater than 200-300 mg is useless because it "cannot be absorbed" by the body is simply wrong. I'll repeat it again, because separating truth from falsehood is essential, and I apologize if this sounds obvious to some: oral doses > 200-300 mg, that is, non-dietary doses, can significantly increase plasma levels and tissue concentrations (as clearly shown in the graph above, where 3 grams can yield a plasma level of 220 micromoles/L). The point is that, unlike dietary doses (< 300 mg), they do so temporarily (as an acute spike, in fact) and in a manner mathematicians call nonlinear. What does "nonlinear" mean?

The term "nonlinear" refers to an absorption model that differs from linear models. A linear model describes a dynamic in which doubling the dose results in what one would normally expect, that is, a doubling of the plasma concentration (it should be noted that the absorption of dietary-level doses follows a perfectly linear model). Nonlinear models, on the other hand, describe a situation in which doubling (or tripling, if you prefer) the dose leads to a sub-proportional increase in plasma concentration. The values reported in reference (22) are clear examples of nonlinearity:

1 gram = 187 micromoles/L;

3 grams = 220 micromoles/L.

If the system were linear, 3 grams would have produced a concentration of 561 micromoles/L (3 × 187), which is far higher than the actual concentration achieved, 220 micromoles/L.

With non-dietary dosing, what occurs is essentially a shift caused by the atypical bioavailability of vitamin C (a direct result of SVCT1 saturation): a transition from linearity to nonlinearity. As a result, excessive use of a single non-dietary oral dose can lead to a plateau, and even cause mild gastrointestinal symptoms, especially under physiological conditions, where metabolic demand is presumed to be much lower than in pathological states. This has led many scientists to a rational, though often misunderstood, conclusion: the establishment of a tolerable upper limit for oral vitamin C intake, typically set at 2-3 grams per day.

It is important to clarify this point, as it is a fundamental concept: the notion of a "tolerable upper intake level", as it is commonly presented, appears inconsistent, much like a street name would be confusing if not properly contextualized within its city. In fact, the definition of "tolerable upper intake level" should also account for the duration of time that the vitamin C actually remains in the body, that is, the very short period dictated by rapid renal excretion. This implies that associating the term "daily" (typically used by health authorities to describe RDAs and tolerable upper intake levels of nutrients) with the established single well-tolerated dose of 3 grams is scientifically inaccurate, since the biological effects of a high oral dose of ascorbic acid, including any potential side effects, tend to disappear well before 24 hours have passed.

We can't drink more than half a liter of water in just a few seconds without experiencing some issues. But we can drink just under half a liter every four to six hours without any problems, in fact, we should! So, that half liter is not the ideal daily amount!

Alongside the issues of nonlinearity and maximum tolerability, the key point to emphasize is the difference in plasma residence time between non-dietary and dietary doses: only a few hours for the former, versus about 24 hours for the latter. And I stress in plasma, because we are by no means certain that a high dose is entirely excreted at the end of its short plasma residence. This leads us to hypothesize, as we will explore later, that other areas of the body may absorb part of the high dose before urinary excretion occurs.

What has been illustrated should not come as a big surprise, as it has already been mentioned during the discussion on the common cold. The reference is mainly to the statements by Hickey and Roberts: "A large oral dose raises blood plasma levels briefly: they reach a peak after two to three hours, before decaying back to baseline. Frequent repeated doses allow sustained high plasma levels of about 250 micromoles/L" (23).

Despite the now solid pharmacokinetic evidence, this concept continues to be overlooked in clinical research: references to the clinical applications of dynamic flow are so rare in the literature that they raise doubts about its real usefulness. After all, why should we support the unnatural idea of bypassing the strict intestinal-renal control through an artificial system of high and frequent doses?

An intriguing question: is it really so strange to imagine that something unnatural might be needed to compensate for the unnaturalness caused by the genetic loss of the GULO enzyme?

Let's try to build a logical argument, starting with the assumption that we are in perfect health and not under stress, since the presence of factors such as disease or severe stress, which increase the need for ascorbic acid (63), would make the reasoning self-evident. Assuming no SVCT polymorphisms are present, we can associate a rich intake of fresh vegetables with stabilized plasma concentrations around 70 micromoles/L. Now, a few questions arise:

What would happen if we came into contact with a dangerous pathogen, or were exposed to a significant source of pollution, or suffered a major physical trauma?

And going a step further: what would happen in the event of an acute pathological incident, such as a severe allergic reaction or a major cardiovascular disorder?

It is worth noting that a series of highly stressful situations have just been listed. Unlike our bodies, such events would trigger a significant increase in ascorbic acid biosynthesis in animals, highlighting the metabolic gap repeatedly emphasized by Stone. This gap is so striking that it strongly supports the following thesis: allergic reactions, cardiovascular attacks, trauma, environmental stressors, and infections are among the many "ascorbic drains" capable of substantially lowering the 70 micromoles/L equilibrium that can be achieved through a robust diet. This makes the prospect of a subsequent ascorbic acid insufficiency quite realistic, one that could critically impair the vitamin's many physiological functions.

Therefore, no matter how impeccable it may be, diet alone may not be sufficient to ensure the integrity of the biochemical processes linked to vitamin C, including the stress response, which occurs spontaneously only in the lucky mammals that can synthesize it. This endogenous response optimizes key processes such as catecholamine synthesis and cortisol modulation.

It is plausible that the impairment of these vital processes, which are truly fundamental for sustaining the body under stress, could have a very negative biological impact. On that note, let us not forget Paul Marik's observation: "Due to an unfortunate evolutionary mutation, humans have lost the ability to synthesize vitamin C (Homo Sapiens Ascorbicus) and consequently have an impaired stress response. The inability to produce vitamin C during stress increases the vulnerability of humans to infectious disorders" (25).

It is also important to highlight the difficulty of replenishing depleted levels of vitamin C, replenishment that may require high oral doses or, as is commonly the case in critical illness, intravenous administration.

Finally, it will be shown that chronically inadequate levels of vitamin C can expose the body to a range of diseases.

In essence, several rational elements suggest that 70 micromoles/L may not be fully adequate to meet the needs of our bodies, bodies that are increasingly immersed in a world full of stress, threats, and unnatural conditions.

What has just been outlined is clearly only a tantalizing appetizer. The topic will soon be enriched with valuable insights regarding intracellular concentrations, where the dynamics appear to behave differently than they do in plasma. I also preview that later on, some elements will be presented that will shape a rather disorienting hypothesis: namely, that plasma concentration may not be a sufficiently reliable indicator for effectively assessing the systemic presence of vitamin C in the body.

Pharmacokinetics of the intravenous route

Some articles already illustrated (22), (62), (65) also contain an accurate description of the dynamics governing the pharmacokinetics of the intravenous route.

In general, the administration of drugs by intravenous infusion is more effective than the oral route, achieving plasma concentrations with 100% bioavailability.

As far as vitamin C is concerned, the preference for the intravenous route may seem surprising. In fact, intravenous administration completely (I repeat, completely) bypasses the saturable absorption mechanisms that strongly influence the oral route, allowing plasma concentrations to be reached that would otherwise be impossible. Consider the theoretical limit (never formally demonstrated) of the maximum plasma concentration obtainable by the oral route, estimated by some authors at 220-250 micromoles/L. This is a barrier that intravenous administration easily overcomes, even with the use of small amounts. This identifies parenteral administration (typically associated with intravenous infusions, although Klenner also used another route, the intramuscular one, which is no longer used today for technical reasons) as a valuable tool capable of broadening the therapeutic horizon of vitamin C, allowing the treatment of clinical conditions that are difficult to treat with the oral route.

At this point, some may wonder how big the differences are between the two routes of administration. They are so great that vitamin C, in the vast world of pharmacology, is considered one of the main substances capable of maximising the pharmacokinetic gap between the oral and intravenous routes. The bypassing of saturation mechanisms, therefore, opens up scenarios that the oral route cannot explore, allowing plasma concentrations of up to 150 times higher than the maximum levels achievable via the oral route (22), (66). This corresponds to plasma levels up to 30 millimoles/L (30000 micromoles/L). Interesting, isn't it?

However, one small problem still arises. Even the levels obtainable from the intravenous route, in fact, obey the law of short stay, expressing peaks that are as extraordinary as they are transient due to the usual intervention of renal excretion. In particular, the so-called half-life (the half-life is a pharmacokinetic parameter that indicates the time required for a 50% reduction in the plasma concentrations of a given compound) of a high intravenous dose of vitamin C is estimated to be 60-120 minutes (66), a very short time compared to dietary intake, which is characterized by a much longer half-life, ranging from a minimum of 48 hours to several days depending on plasma concentration (23), (62).

It may be useful to reinforce the theory by presenting an interesting comparison between oral and intravenous administration. Unlike the plasma peak of 220 micromoles/L reached with an oral dose of 3 grams, the same amount administered intravenously results in a peak plasma concentration of 1760 micromoles/L, approximately 8 times higher. The gap widens further with increased dosage: for example, the plasma concentration of 13350 micromoles/L resulting from a 50 g intravenous dose is of an entirely different order of magnitude than the concentration achievable with the same oral dose, a value which, although never precisely calculated, would presumably not exceed 300-400 micromoles/L (22). These differences are so substantial that they clearly separate the two routes of administration. Here, we touch on a critical point. At this stage, it is worth reflecting on the ambiguities that have clouded the long history of vitamin C and led to unfair criticism of Pauling and Cameron. It is evident that the enormous disparity between the two routes of administration necessitates specifying the method used in any clinical trial, as the effects of the two routes could lead to very different outcomes. Would one expect to successfully treat a bacterial infection using one-hundredth of the recommended antibiotic therapy?

This provides a first demonstration of the theorem referenced in the introduction. The reference is to the often-heard verdict “Vitamin C does not cure disease M”, a statement that lacks logic unless it is properly qualified by information regarding the type of therapy employed.

In any case, it is clear that the greater effectiveness of the intravenous route has opened up unimaginable possibilities, reigniting scientific research that at one point seemed to have stalled. The importance of the intravenous route, empirically explored by Klenner but only scientifically recognized in the early 2000s, is now finding application, at least experimentally, in the treatment of cancer and other complex clinical conditions such as infectious diseases, ischemia, burns, sepsis, and postoperative care.

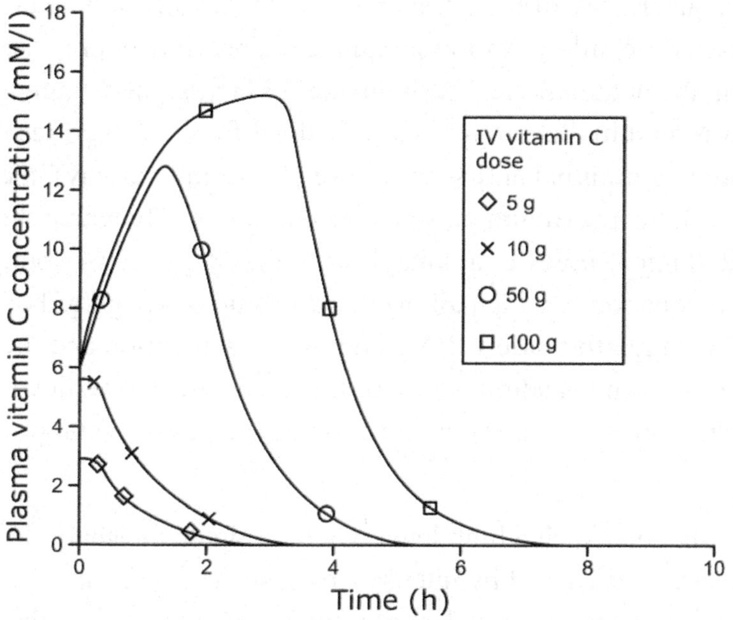

graph adapted from (22)

A technical note: the graph reveals a data point that confirms the rapid renal excretion. For any dosage (from 5 to 100 g administered intravenously), it is evident that after a certain period, approximately 12 to 16 hours, the various plasma concentration curves tend to converge and eventually return to baseline levels. This suggests that, under physiological conditions, 24 hours are more than sufficient to eliminate the vitamin C load (424).

The dynamics appear to differ significantly in the presence of cancer cells: vitamin C is retained for a longer time by these cells, and we will understand why in the dedicated chapter. One of the demonstrations comes from an important pharmacokinetic study in which a comparison between healthy individuals and cancer patients showed a difference in the amount of vitamin C excreted 24 hours after a high-dose intravenous administration (424). Unlike the 99% of vitamin C excreted by healthy subjects after 24 hours, cancer patients excreted only 89%, indicating that a significant portion of the vitamin C tends to persist in cancer patients. This is likely the result of increased cellular uptake, as suggested by some researchers: "The difference in the amount excreted is presumably due to tissue utilisation of ascorbate in cancer patients" (424).

The clear superiority of the intravenous route, already anticipated in Cathcart's discussion, allows us to rationalize the previously proposed framework for identifying the potential ideal daily intake. In fact, at the beginning of the book, there was an initial attempt to classify the different categories of vitamin C supplementation: a minimal anti-scurvy dose (10-15 mg per day), the RDAs (70-100 mg per day), the maximum plasma concentrations achievable through oral intake (220-250 micromoles/L, attainable with the "3 g every 4 hours" regimen), and the intravenous route, which allows for doses up to 1.5 g/kg/day to be administered with relative safety. Based on this classification and the undeniable superiority of intravenous administration, it is plausible that achieving millimolar plasma concentrations (i.e., through intravenous infusions) could provide benefits. But how?

It is plausible that such a high level would mitigate the sharp decline in plasma concentrations caused by intense stress, such as an acute illness (e.g., infectious, allergic or cardiovascular) or a severe trauma. In fact, the drop in plasma levels would be counteracted by the previously accumulated high concentration in the plasma, which would keep the levels for some time above the oral maximum, i.e., the 220–250 micromoles/L threshold achievable through the dynamic flow. Therefore, a millimolar concentration would effectively manage the steep decline in plasma levels caused by a major insult, maintaining levels far from deficiency. This would ensure the normal physiological functions of vitamin C during the acute phase of the insult, offering a degree of protection from the multiple metabolic dysfunctions that may result from it.

Although theoretically sound, this concept faces a significant practical limitation: the extreme effectiveness of intravenous infusions is offset by their low practicality. After all, who would be willing to undergo constant intravenous therapy?

The answer, therefore, points to using the intravenous route only in selected cases, for example, certain acute conditions where a temporary intervention is generally required. And, of course, this must always be accompanied by essential medical supervision.

Therefore, at least in terms of prevention, the oral route seems to be a necessary fallback to the more powerful but inconvenient intravenous route. Oral supplementation, which can be optimized through a high and frequent dosing schedule, fits well with the basic concepts of "something is better than nothing" or "doing the best I can". It represents a valid strategy for raising plasma concentrations, one that mimics, albeit imperfectly, the spontaneous mechanisms seen in more fortunate animals. The repetition of high oral doses appears to be a reasonable compromise between the dietary intake and the powerful intravenous approach. It is a compromise through which hypoascorbemia could be corrected, a compromise that may allow us to narrow the gap that leaves us far behind the animal world.

Two clarifications before concluding: the arguments presented here are only one element of a wider framework, whose full scope will emerge later on as further knowledge is introduced to enrich the discussion. I therefore ask for a bit of patience if something appears temporarily unclear.

Second: the safety profile of intravenous vitamin C, which remains excellent even at supraphysiological concentrations. A large body of research has provided sufficient data to paint a largely reassuring picture of the entire therapeutic profile, ranging from moderate doses (1-10 g) to true megadoses (100-125 g). Laboratory tests, vital signs, electrocardiographic evaluations, and physical examinations have never been negatively affected by intravenous infusions (even at very high doses) in the studies conducted, including a recent clinical investigation published in the specialist journal "Clinical Pharmacokinetics" in 2022, entitled "Pharmacokinetic Evaluation of Intravenous Vitamin C: A Classic Pharmacokinetic Study" (424). At the end of the abstract, one can appreciate a reassuring and at the same time paradigmatic assertion: "Intravenous vitamin C up to 100 g elicited no adverse effects or significant physiological/biochemical changes and appears to be safe. These data can be used to rectify existing misinformation and to guide future clinical trials".

According to Ping Chen, Reed, Jiang, Wang, Sunega, Dong, Ma, Esparham, Ferrell, Levine, Drisko and Qi Chen, therefore, a certain amount of "misinformation" about pharmacological vitamin C still persists. It seems like an effective portrayal of the state of confusion that can no longer be tolerated.

Distribution in the tissues

As previously mentioned, vitamin C is distributed throughout the body in a highly compartmentalized manner. Tissue concentrations range from 0.2 to 12 millimoles, displaying a heterogeneous localization that can resemble population density on a geographical map (62). This range is so extensive that the physiological plasma levels observed in healthy individuals, typically 50-250 micromoles/L, are, by comparison, quite low, highlighting the strong tissue preference for vitamin C.

The influx into tissues reflects the high affinity of the SVCT2 transporter for ascorbic acid. Excluding red blood cells, which obtain a small but vital amount through intracellular recycling of DHA (leading to a local concentration of 50-60 micromoles (62)), nearly all tissues receive AA via the SVCT2 transporter, typically resulting in tissue accumulations in the millimolar range.

Area	Local concentration (mM)
Heart	0.2-0.4
Liver	0.6-0.9
Adrenal glands	1.7-2.3
Kidneys	0.4-0.8
Muscles	1.4-1.8
Lungs	0.5
Eyes	2.0-4.0
Brain	1.0-2.0
Neurons	5.0-10.0
Pituitary gland	2.3-2.8
Lymphocytes	3.8
Platelets	2.8
Neutrophils	1.4
Erythrocytes	0.05
Plasma	0.05

Under physiological conditions, the body is generally able to retain between 1.5 and 3 grams of ascorbic acid (67). These values, seemingly modest, are in fact quite substantial when compared to the much more dangerous threshold of only 400 mg of total body reserves, a level statistically associated with deficiency (plasma level < 11 micromoles/L) and thus a high risk of scurvy.

Which areas are richest in vitamin C?

As shown in the figure, leukocytes (white blood cells, represented in the table by lymphocytes and neutrophils), the adrenal glands, and especially the brain exhibit very high concentrations. The brain, in particular, possesses a sophisticated defense mechanism capable of ensuring significant ascorbic acid retention during times of deficiency. This cerebral retention mechanism is considered crucial for several reasons, including the preservation of key processes such as maintaining brain function and protecting internal structures (68).

It is now time to introduce a personal definition that effectively captures vitamin C's behavior. The brain seems to represent the tip of the iceberg in a physiological dynamic that also involves other areas with unique properties. Specifically, the adrenal glands, leukocytes, and the brain, which I personally refer to as "favourite sites", are particularly tied to vitamin C. In addition to exhibiting unmatched concentrations, the cells in leukocytes, the adrenal glands, and the brain appear to overcome local deficits through a dynamic redistribution of the body's total AA pool (62), (495). This phenomenon has been demonstrated in several experiments, where local upregulation of transporters was also observed, presumably to ensure an adequate supply of ascorbic acid to these favourite sites when systemic concentrations begin to fall.

Therefore, the concentration of ascorbic acid in the favourite sites (adrenal glands, leukocytes, and brain) appears to be regulated by strict defensive mechanisms, suggesting a regulatory mechanism comparable to that governing other vital substances, such as glucose, which is strictly controlled by the hormones insulin and glucagon.

The brain, in particular, is considered the last stronghold. This means that, in the event of deficiency, it tends to sequester vitamin C beyond all limits, with the implication that ascorbate levels in the brain are depleted only after all other bodily reserves have been exhausted. This mechanism is justified by the priority of ensuring antioxidant protection in cases of severe deficiency, a situation in which oxidants could cause irreversible damage to brain structures.

Therefore, it is plausible that the extremely high levels of cerebral ascorbate and the mechanisms developed to protect the brain represent two evolutionary countermeasures designed to ensure cellular integrity in a vital area that is highly rich in oxidants, and thus at high risk for oxidative damage.

Lind's observations on the mental clarity of his sailors seem, in this light, to find a rational explanation. The reader may recall that the final manifestations of scurvy include a range of neurological disturbances, consistent with the meaning of the adjective "scorbutic", which is commonly used to describe irritable or bad-tempered individuals. It now becomes clear why Lind described his sailors as generally maintaining a certain degree of mental clarity, even while suffering from severe infections and devastating hemorrhages: evidently, their brains were stoically attempting to retain as much vitamin C as possible.

Descriptions of the intracellular distribution of vitamin C offer numerous points of interest, not only from a historical but also a highly topical perspective, some of which highlight the difficulties that persist in understanding certain dynamics of theoretical and potentially even clinical value. For example, although our knowledge is well advanced on many aspects, the mechanisms underlying different tissue concentrations remain largely unknown. The existence of multiple tissue-specific variants of SVCT2 has never been confirmed, lending credence to the hypothesis that the degree of individual expression of SVCT2 in tissue cells may determine levels that are closely linked to plasma availability. However, the issue is still highly controversial due to a number of counterexamples, including the marked heterogeneity of ascorbate concentrations among different brain cell types.

A number of researchers have expressed misgivings about the interconnection between plasma availability and tissue expression. "Tissue concentrations of vitamin C, which are frequently millimolars, are far in excess of what is required for its actions as a coenzyme. Millimolar concentrations of intracellular vitamin C may simply serve as a reservoir of the vitamin, or may have other unknown functions", reads an important report published in the journal "Oral Diseases" (67). These elements will combine with later information to weaken the reservoir hypothesis, thus supporting the possibility of additional unknown functions. It seems more likely, in fact, that the enormous tissue accumulation of AA may be involved in some functions that still elude our understanding, in addition to the known ones including neuroprotection, neurotransmission and neuromodulation (nervous system), immune cell support (white blood cells), stress reactivity (adrenal glands) and systemic antioxidant defence. To this impressive list must be added a further systemic involvement, the very important cofactor activity, which is indispensable for many crucial metabolic pathways.

Overall, the topic of intracellular distribution remains a largely unexplored and uncertain field. Human studies investigating the impact of administration on the amount of vitamin C distributed throughout the body are scarce and limited to just a few tissues, failing to provide a clear and effective interpretation, and leaving many important questions unanswered. For example, in the case of deficiency (plasma level < 11 micromoles/L), what would the ascorbic acid level be in leukocytes? And in the brain? In the liver?

And at plasma levels considered optimal (the point of plasma saturation), what would AA concentrations be in various tissues? Would there be tissues saturated with vitamin C at the point of plasma saturation?

Furthermore, in the event of illness or acute stress, which area would go into vitamin C deficiency first? Cathcart, for example, put forward a hypothesis that has never been explored further, according to which the depletion of the area affected by the disease would take precedence over the plasma and any other site.

These questions have found partial clarification in some animal experiments. Prominent among these is a study published in "The Journal of Nutrition" in 1987 (69), in which researchers, using six percentages of dietary intakes of AA (0, 0.076, 0.5, 1, 5 and 8%), examined the concentrations in the blood and tissue of mice. What specifically did they find?

Ascorbic acid in plasma increased proportionally when AA intake varied from 1% to 8%. Mice fed 5 or 8 per cent ascorbic acid expressed much higher concentrations than control mice (0 per cent group) in the heart, kidneys, lungs, muscles and spleen; mice fed 1 per cent AA also outperformed the control group, at least with regard to concentrations in the heart, kidneys, lungs and spleen.

It is extremely interesting to note that ascorbate concentrations in the brain, adrenal glands and leukocytes (which are the favourite sites) showed no significant changes in each of the experimental groups.

But that's not all: ascorbic acid levels in the eyes were slightly increased in the 8% group, while strangely, a 0.076% diet slightly reduced concentrations in the liver, lungs, muscles and spleen. The same was true for mice fed a 0.5% diet: compared to controls, they had lower levels in the liver and muscles.

This study allows the formulation of intriguing conjectures, which are also useful in identifying an appropriate daily dosage. Overall, the results provide three relevant considerations. Firstly, the favourite sites (let us again recall: brain, adrenal glands and leukocytes) showed no variation from the control group in all supplementation groups (let us not forget endogenous biosynthesis!). This suggests that biosynthesis is sufficient to ensure saturation in the favourite sites. In fact, the favourite sites appear to reject any dietary supplementation, in line with the already highlighted concept of local homeostasis.

A note: it cannot be ruled out that these results, and also the subsequent points we will discuss, may only occur in the presence of physiological conditions, leaving open the hypothesis that pathological patterns produce different responses.

Secondly, a high dose of AA (5% or 8%) significantly increased the level of ascorbic acid in the heart, kidneys, muscles, spleen and lungs, suggesting the non-saturation of these organs. Therefore, it is plausible to assume that the ascorbic concentration of these organs may respond very reactively to supplementation, expanding proportionally; in the case of an animal model, the contribution of supplementation would clearly add to that of biosynthesis.

The third point is an unexpected result that illustrates the potential drawbacks of going against nature: mild supplementation (0.076%) unexpectedly reduced ascorbic acid levels in several organs (liver, lungs, spleen, and muscles), suggesting that it can inhibit endogenous biosynthesis. This indicates that AA supplementation in animals capable of biosynthesis may be unnecessary or even counterproductive, particularly if administered at very low dosages (69).

This is an animal study, which calls for caution when interpreting the results in humans, especially given the disparity in biosynthetic capabilities. However, the distinction appears plausible: favourite sites may reach saturation much more easily than other organs, i.e. at low doses. In other areas, including vital organs such as the heart, lungs, and kidneys, larger doses may be required to achieve a full reservoir of ascorbate. It is worth noting that a full reservoir could be advantageous. Although this will be discussed later in more detail, it is already reasonable to hypothesize that a fully stocked local reservoir might strengthen the so-called “non-favourite sites” in terms of antioxidant capacity, increasing the antioxidant protection provided by intake that saturates the favourite sites and plasma.

Some vital organs, therefore, could benefit from increased antioxidant protection if saturated with vitamin C. This is significant!

Confirmation that vital organs, such as the heart, liver and kidneys, require larger amounts to reach saturation than the favourite sites, came from a subsequent study based on a comparison between wild animals and animals with altered GULO (363). This study, it should be noted, was published in the prestigious "The American Journal of Clinical Nutrition". "The heart, liver, and kidneys in particular require a much higher dose to reach optimal ascorbate concentrations. Notably, we found that the daily dose deemed to be sufficient for the GULO–/– mouse (1.65 mg/day), which results in almost normal brain concentrations, actually corresponded to very low liver, heart, and kidney concentrations and that up to 10 times the recommended dose was required to reach the concentrations seen in the wild-type littermates. If a similar situation occurs in humans, then an increase in the RDA should be recommended to intakes that achieve saturated plasma concentrations to ensure adequate tissue concentrations throughout the body", the authors report (363). In other words: in GULO-deficient mice, the minimum amount needed to saturate the brain provided very little vitamin C to the liver, heart, and kidneys.

Therefore, based on the extensive data collected, the researchers arrived at a calculation that leads to intriguing interpretations: an amount greater than the RDA, perhaps even 10 times the recommended dose, would be necessary for a mouse lacking biosynthesis to match the liver, heart, and kidney levels of a wild-type mouse (363). This appears to be a definitive verdict in favor of Stone, and it can be interpreted as paradigmatic: the human RDA equivalent is far lower than the biosynthetic capacity of animals.

This valuable study highlights a significant asymmetry between the saturation of favourite sites and that of certain vital organs, suggesting the insufficiency of the RDA and thus lending support to Stone and proponents of the "total saturation" concept. This concept emphasizes the biological importance of saturating all tissues, not just the favourite sites, which are easier to saturate because this can also be achieved by dietary intake. "The recent identification of an extended role for ascorbate in regulating the hydroxylation of HIF-1 and histone demethylases highlights the necessity for the maintenance of adequate ascorbate in all body tissues to control cell metabolism and gene expression", the authors argue (363).

Overall, animal studies have revealed a discrepancy between the favourite sites and certain vital organs in terms of local uptake, offering a rational perspective suggesting that saturating the plasma and/or favourite sites may not be sufficient to achieve the full biological benefits of vitamin C. If confirmed in humans, this would represent a small revolution, as it is precisely the saturation of plasma and/or leukocytes that constitutes the official model adopted by the scientific community to estimate the optimal daily intake of vitamin C.

What do the human studies indicate?

As previously mentioned, human studies analyzing the relationship between intracellular and plasma concentrations are few and limited. One particularly interesting study dates back about 20 years and focused on apparently healthy young women (70). This study, which analyzed concentrations in neutrophils, monocytes, lymphocytes, and platelets, revealed findings consistent with the dynamics of plasma saturation, identifying 200-400 mg as the saturation point for these cells (again, under healthy conditions). In fact, similar to plasma concentrations, single doses above 400 mg produced increasingly smaller local increases, forming what mathematicians refer to as a sigmoidal curve (see figure).

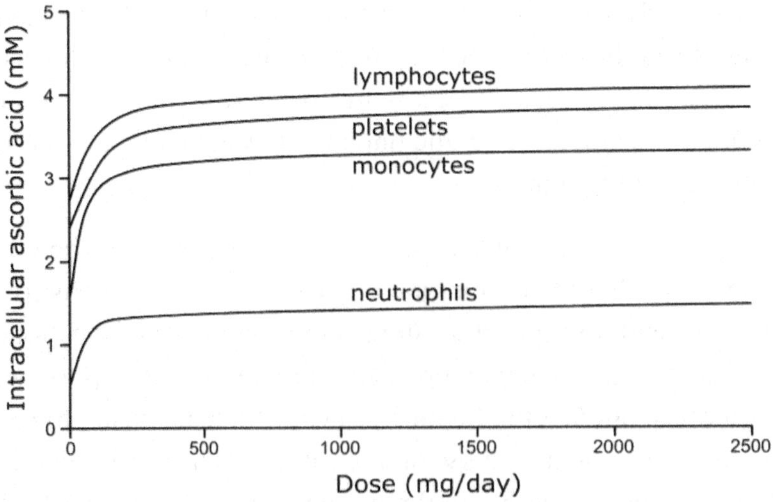

graph adapted from (70)

Therefore, under typical assumptions of perfect health, absence of stress, and no AA deficiency, there is strong evidence suggesting that 200-400 mg is the appropriate amount to saturate plasma and leukocytes (lymphocytes, monocytes, and neutrophils all belong to the broader leukocyte category).

Before moving on with an acute observation, it is useful to ask why the RDAs are still stuck at 70-100 mg (generally: 90 mg for men, 75 mg for women). "On the basis of criteria for ideal vitamin C intake, these data provide evidence that the recent RDA of 75 mg for young women should be increased", stated the authors of the previous study, which was published in the authoritative journal "Proceedings of the National Academy of Sciences of the United States of America" (70) in the scientifically distant year 2001. It is curious to note that the same journal had reported similar findings five years earlier, which shows that the results of (70) only reinforced certain perceptions already present in the 1990s (516): "Based on these data and Institute of Medicine criteria, the current RDA of 60 mg daily should be increased to 200 mg daily" (516).

After more than 20 years, little has changed. Even the narrow pharmacokinetic view of the plasma-white blood cell pair, according to which the RDA should be raised to 200 mg, continues to be ignored.

The perplexity increases when one "acutely" notices that our body is much more than plasma and white blood cells, thus widening the pharmacokinetic view to 360 degrees: the question thickens with interesting questions. What happens in other tissues? Does something similar happen to what happens in the animal world?

In the muscles, for example, the data show a markedly different trend. A randomized placebo-controlled study (401) published in the highly regarded journal "Free Radical Biology and Medicine" assessed the effects of a modest oral supplementation (500 mg twice a day, for 42 days) on the skeletal muscle of some healthy individuals. A marked asymmetry emerged with respect to what was observed in leukocytes, because those who received supplementation expressed significantly higher muscle concentrations than those who obtained AA exclusively through dietary intake (approximately 200 mg). This is clearly at odds with leukocyte dynamics, for which a robust dietary intake should readily achieve local saturation.

One note: the increase in muscle concentration was substantial but rather gradual, since it took 7 days of supplementation to observe a significant increase in muscle vitamin C concentration. It is not trivial to note that this contrasts with what occurs in plasma, where concentrations increase rapidly in response to supplementation. A striking question arises: what would have emerged if this study had been based on a shorter time frame, such as 3-4 days?

In all likelihood, the results would have been unrealistic and would have contributed to confusing the understanding of the pharmacokinetics of vitamin C.

Further confirmation in support of the high receptivity of muscles comes from the prestigious "The American Journal of Clinical Nutrition" through a clinical evaluation in which Carr and co-workers were able to clearly state the following: "Human skeletal muscle is highly responsive to vitamin C intake and plasma concentrations and exhibits a greater relative uptake of ascorbate than leukocytes" (537).

As for the other tissues, we are almost groping in the dark. Almost, in fact, because the question has been made less obscure by an organ directly involved in vision: the crystalline lens, a natural lens of the eye that helps focus light rays on the retina. The conclusions of a surprising study published in 1997 (410) have very interesting practical implications. With 265 participants, it was possible to demonstrate that no dietary intake is capable of producing vitamin C saturation in the crystalline lens. This is consistent with the results obtained in animal studies, but has more value given the clinical characterisation of the study.

Even with regard to the aqueous humour, an important saline fluid located between the cornea and the crystalline lens, clinical evidence does not support dietary intake as sufficient. A series of studies conducted from the 1990s to 2017 (431) showed optimal results, indicating that 2 grams are required to saturate the human aqueous humour. This finding reinforces the notion that both dietary intake and typical supplement doses (500-1000 mg) are insufficient to achieve vitamin C saturation in all tissues.

While waiting for further clinical research to improve understanding, let us try to produce a rational argument based on what is known. As has already been documented, it appears that the liver, kidneys, heart and lungs, organs which, moreover, start from a very low physiological concentration, do not easily reach saturation, showing a much higher capacity for local absorption than the favourite sites. What local benefits might arise from intracellular concentrations higher than what is considered "ordinary" (with "ordinary" defined as the levels achieved by the dose that saturates leukocytes and plasma)?

Although it is impossible to provide a definitive answer, logic suggests that higher concentrations could offer a more effective response to localized pathological challenges.

What do I mean by that?

It has been widely demonstrated that the level of ascorbic acid in the heart generally ranges between 0.2 and 0.4 millimoles (where "generally" refers to a concentration achieved through dietary intake, which is sufficient to saturate plasma and leukocytes under physiological conditions). It is plausible that this level could be increased through vigorous supplementation, though to what extent is unknown, as we lack specific studies on the matter. Let us therefore assume, without exaggeration, that high-dose supplementation might raise cardiac levels to 0.6 millimoles. It is known that severe cardiac conditions, such as myocardial infarction, myocarditis or arrhythmias, can drastically reduce local ascorbic acid concentrations. Unlike the well-known favourite sites, the heart does not appear to possess homeostatic mechanisms capable of compensating for ascorbic acid levels during emergencies. Would a cardiac level of 0.6 millimoles prior to disease onset be more beneficial than a level of 0.2 millimoles? Is it rational to deduce that a higher concentration could provide greater biological resilience against certain acute pathological events?

In essence, a new scientific perspective is emerging: vitamin C as a prophylactic model. This model, whose full effectiveness may require an intake much higher than what is needed to maintain normal metabolism, appears to be natural, almost as if it were an evolutionary extension aimed at aligning humans with the animal kingdom, where vitamin C functions not only as a dietary component but also as a fundamental regulator of stress (the "stress hormone").

A second observation concerns leukocytes, which can be saturated through robust dietary intake under physiological conditions. Suppose an infectious disease occurs: there would likely be a rapid depletion of ascorbate in the leukocytes (71), which, unlike the heart, would trigger compensatory mechanisms. This would imply a withdrawal from systemic concentrations, thereby increasing the risk of deficiency due to the redistribution of ascorbate toward infected tissues and white blood cells. Once again, the prevailing philosophy seems to be that it is better to err on the side of excess rather than deficiency. And it is not just logic that supports this: another point already mentioned on several occasions, the very low toxicity of vitamin C, emerges as a strong justification. This non-toxicity, it should be noted in advance, appears to characterize every therapeutic approach, from high oral doses to intravenous administration (72), (73).

Would a reservoir full of vitamin C in all areas of the body only be useful as a defence against acute damage?

Probably not. According to data from (363), even under physiological conditions, the full functionality of vital organs such as the heart, kidneys and liver may require saturation, and therefore a higher intake than normal. It is thus reasonable to state that cardiac saturation could provide at least two benefits: limiting the effects of potential acute damage and maximizing the biological functions of vitamin C within cardiac tissue. We can therefore observe a clear connection with the statements made by Padayatty and Levine in (67), who noted that "Millimolar concentrations of intracellular vitamin C may simply serve as a reservoir of the vitamin, or may have other unknown functions". In fact, it cannot be ruled out that a higher-than-normal local concentration, namely (pardon the repetition) one exceeding the levels required to saturate plasma and leukocytes, and thus surpassing the official reference point, may give rise to such "unknown functions", potentially enhancing the metabolic efficiency of the organ involved.

Therefore, I believe it is appropriate to conduct studies aimed at identifying the saturation levels of various tissues and the compensatory mechanisms that modulate tissue distribution during pathological states, a circumstance in which the pharmacokinetics of vitamin C, as has been partly observed and as we will soon demonstrate, tends to change. In essence, it is necessary to characterize the dynamic relationships that different organs and their saturation thresholds establish depending on whether the body is in a physiological or pathological state. This is an ambitious project that could shed full light on a range of issues concerning both prevention (determining the correct dosage to ensure good health) and clinical practice, where vitamin C is increasingly emerging as a promising and multifunctional pharmacological agent.

This raises the final question: what rationale led health institutions to calculate the RDA for vitamin C based on leukocyte and/or plasma saturation levels, setting it, moreover, at half of what it should be according to that very model?

Renal excretion

The kidneys and SVCT1 are the main elements that regulate ascorbate homeostasis, a function that SVCT1 is able to coordinate by modulating several key mechanisms such as intestinal absorption, renal reabsorption, and renal excretion (62).

We can imagine the excretion mechanism as a smart faucet, ready to open when SVCT1 is saturated and able to shut quickly in case of deficiency. Unfortunately, certain abnormalities can impair this intelligence, leading to significant imbalances not only in renal excretion. This is due to the fact that a dysfunction of SVCT1, which can be caused, for example, by a disease or a genetic polymorphism, may alter intestinal absorption or impair renal excretion and reabsorption, with potentially significant consequences. As previously mentioned, the importance of SVCT1 has been highlighted in various animal studies, where alterations in SLC23A1 often increased renal excretion, leading to massive urinary losses, sometimes up to 20 times higher than normal (62). One such example is a particular polymorphism known as A772G RS35817838, which is believed to reduce plasma concentrations to below 20 micromoles/L, regardless of dietary intake (62). This would result in a permanent and refractory deficiency, for which the only effective solution might be intravenous supplementation or dynamic flow.

Over the years, other genetic polymorphisms have been identified that can drastically reduce plasma and cellular concentrations, confirming that the issue of polymorphisms is significant. For example, the genetic variant RS33972313 is believed to reduce intracellular concentrations in various tissues by half (60). It is important to note that an alteration capable of reducing intracellular absorption could be a significant problem and difficult to detect. This is due to the challenges of monitoring intracellular levels and, especially, to the fact that a local deficiency could be masked by the presence of a normal plasma concentration. This indicates that dysfunction of SVCT2 may be more insidious than that of SVCT1.

The dysregulation of transporters is a topic of considerable importance because, although its prevalence in the global population is unknown, it raises multifaceted considerations involving vitamin C homeostasis and casts doubt on whether plasma is the optimal site for assessing its systemic concentration. It is worth emphasizing that renal reabsorption and renal excretion, being processes that vary depending on underlying conditions, are highly fluctuating. For example, during illness, prolonged stress or deficiency, certain changes may occur: as previously mentioned, the body attempts to drastically reduce renal losses in order to conserve residual vitamin C. It was Hoffer who first observed in the 1980s that the kidneys of schizophrenic patients tend to retain large amounts of ascorbic acid in response to high-dose supplementation, contrary to the pharmacokinetic rules seen under physiological conditions (74), (75).

Two examples can help clarify this concept. The results of a 1990 clinical study (76) showed that diabetes can alter the renal excretion of AA, leading to urinary losses that are inversely correlated with glycated hemoglobin levels (a form of hemoglobin used to assess the average plasma glucose concentration over an extended period). In practice, high blood glucose levels appear to force the body to limit renal losses of ascorbic acid. This behavior seems to be common to several diseases, including the common cold. In fact, urinary AA levels are generally reduced during this illness, a clear sign that the body tends to retain a molecule considered essential for counteracting the development of the common cold. Notably, at the end of the infection episode, urinary AA levels return quickly to normal (378), (545).

Therefore, the presence of disease alters the rules of pharmacokinetics: during illness-induced deficiency, the body tends to sequester as much vitamin C as possible, primarily by reducing renal excretion.

However, this also appears to occur under physiological conditions. In an interesting 1988 study (396), renal excretion was analyzed after a single oral supplementation of 1 gram. The two groups examined, young and elderly subjects, yielded a result consistent with previous findings: urinary ascorbate levels in the elderly were much lower than in the younger individuals. This outcome may be attributed to certain disturbances that can affect transporters, particularly disadvantaging elderly subjects. As already noted, aging can substantially impair the function of SVCTs (63).

Overall, a growing number of studies attribute to the kidneys the ability to modulate ascorbate homeostasis, while also suggesting an intriguing perspective: in an emergency, the body would "greedily" accept any input capable of alleviating the depletion caused by the crisis.

We can therefore propose two general principles, to be added to the established law of short stay:

1- During illness, renal excretion of AA is inversely correlated with disease severity;

2- During illness, the metabolic requirement for AA increases in direct proportion to the severity of the condition.

Principle 2, which could be redefined as the "Fundamental Theorem of Vitamin C", states that ascorbate depletion is directly associated with disease severity. This is a theorem with potential clinical implications, considering the high global prevalence of diseases and the many factors that can deplete vitamin C stores. Consider, for instance, SVCT dysregulation, whose etiology is clearly multifactorial, or the increased cellular metabolism typical of illness, two important "destroyers" of vitamin C (62), (63). Not to mention what might be the central component: the disruptive action of oxidative stress, which characterizes every pathological state and against which vitamin C serves as the first major antioxidant defense. Indeed, vitamin C is the first antioxidant to counteract oxidative attack, thus highlighting one of the many unique properties that make it exceptional.

Chapter 4
Vitamin C Physiology

'Many people place their trust in vitamin C only at sunset, when they should be doing so at dawn'

Angelica Paradiso

Introduction

Over the years, scientific knowledge about vitamin C has led to an evolving centrifugal model, historically focused on scurvy and free radical antagonism. Subsequent studies have uncovered important new biochemical implications in which it acts as an enzyme cofactor. Collagen synthesis, the production of those stress mediators known as catecholamines, and gene transcription are just some of the processes that are impossible without the presence of vitamin C as a cofactor.

What we are about to examine is a truly crucial chapter, in which certain singularities will be revealed that clearly demonstrate the uniqueness of vitamin C. For example, it will be noted that its marked antioxidant activity provides certain biologically crucial compounds with strong protection against oxidants, as well as a notable sparing effect.

The chapter will also examine the various fundamental roles that vitamin C plays in the immune system, in iron absorption, in cholesterol metabolism, and in the synthesis of several hormones with significant metabolic impact, not to mention its remarkable potential that has recently opened up promising avenues in the fight against cancer: the modulation of HIFs, the so-called oxygen sensors. However, before exploring the multidirectional actions of vitamin C, attention will first be given to its operational core, the point of balance that sustains the entire system of actions: its antioxidant function.

Oxidative stress and antioxidant function

Everything begins with the concept of a free radical. A free radical is defined as a molecular entity characterized by the presence of a destabilizing element: an unpaired electron. An unpaired electron is one that occupies a given atomic or molecular orbital alone. Since orbitals usually contain either zero or two electrons, the presence of a single unpaired electron represents a chemical anomaly. This anomaly forces the molecular entity to seek stability by "stealing" electrons from nearby molecules.

Free radicals, in short, are highly unstable and reactive molecules, characterized by a very short lifespan and a continuous search for stability.

Stated this way, it might sound like the description of a monstrous entity with deceptive traits. But the reality is more nuanced: free radicals, which regulate various metabolic processes and responses to external stimuli, are often considered "two-faced compounds". The production of free radicals is actually essential for several physiological functions, including intracellular communication and immune response. However, they can also be generated in response to environmental or other external stimuli, thereby displaying potential toxicity. Among the main factors that can trigger the uncontrolled formation of free radicals are illnesses, pollution, radiation, intense physical activity, smoking and some medications.

It is therefore the dose that makes the poison, as the legendary Paracelsus claimed. If not neutralised, an overload of free radicals can cause the well-known condition of oxidative stress, a condition characterized by an imbalance between the formation of free radicals and the ability to protect against them. In such cases, internal defences are insufficient to counteract the damage, requiring external (antioxidant) support, foreshadowing the intimate relationship between vitamin C and oxidative stress.

Oxidative stress is widely recognized as a harmful imbalance in the body, as it can lead to the development of various chronic diseases such as cancer, autoimmune disorders, and neurodegenerative diseases (77).

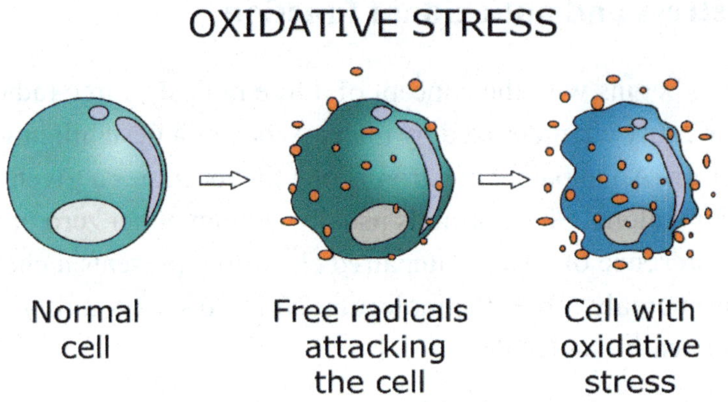

We are therefore introduced to antioxidants, many of which act as reducing agents, special molecules capable of preventing the oxidation of other molecules by generously donating electrons.

Oxidation occurs when an element gives up electrons to another substance (this element is said to be "oxidized"), which is then reduced by this transfer (this substance is said to be "reduced"). This describes the well-known oxidation-reduction, or redox, reaction, in which, depending on the flow of electrons, a compound can shift from its oxidized form to its reduced form. Oxidizing agents, therefore, are substances that tend to acquire electrons from others, which is why free radicals must be classified as oxidizing agents.

As previously discussed, preventing oxidation is extremely important, as oxidation can trigger chain reactions that irreversibly damage cells, with potentially serious consequences for the organism. The mechanisms by which an uncontrolled presence of free radicals, a condition known as oxidative stress, disrupts the body's equilibrium are mainly linked to the formation of reactive oxygen species (ROS). ROS, which include both oxygen-containing free radicals and non-radical species, are among the most reactive oxidizing agents; at high concentrations, they can directly lead to cell death. In short, they are the most aggressive type of oxidants.

How much does oxidative stress really affect health?

Although the exact role of oxidants in the pathogenesis of disease has not yet been fully defined, there is no doubt that oxidative stress can be an influential factor. Given the limited evidence for a predominant role in disease development, it is currently regarded as one of several concomitant causes. Nonetheless, it is dangerous, as it tends to intensify during the course of illness. Thus, oxidative stress can be both a cause and a consequence of disease.

This aspect must not be misunderstood, but rather integrated into a rational analysis. Although antioxidant therapy may prove insufficient to halt the progression of a disease, as other factors may play a central role in its course, it can still be beneficial. In fact, antioxidant treatment may help slow disease progression and support more specific therapeutic approaches. Consider, for example, a condition linked to the triad of poor nutrition-oxidative stress-inflammation, which promotes the formation of oxidants: hyperglycemia. It is well known that physical trauma, surgical procedures, poor diet, and intense physical activity, all major sources of oxidative-inflammatory stress, can lead to a spike in blood glucose levels, often sharp and temporary. This increase tends to exacerbate the oxidative-inflammatory overload caused by the initial event, creating a vicious cycle that can be interrupted by antioxidant action.

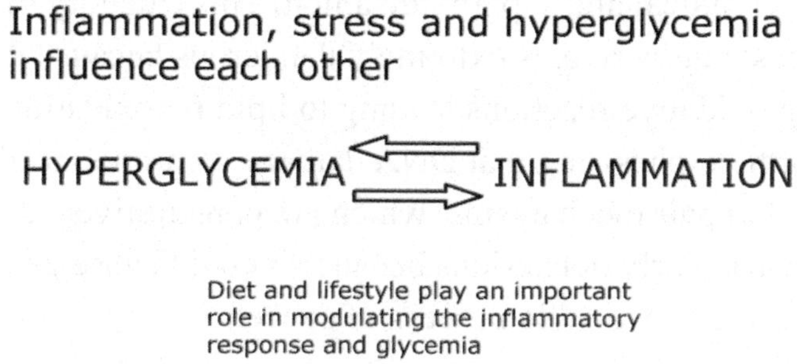

Another interesting example is the so-called ischemia-reperfusion injury (more on this later), a condition that follows an ischemic event in which oxidative stress, often massive, leads to important consequences. Mechanistically, oxidative stress promotes inflammation, impairs mitochondrial function and induces oxidative damage to lipids, proteins, and DNA. Therefore, without effective antioxidant strategies, these effects could increase ischemic tissue damage and functional decline.

How can we stem the damage of oxidative stress?

In response, it is useful to point out a paradox of metabolism: while it is well known that most complex organisms require oxygen for their existence, it must be emphasised that oxygen can induce a highly reactive environment. This sets up a delicate balance, the disruption of which would cause damage through uncontrolled production of reactive oxygen species. This danger has forced humans to develop a fundamental countermeasure in the course of evolution, namely a network of compounds highly specialised in protecting against oxidative damage. What are they?

The main internal (endogenous) defence compounds include glutathione, catalase (an enzyme primarily involved in the anti-tumour mechanisms of ascorbate), coenzyme Q10, the class of superoxide dismutase enzymes (which has recently gained importance because it is probably implicated in the pathogenesis of amyotrophic lateral sclerosis (538)), peroxiredoxins, uric acid and melatonin (a hormone known mainly for regulating circadian rhythm, but with remarkable antioxidant properties). These elements are capable of acting in a complementary manner, whose synergy determines a protective structure essential for survival.

It should come as no surprise that this protective structure is particularly efficient against reactive oxygen species, mainly represented by hydrogen peroxide, hydroxyl radical and superoxide anion. This category of oxidants, essentially the most aggressive, is extremely dangerous because it can damage cells by initiating oxidative reactions leading to lipid peroxidation or DNA damage. It is worth emphasising that DNA damage so pronounced as to override the so-called DNA repair mechanisms, which are constitutively active in human cells, would be particularly deleterious because it could cause genetic mutations that would trigger the irreversible process of cancer.

Let us now describe the variety of antioxidants, a vast and heterogeneous family in which there are several specialisations. Let us introduce a classification useful both to develop an effective description and to provide the demonstration of an often instrumentalised thesis: "Not all antioxidants act in the same manner".

A first classification of antioxidants is based on their "preference" for water. This leads to two broad categories: hydrophilic or water-soluble antioxidants, such as vitamin C, and hydrophobic or fat-soluble antioxidants, such as vitamin E. Water-soluble antioxidants generally react with oxidants in the plasma and in the cytoplasm, the part of the cell between the membrane and the nucleus, which consists mainly of an aqueous compartment known as the cytosol. Fat-soluble antioxidants, by contrast, protect cell membranes from the damaging effects of lipid peroxidation, a process in which fatty acids in the membrane are oxidised by specific types of free radicals.

A second classification of antioxidants is based on their origin. In addition to being synthesised endogenously, antioxidants can also be obtained from food or supplements. A well-known example of exogenous antioxidants is the triad formed by vitamins A, C, and E.

Vitamin C stands out in the antioxidant family for a number of reasons, displaying unique biochemical properties. In fact, it is considered the most important water-soluble antioxidant defence, so much so that it can neutralise oxidative damage much better than glutathione and vitamin E; for example, vitamin C can in some circumstances neutralise superoxide much faster than glutathione (149).

Leaving aside the speed aspect, ascorbic acid is characterised by a fundamental property called "first-line ROS sink". This term, used by some specialists, indicates a unique feature with profound biological implications, which places AA at the forefront of antioxidant defences. AA, in fact, establishes the systemic antioxidant first line of defence (67), (427), (78), (160), (528), i.e. a robust antioxidant barrier that comprehensively and readily defends the aqueous compartments and, by extension, the plasma membranes. What is meant by "first line of defence"?

In many in vitro experiments, it has been consistently observed that the oxidation of vitamin C precedes that of all other endogenous and exogenous antioxidants, including the two powerful antioxidants glutathione and vitamin E (67), (427), (528). This highlights a distinctive property of vitamin C: it intervenes with full urgency and top priority, as one might say using police jargon, to neutralize reactive oxygen species (ROS). This priority does not appear to be confined to the laboratory setting. Although in vivo studies are relatively limited, there is a certain scientific consensus supporting the validity of this dynamic at the clinical level as well (427), (528).

The evidence, while indirect, is compelling: numerous clinical studies have shown a predominant depletion of vitamin C, a clear sign of what might be called an "ascorbic preference". As will be discussed below, many studies have revealed an asymmetric situation in which, unlike other potent antioxidants such as glutathione, vitamin A and vitamin E, vitamin C levels are drastically reduced in response to disease, surgical interventions, or trauma (526). It is therefore plausible to hypothesize that during conditions capable of triggering massive oxidative stress, such as ischemia or sepsis, ascorbic acid serves as the first line of antioxidant defense, acting as the initial responder to the ROS assault. As a kind of collateral benefit, this early intervention can spare other vital molecules such as glutathione and vitamin E.

Let's pause for a moment, because what we have illustrated provides insight into one of the main reasons behind the ascorbic depletions that occur systematically following illness or highly stressful circumstances: these, as is well known, have the capacity to generate oxidative stress, thereby depleting the primary agent responsible for neutralizing excess free radicals.

Illness, or more generally severe stress, can trigger a metabolic conflict in which an excess of reactive oxygen species overwhelms the commendable self-sacrificing nature of ascorbic acid, depleting it throughout the body. The situation would be different in the presence of a timely and adequate intake of ascorbic acid, similar to the steady optimal concentrations typically maintained in animals. High levels of AA, in fact, may spare glutathione and vitamin E, which are also involved in the neutralization of ROS, particularly in areas less accessible to AA, such as the plasma membranes. It should be noted that glutathione and vitamin E play important physiological roles beyond their antioxidant function alone.

In any case, it is worth anticipating that antioxidants act in different ways, especially when comparing water-soluble compounds with fat-soluble ones. Vitamin C, for example, acts both inside and outside the cell, primarily in aqueous compartments, where it fits perfectly due to its water-soluble nature. By neutralizing free radicals quickly and effectively, it is therefore characterized by a fast and versatile action, qualities that not all antioxidants possess.

Vitamin C's action is also well-integrated, as it can work synergistically with certain "competing antioxidants". A particularly interesting example of this cooperation is the synergistic antioxidant shield formed with vitamin E. Technically, vitamin C is able to recycle vitamin E by effectively "repairing" oxidized vitamin E (79). Given the differing natures of the two molecules, one water-soluble, the other fat-soluble, this dynamic is extremely valuable for the cell: vitamin C scavenges ROS in the cytosol, while vitamin E does so in the plasma membranes (80). In essence, vitamin C is capable of regenerating vitamin E. This regeneration occurs when vitamin E has participated in defending cellular membranes and becomes oxidized; vitamin C then reduces the oxidized form of vitamin E, restoring its antioxidant function (80).

Therefore, it is plausible to assume that the combined administration of the two powerful antioxidants can provide great benefits. In fact, more and more research has suggested that vitamin C-E combination can markedly counteract oxidative stress caused by disease or intense stress (81), (82). We will illustrate two clinically different examples. The first concerns endometriosis, an inflammation caused by the presence of endometrial tissue (the mucous membrane lining the inner cavity of the uterus) in organs other than the uterus or in inappropriate portions of the uterus. In a randomized, placebo-controlled clinical trial, published in 2021 in the journal "Pain Research and Management" (82), the combination of vitamin C and vitamin E was effective despite the use of low dosages. The combination therapy, with daily doses of 1 g vitamin C and 800 IU vitamin E, alleviated dysmenorrhoea (menstrual pain) and improved pelvic pain control, while also demonstrating strong antioxidant capacity. The authors wrote: "After treatment with vitamin C and vitamin E, we found a significant reduction in MDA and ROS compared to the placebo group" (82); the acronym MDA stands for one of the most reliable biomarkers of oxidative stress (more precisely, of peroxidative damage), the so-called malondialdehyde.

Before moving on to the second example, it is worth noting the strong evidence supporting the effectiveness of the vitamin C-vitamin E combination in managing endometriosis-related pain, as recently demonstrated by a meta-analysis of randomized controlled trials (589). A meta-analysis is a statistical method that combines results from multiple clinical studies on a treatment, providing a cumulative and therefore more robust assessment than individual trials. It shares similarities with systematic reviews but includes a quantitative synthesis of data.

The second example concerns the increasingly emerging phenomenon of intense physical activity, a source of high oxidative stress. Many studies have come to one conclusion: C-E synergy is very protective against oxidative damage caused by intense physical exercise. "The obtained data underline the necessity of intensifying the means of endogenous antiradical defence with exogenous antioxidant vitamins C and E. This study highlights the need of a proper vitamin supplement in organism under stress", reads the end of one of many papers (83).

Vitamin C, however, also clearly exhibits its own antioxidant activity, independent of other compounds. One of the many lines of evidence for this comes from the field of physical exercise. A recent meta-analysis of randomized clinical trials (400), published in 2020 in the reputable journal "European Journal of Nutrition", indicated that vitamin C supplementation can be highly beneficial in reducing two common consequences of high-intensity exercise: oxidative stress and inflammation.

In combination or alone, therefore, but also as a substitute. Interestingly, vitamin C can replace other antioxidants, vitamin E in the first place, in certain tasks. An article published in "The Journal of Nutrition" (84), for example, focused on the impact that ascorbic acid may have on the famous good cholesterol (HDL), the oxidation of which is implicated in triggering atherosclerosis. This interesting research filled a small scientific gap, as the relative ascorbic acid contribution has been little explored compared to the well-characterised efficacy of vitamin E. Hillstrom, Yacapin-Ammons and Lynch provided the first positive evidence in 2003: vitamin C can also inhibit lipid oxidation in HDL (84).

The countless examples should not distract us from the overall meaning of antioxidant activity: vitamin C provides rapid, robust and multifaceted protection against conditions associated with excessive free radical production, including complex diseases, surgical procedures, trauma, environmental pollution, radiation, smoking and more. Organs and tissues such as the heart, liver, lungs, thyroid, kidneys, pancreas, spleen, stomach, adrenal glands, white and red blood cells, skin and eyes are particularly sensitive to ascorbic defense. This is especially true for the nervous system, where the essential role of vitamin C is most pronounced.

Whether acting alone or in synergy with other antioxidants, vitamin C is therefore fundamental in neutralizing oxidative stress and all processes involving extensive oxidative damage, willingly sacrificing itself on the front lines of the ROS assault. As we will explore in later chapters, this self-sacrifice may bring significant benefits in the clinical management of many diseases.

Vitamin C as a prooxidant

Many health professionals express concern about a supposed dark side of vitamin C, advising against any form of supplementation beyond routine use. This refers to the scenario in which vitamin C behaves atypically as a prooxidant, thereby promoting the formation of oxidizing substances. A dark side that we will seek to clarify with scientific rigour.

It is widely believed that high doses of antioxidants can cause serious damage. This is a superficial and unfounded belief, as it is impossible to consider the heterogeneous family of antioxidants as a single group. Vitamins A, C, E, alpha-lipoic acid, NAC (N-acetylcysteine), glutathione, coenzyme Q10, epigallocatechin gallate, resveratrol, astaxanthin and curcumin, among the main known antioxidants, possess very different characteristics, which is why it is clear that an excess of one antioxidant may have different consequences from those of another. The accumulation of water-soluble compounds, such as vitamin C, is much more difficult than that of fat-soluble substances. Take vitamin E, for instance, a strongly fat-soluble compound: when consumed in excess, it can cause effects such as altered blood coagulation, which are not typically observed even at high doses of vitamin C or of most other antioxidants. Furthermore, some evidence has linked high doses of vitamin E to a statistically significant increase in mortality (543).

Therefore, although it is true that some antioxidants, and I emphasize some, can cause problems, it is important to highlight that vitamin C has amply demonstrated its safety, as we will explore further.

As for the phenomenon of prooxidation, you will notice that, although the nature of ascorbic acid is dual (antioxidant-prooxidant), the prooxidant action is only possible through intravenous administration. Does this mean that intravenous administration can potentially be dangerous?

Perhaps there is something almost magical about all this, something that philosophically seems to justify the pro-oxidant side of vitamin C, and thus the absolute perfection of Nature itself. In the chapter on cancer, in fact, it will be shown that it is precisely this pro-oxidant action that reveals its most potent anticancer properties.

The pro-oxidant action of ascorbic acid, now well characterized from a biochemical perspective, depends on its natural ability to initiate a reduction reaction with certain highly reactive transition metals, particularly copper and especially iron. At millimolar concentrations, this dynamic appears to trigger the sequential formation of two oxidants, superoxide and, ultimately, hydrogen peroxide, culminating in the so-called Fenton reaction.

Therefore, does ascorbic acid supplementation pose a danger?

Can the use of dynamic flow induce oxidative stress?

Once again, we turn to the scientific literature for answers. Several authors (85) have investigated the effects of various oral dosages of vitamin C in terms of oxidative risk, conducting analyses within the 500-5000 mg range. The parameters assessed included DNA integrity, natural killer cells (a type of lymphocyte with tumor- and virus-fighting capabilities), and the process of cellular apoptosis (programmed cell death). The results were clear: after the two-week study period, the 20 participants showed no DNA alterations, no negative effects on immune cells or apoptosis. Therefore, across the entire dosage range, vitamin C exhibited exclusively antioxidant properties.

Further reassurance comes from a 2013 systematic review (86), whose 17 incorporated studies associated the manifestation of prooxidant effects with a plasma concentration of an order of magnitude typical of intravenous administration, i.e. the millimolar order of magnitude. It is useful to remember that pharmacokinetic models have identified the barrier of 250 micromoles/L, which seems impossible to exceed with oral supplementation, thus tending to rule out the possibility that the oral route could produce pro-oxidative effects.

Moreover, according to the numerous authors of the review, there is much more: "In vitro, animal and ex vivo studies of pharmacologic ascorbic acid (AA) have yielded meritorious results proving vitamin C as an effective cytotoxic agent against oral neoplastic cells with potentially no harmful effects on normal cells" (86). The review is therefore quite clear: oral administration, regardless of the dosage, cannot induce oxidative effects, as it is unable to achieve millimolar concentrations in the plasma. Intravenous administration, by contrast, allows vitamin C to reach such levels, enabling it to act as a pro-oxidant. However, when this occurs, its potentially harmful, or rather, cytotoxic, action appears to be directed selectively against cancer cells.

What has just been described is important because it outlines an extraordinary mechanism by which an infallible sniper would target tumor cells while completely sparing healthy ones, a mechanism that no other conventional anti-tumor approach appears capable of achieving.

At this point, the focus of the discussion naturally shifts to another question: what is the minimum dosage, clearly to be administered intravenously, capable of generating oxidants?

An important study published in the prestigious journal "Nature" in 2004 helped clarify the issue by identifying a reassuring limit. This study (87) was conducted on volunteers who were given daily infusions of 750 mg or 7500 mg for six consecutive days. The results revealed no evidence of pro-oxidative effects, indicating that intravenous vitamin C, at doses up to 7500 mg, does not induce oxidative stress.

What can we say regarding children?

Even in the pediatric field, no concerning signals have emerged. A 2021 review published in the specialized journal "Pediatric Critical Care Medicine" (88), for example, confirmed its safety, in line with the rest of the literature. The review reported that doses ranging from 100 mg/kg/24 h to as high as 1500 mg/kg/24 h were not associated with toxicity, either in terms of potential oxidative risks or overall safety.

The topic of "pro-oxidant risk" deserves a final clarification, which can be presented through a theorem with potential clinical implications. Intravenous administration of ascorbic acid in a healthy individual could produce markedly different outcomes compared to a critically ill patient. The reasoning is simple: it is plausible to hypothesize that the plasma and tissue concentrations in a critically ill patient are involved in countering the massive oxidative stress associated with their condition, thus displaying a very low level of ascorbic acid. This could result in lower concentrations compared to a healthy individual, even with the same dosage. An example based on a 3 g dose will be illustrated below in the context of critically ill patients. This reasoning leads to a practical suggestion: the parameter to consider when assessing the potential for a pro-oxidant state should not be the administered dosage, but the plasma concentration achieved.

This is the context for my personal hypothesis, which proposes the existence of a threshold L (related to plasma concentrations) that would distinguish the potential for pro-oxidant effects from antioxidant action. In other words, pro-oxidant phenomena may only occur when plasma concentrations exceed a well-defined threshold. Beyond this hypothetical limit L, it is also plausible that the infusion rate could become a critical variable, as some preliminary data have associated the speed of infusion with the generation of oxidant molecules. These are truly fascinating technical issues, and a full understanding of them could support experimental and clinical practice, improving the manageability of intravenous vitamin C. Therefore, dose and infusion rate appear to be very useful parameters for modulating intravenous administration of vitamin C. Their functional modulation can, in fact, steer the biological effects according to therapeutic goals, either toward the creation of a highly oxidative environment potentially harmful to cancer (and likely only to cancer cells), or toward the classic antioxidant effect.

The conclusion of this paragraph is emblematic. It refers to a randomized prospective study (181) conducted in Japan (which will be analyzed in more detail later), in which a continuous intravenous infusion at a rate of 66 mg/kg/h, maintained for 24 hours, provided a range of insights, including a reassuring antioxidant effect. This is an astronomical dosage, equivalent to over 110 grams intravenously for a 70 kg individual. However, this high dosage was slowed down by being administered over 24 hours, that is, about ten times more slowly than in oncology studies where a pro-oxidant effect is sought through "flash" exposures of 2-3 hours. Although this therapy was theoretically compatible with a pro-oxidant scenario, the data collected ruled out such an effect, as a clear reduction in oxidative markers was observed. This reinforces the idea that vitamin C has a form of redox adaptability, enabling it to modulate its pharmacological actions depending on the clinical context.

We have reached the conclusion. We have sought to shed light on the pro-oxidant side of vitamin C with the utmost transparency. The hope is that this will be enough to distinguish truth from falsehood, no matter how authoritative the latter may appear under unclear circumstances.

The important role as a cofactor

In addition to its antioxidant function, much of the importance of vitamin C lies in its immunomodulatory nature. However, it would be a mistake to marginalize its role as an enzymatic cofactor, a function in which it plays a crucial part in the production of several biologically essential molecules.

What is a cofactor?

An enzymatic cofactor is a non-protein chemical compound or ion that binds to an enzyme and is necessary for its biological activity. An enzyme is a protein that accelerates a specific chemical reaction without being consumed or permanently altered. It is important to emphasize that enzymes requiring a cofactor are inactive in its absence or when the cofactor is non-functional. Essentially, the cofactor enables the enzyme to perform its catalytic function properly.

An important subclass of cofactors is represented by the so-called coenzymes, molecules that contain a vitamin or a vitamin-derived structure. We are now at a crucial point, as this highlights the relationship between cofactors and vitamins, a relationship in which many vitamins act as coenzymes or as precursors to coenzymes. Typical examples include vitamin B1, the precursor of the coenzyme thiamine pyrophosphate (the biologically active form of thiamine); vitamin B5, the precursor of the essential coenzyme A; and vitamin C, which also functions as a cofactor.

Without delving into the more technical aspects, we will first highlight the numerous activities in which vitamin C functions as a cofactor, followed by its most influential biological implications. There are two large families of enzymes that require vitamin C as a cofactor: monooxygenase enzymes (such as dopamine beta-hydroxylase and peptidylglycine alpha-amidating monooxygenase) and dioxygenase enzymes (such as prolyl 4-hydroxylase, prolyl 3-hydroxylase, lysyl hydroxylase and gamma-butyrobetaine hydroxylase).

We begin with the enzyme dopamine beta-hydroxylase, which synthesises noradrenaline. This synthesis, which takes place in the nervous system and adrenal glands, involves the conversion of dopamine into noradrenaline and requires molecular oxygen, copper and ascorbate (67). We are now entering a crucial point: the fundamental role of catecholamines (dopamine, but above all noradrenaline and adrenaline) in stress management, and the reaction systems that allow animals to dynamically modulate their biosynthesis under stress, a countermeasure that is impossible for humans, suggest that managing stress in humans requires large amounts of vitamin C.

With regard to catecholamines, there are other metabolic pathways in which AA acts as a cofactor, technically through hydroxylation and decarboxylation processes. One of these pathways involves the degradation of an important amino acid called tyrosine, the precursor to catecholamines. This degradation, known as tyrosine catabolism, has as its product a particular compound called fumaric acid (89); in addition to degrading tyrosine, AA, as will be seen in more detail in a moment, also comes into play in two segments of the metabolic pathway through which tyrosine (or its precursor, phenylalanine) forms catecholamines, potentially leading to adrenochrome (67), (89).

The centrality of vitamin C in the biosynthetic pathways of catecholamines is an indisputable fact that can be deduced from various elements. Prominent among these is the fact that catecholamines are produced in two tissues known for their high concentrations of vitamin C, namely the adrenal glands and the brain. It is also believed that the antioxidant value of vitamin C is so strong that it prevents the oxidation of catecholamines while helping to eliminate excessive levels of adrenochrome (89). In essence, vitamin C contributes to the synthesis of catecholamines and can prevent their oxidation.

Overall, there are two vitamin C-dependent processes: a broader one that supports the synthesis of all catecholamines, and a more specific one that directly involves the conversion of dopamine to noradrenaline.

It is important to note a distinction, as the role by which ascorbic acid promotes the conversion of phenylalanine into tyrosine and subsequently into catecholamines, unlike the direct synthesis of noradrenaline from dopamine, is not strictly related to its function as a coenzyme, but rather to its role as a "protector of coenzymes". Tyrosine metabolism, in fact, involves another key coenzyme closely linked to vitamin C: tetrahydrobiopterin (BH4). This biologically valuable compound plays a crucial role in several critical enzymatic reactions and is present in all tissues of the body. BH4 also serves as a cofactor in two other fundamental biosynthetic pathways: the conversion of the amino acid tryptophan into serotonin, and the conversion of arginine into nitric oxide, a reaction regulated by nitric oxide synthase, an enzyme that exists in three forms: neuronal, inducible, and most notably, endothelial.

As in tyrosine metabolism (where BH4 acts as a cofactor in two distinct processes, first converting phenylalanine into tyrosine, and then tyrosine into the dopamine precursor, levodopa), also in the tryptophan-serotonin and arginine-nitric oxide pathways, AA does not play a direct cofactor role, but rather ensures that the cofactor BH4 remains in its reduced form, recycling it when necessary. In short, AA strives to keep BH4 efficient by protecting it from oxidation, thereby helping to preserve it in its reduced form, which is essential for enzymatic reactions to function properly.

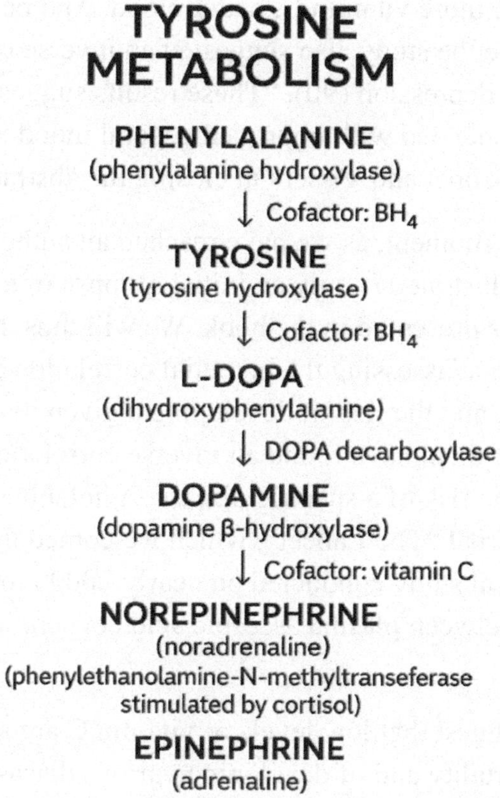

Tyrosine metabolism

The protection that AA provides to BH4 is therefore not only fundamental but also unique, as no other antioxidant is known to replicate this specific function

(149), (565). As a result, low levels of AA may impair the synthesis of catecholamines, serotonin and nitric oxide, potentially leading to very negative physiological impacts (67), (89).

Here is a first relevant implication: AA plays a significant role in the synthesis of the well-known “happiness hormone”, serotonin. Its deficiency has been widely linked to depression, highlighting the importance of vitamin C both in mood modulation and in the pathogenesis of depressive disorders. Although the topic of depression will be addressed later on, it is still useful to introduce it by presenting a recent study (90) that examined the relationship between plasma levels of AA and mood. This study, based on a group of one hundred students, showed an inverse correlation between plasma concentration and mood disorders, and also showed that plasma levels > 50 micromoles/L were associated with better mood. In short: more vitamin C, better mood. And perhaps not only an improved mood, since the study also suggested an inverse correlation between AA levels and the risk of depression (90). “These results suggest that a high level of vitamin C may be associated with improved general mood in young adult males”, write Pullar, Carr, Bozonet and Vissers in closing the abstract of their paper (90).

Let’s pause for a moment, as we have reached an authoritative presentation. What has just been illustrated is only an initial glimpse of a large number of statistical correlations presented in the book. We will thus discover that the various studies aimed at assessing the potential correlation between plasma concentrations of AA and the risk of developing a given disease have valued vitamin C, as most of them have found an inverse correlation between its plasma concentrations and the risk of a specific disease. A notable example can be found in the prestigious journal “The Lancet”, which welcomed the results of a large 48-month epidemiological study conducted on nearly 20000 individuals, finding an inverse association between plasma ascorbic acid concentration and all-cause mortality (334).

These results suggest that low levels of vitamin C are associated with an increased risk of mortality and of developing various diseases: “Risk of mortality in the top ascorbic acid quintile was about half the risk in the lowest quintile”, the authors of the paper report (334). In short, one of many pieces of evidence supporting the insights of Stone, the man who first correlated the pathogenesis of many diseases with vitamin C deficiency.

We now return to BH4, illustrating its role as a cofactor of the enzyme endothelial nitric oxide synthase (eNOS), an enzyme involved in the production of nitric oxide (NO) at the endothelial level. Considering the unparalleled protection AA can give to BH4, this role is significant because it allows AA to protect the endothelium, thus contributing to the prevention and treatment of a condition called endothelial dysfunction (67), (149). Nitric oxide is a molecule of great biological value, best known for its vasodilating activity. However, nitric oxide (an oxidant, confirming that only a redox imbalance can trigger oxidative stress) is not exclusively involved in controlling arterial tone. Its involvement in neurotransmission, immune response and platelet aggregation inhibition processes suggests that it is polyfunctional and goes beyond endothelial physiology, as can be deduced from the multifaceted nature of the NO-generating enzyme, nitric oxide synthase (in addition to the endothelial eNOS form, there are the "neuronal" and "inducible" forms).

We now turn to the enzyme peptidylglycine alpha-amidating monooxygenase (PAM), which requires molecular oxygen, copper and the cofactor ascorbate (67). PAM is involved in the synthesis of many hormones, mostly of hypothalamic origin, and prominent among them is vasopressin, also called ADH or antidiuretic hormone (67). The dual abundance that characterises the pituitary gland, where PAM expression and AA concentration abound, seems to reinforce the importance of vitamin C as a cofactor (91). This pituitary gland-PAM-AA axis effectively forms a biochemical "laboratory" for the production of key hormones, some of which have demonstrated their clinical relevance even in the difficult management of pain.

It is with vasopressin, however, that vitamin C seems to have an extra edge. Synthesised mainly by the hypothalamus and deposited in the pituitary gland, vasopressin is essential for regulating plasma volume and helping maintain homeostasis in critical conditions. In fact, its secretion is stimulated in the presence of situations of great clinical complexity. Typical examples are dehydration, in which ADH can retain fluids and exert a vasoconstrictive action and consequently hypertensive action, and especially sepsis, a complex systemic pathology in which there is a dysregulated inflammatory response to the presence of an infection; ADH also appears to influence the nervous system, and is thought to be involved in neurotransmission and neuromodulation (559).

Let us return to the topic of sepsis: the goal is to provide concrete evidence of the true value of vitamin C as a cofactor. The chosen model is the sepsis-vasopressin-noradrenaline triangle, which, however, will be revisited and explored in greater depth later on. Let us begin with a premise: during sepsis, it is common to develop a serious condition known as refractory hypotension. This form of hypotension is particularly challenging because it is resistant to many pharmacological treatments, including fluid resuscitation, a technique that involves administering large volumes of fluids to expand blood volume (volemia) in an attempt to raise blood pressure. Refractory hypotension, therefore, is typically managed in intensive care units, and may require aggressive therapies based on so-called vasopressors, agents with strong hypertensive action; among the most powerful vasopressors are vasopressin and, in particular, the catecholamine noradrenaline.

We have reached a crucial point. As previously discussed, the enzymes dopamine beta-hydroxylase and peptidylglycine alpha-amidating monooxygenase (PAM) are involved in the synthesis of noradrenaline and vasopressin, and cannot function without the presence of the cofactor AA. This leads to an inevitable question: could AA supplementation improve refractory hypotension?

An affirmative answer appears plausible, especially considering the ascorbic acid deficiency observed in many septic patients (34). It is therefore entirely logical to hypothesize that AA supplementation could reduce the need for vasopressors in septic patients. Indeed, several researchers have identified the biosynthesis of vasopressors as a physiological mechanism by which ascorbate may serve as an effective adjunct in the management of sepsis and septic shock, the most feared complication of sepsis (91). It is worth noting, as will be further explored in a dedicated section, that this mechanism is not the only one with potentially relevant clinical implications. Endothelial preservation (the AA-BH4-NO axis), cortisol modulation (the anti-stress function of AA), and its potent antioxidant action represent further elements that support a therapeutic role in the treatment of sepsis. Indeed, based on the additional aspects that will be progressively presented, we will identify sepsis as the most appropriate model to illustrate the multifaceted biochemistry of vitamin C.

Let us continue by describing the implications involving the amino acid derivative carnitine, which is produced through the activity of two dioxygenase enzymes: trimethyllysine hydroxylase and gamma-butyrobetaine hydroxylase (67). Carnitine synthesis involves the amino acids lysine and methionine and requires iron and a reducing agent, with AA recognised as the most effective reducing agent. This comparison is particularly interesting because it highlights that the role of AA as a coenzyme appears to be linked to its antioxidant nature. Although the issue has not been fully clarified, it is believed that all enzymes requiring AA, as they are characterised by the presence of a metal ion (iron or copper), need AA to maintain these metals in a reduced state, which is essential for enzymatic activity. While one might hypothesize that other reducing agents could fulfill this role, several studies have demonstrated that vitamin C uniquely protects the iron-copper pair from oxidative inactivation. Thus, vitamin C appears to be irreplaceable even in its function as a cofactor (67).

Returning to carnitine biosynthesis, it's useful to note that the role of ascorbic acid in this process may help explain why fatigue is one of the symptoms of scurvy. This stems from the fact that carnitine regulates the transport of fatty acids into the mitochondria, where a process known as beta-oxidation converts fatty acids into usable energy. It is therefore not surprising that carnitine has shown potential to significantly enhance physical performance (560).

As for the symptomatology of scurvy, it is important to emphasize that the tendency to bleed and delayed wound healing result from connective tissue defects. These are directly linked to the role of ascorbic acid as a cofactor for a subclass of dioxygenase enzymes that hydroxylate the amino acids proline and lysine, converting them into hydroxyproline and hydroxylysine, two key components of collagen (67). Thus, the synthesis of collagen, the main structural protein of connective tissue in animals, requires vitamin C. Collagen is a fundamental and predominant protein, providing tensile strength to connective tissues much like a supportive scaffold. It is also the most abundant protein in the mammalian body, accounting for about 25% of total protein mass. Tendons, ligaments, skin, blood vessels, bones, heart valves, intervertebral discs, cornea, and lens are just some of the areas where collagen is found in high amounts, further underscoring its essential role in human health.

Let us try a small experiment: suppose we replace AA with another antioxidant in what is believed to be AA's central role in collagen synthesis, specifically, the reduction of iron. The outcome would be negative for any attempted substitution. It is, in fact, plausible that irregular collagen fibers would form, leading to skin lesions and blood vessel fragility, two early signs of scurvy (67). This provides practical evidence of the irreplaceability of AA and highlights its fundamental physiological link with collagen.

The widespread presence of collagen in many organs and its dependence on ascorbate suggest crucial biological implications for human health. Consider collagen deficiency and hemorrhagic stroke (a type of stroke that occurs when a blood vessel in the brain ruptures and bleeds), two elements in a direct causal relationship. Findings from an epidemiological study (92) conducted in a small Japanese community, which examined the relationship between stroke and vitamin C between 1977 and 1997, provide compelling evidence supporting the "structural" role of vitamin C. The statistics revealed an inverse association between plasma vitamin C concentrations and the incidence of all forms of stroke, an association the study's authors described as "strong", and which was published in the prestigious journal "Stroke" (92). A "strong" inverse association that is clearly consistent with the pathophysiology of the AA-collagen-haemorrhagic stroke triangle.

Vitamin C thus appears to play an important role in the prevention of stroke and ischemia. To this prophylactic value, a promising therapeutic perspective can be added: its oxidized form, dehydroascorbic acid (DHA), appears to possess all the biological properties needed to limit stroke progression (216), further confirming the dual prophylactic-therapeutic nature of this highly versatile, safe, and potent vitamin.

This dual nature also seems to emerge in the treatment of trauma. For example, a systematic review (403) provided robust preclinical data highlighting the importance of AA in the management of traumatic injuries, particularly bone fractures. According to the authors, the acceleration of bone healing processes, increased collagen synthesis, and reduced oxidative stress are the main contributions that adequate AA supplementation may offer in this context. "No adverse effects were reported with vitamin C supplementation in either animal models or human participants; thus, oral vitamin C appears to be a safe supplement but lacks clinical evidence compared with controls. Because of the limited number of human studies, further clinical investigations are needed before the implementation of vitamin C as a postinjury supplement" (403).

Vitamin C and HIFs

One of the most remarkable qualities of vitamin C concerns a dominant element in the universe and one that is essential for life: oxygen. Vitamin C is, in fact, involved in the activity of so-called cellular oxygen sensors, technically known as HIFs (hypoxia-inducible factors).

The idea of dedicating an entire paragraph to the relationship between HIFs and vitamin C, a relationship in which it acts predominantly as a cofactor, stems primarily from the potential impact this interaction may have on cancer research, and secondly from the novelty of studies on this topic. It is worth noting that this subject reached peak media attention in 2019, when the Nobel Prize in Physiology or Medicine was awarded jointly to William G. Kaelin Jr., Sir Peter J. Ratcliffe, and Gregg L. Semenza for their groundbreaking discoveries on how cells sense and adapt to oxygen availability.

We have just referred to a fundamental adaptive mechanism essential for our survival, one that allows cells to endure metabolic stress, particularly in conditions of low oxygen availability (hypoxia) (93). The molecules that govern cellular adaptation to oxygen fluctuations are known as hypoxia-inducible factors (HIFs). This group of proteins was discovered in the early 1990s through studies that revealed new insights into the link between red blood cell production and low oxygen levels. The primary function of HIFs is to respond rapidly to hypoxia (whether systemic or local) by modulating the production of red blood cells, the cells responsible for oxygen transport in the blood.

Are oxygen levels dropping? Then the body attempts to optimize available resources by enhancing oxygen transport capacity. That, in essence, is the role of HIFs. To achieve this, HIFs regulate gene expression to stimulate the production of erythropoietin, a hormone that plays a key role in red blood cell formation (94).

Why is oxygen sensing so important?

Hypoxia is a condition in which an inadequate concentration of oxygen occurs, leading to a scenario in which many vital functions may significantly lose efficiency. But our organism, fortunately, is a machine that borders on perfection: for example, to counteract the effects of oxygen deficiency it has developed a series of extremely effective response mechanisms, many of which are modulated by HIF factors. HIFs are therefore a family of transcription factors (proteins that regulate gene transcription) that are essential for maintaining the body's homeostasis. They are particularly responsive during systemic hypoxia as well as during oxygen depletion localized to a specific area, a condition known as local hypoxia.

In summary, HIFs act like a switch that activates in response to oxygen deficiency, whether systemic or local. This latter condition is common in many diseases, most notably cancer, diabetes, heart failure, and ischemic disorders. Consider the example of cancer or ischemic diseases: defective vascularization can create a highly hypoxic environment. In cancer specifically, the uncontrolled expansion of tumor cells can result in large distances between the cells and the blood vessels (which carry oxygen and nutrients), leading to a microenvironment with extremely low oxygen levels. This compels the body to activate HIFs in an attempt to maintain metabolic homeostasis (67).

However, HIFs can also be manipulated by cancer (95), (96). Simply put, cancer is capable of triggering an action-reaction dynamic in which hypoxia and HIFs become key players in promoting its own progression. But why does HIF expression support cancer progression?

To answer this question, we must introduce HIF-1 alpha, a subunit of HIFs that is considered the main transcriptional regulator of the cellular response to hypoxia. It has been shown that overexpression of HIF-1 alpha can increase the gene expression of numerous genes involved in cancer metabolism, thereby promoting tumour growth in various ways (67). A notable example involves genes that encode vascular endothelial growth factor (VEGF), a protein essential for angiogenesis, the process by which new blood vessels develop from existing ones. This process is considered one of the primary strategies by which cancer "cleverly" secures the nutrients and oxygen it needs to grow. In summary, tumor cells exploit HIF activity, particularly the HIF-1 alpha subunit, to survive under the hypoxic conditions typical of cancer.

What role does vitamin C play in this context?

It is necessary to say a few words about HIF-1 alpha, whose fate is strongly dependent on oxygen levels: under normoxic conditions, this subunit is regularly degraded by prolyl hydroxylase (a specific family of dioxygenase enzymes also involved in collagen biosynthesis). However, during hypoxia, certain issues arise that hinder this degradation. In hypoxic conditions, such as in cancer, prolyl hydroxylase is unable to function properly for various reasons, leading to the inappropriate stabilization and overexpression of HIF-1 alpha (67).

A note: in the absence of tumor-related disease, hypoxia itself does not create major issues regarding HIF-1 alpha activity. Although its overexpression and stabilization may promote tumor progression, they are not sufficient to initiate tumorigenesis. In this sense, cancer behaves like a true opportunist, exploiting the commitment with which HIFs manage all oxygen-deficient conditions, including the tumor microenvironment.

Before explaining the reasons behind the difficulties encountered by the prolyl hydroxylase family during hypoxia, it is useful to mention the role played by vitamin C in this context. This role is particularly important, as it has been widely demonstrated that vitamin C acts as a cofactor for prolyl hydroxylase enzymes (67), (96). Alongside iron, another essential cofactor, vitamin C supports the hydroxylation of HIF-1 alpha under normoxic conditions (96). This process, which leads to the rapid degradation of HIF-1 alpha, is biologically important because it helps maintain HIF-1 alpha at physiological levels.

What happens to prolyl hydroxylase under low oxygen conditions?

Let us take cancer as an example, the most insidious model. During oncologic disease, hypoxic stress induces the production of large amounts of ROS, which contribute to disease progression by promoting excessive expression and stabilization of HIF-1 alpha. In fact, ROS can inactivate prolyl hydroxylase, making it unable to hydroxylate HIF-1 alpha under hypoxic conditions (405). Technically, the main destructive mechanism of ROS is thought to act on iron (it is worth noting that iron is one of the essential cofactors of the prolyl hydroxylase family), causing iron oxidation and thereby reducing the enzymatic activity of prolyl hydroxylases (405).

A second major issue can arise during cancer: in addition to the ROS-induced dysfunction of the iron cofactor, cancer is also typically associated with depletion of vitamin C (as previously mentioned (32), (33)), a phenomenon that clearly impairs the physiological functions of vitamin C, including its role as a cofactor. If this were a boxing match, one might say that cancer nearly knocks out both cofactors that support HIF-1 alpha's "regulator", prolyl hydroxylase. In short, cancer can deliver blows capable of overwhelming virtually any opponent. To this devastating one-two punch, one must add the lack of oxygen (since cancer generates local hypoxia due to inadequate vascularization), thus favoring an uncontrollable scenario in which HIF-1 alpha and tumor cells become increasingly aggressive (405).

How can vitamin C be useful?

An adequate intake of vitamin C can have a strong impact on this problem, acting decisively in two key areas. The first involves restoring plasma and tissue levels of vitamin C, thereby reactivating its cofactor functions. This possibility, initially associated with high pharmacological doses (97), has recently been reinterpreted by a number of studies (404) showing that even partial repletion can modulate HIF-1 alpha expression. This has led to a counterproposal challenging the prevailing view, one that is gaining increasing support: cancer progression may be counteracted even with moderate vitamin C intake. To conclude with the study (404), published in 2015 in the journal "Cancer Medicine", it should be noted that this was one of the first studies to demonstrate in vivo (i.e., in animal models) the inverse correlation between ascorbic acid and HIF-1 alpha, a correlation that until then had been observed primarily in in vitro (i.e., cell culture) models.

Summarizing, the inactivation of prolyl hydroxylase enzymes depends on the combination of three phenomena: a low level of AA, oxygen deficiency (oxygen, like AA and iron, is required to hydroxylate HIF-1 alpha) and an excess of ROS, a triad systematically present in cancer (405). And it is precisely the neutralisation of oxidative stress that introduces the second aspect with which vitamin C is useful. In addition to reactivating its role as a cofactor, adequate vitamin C administration can prevent the iron cofactor from being damaged by ROS, thus preserving prolyl hydroxylase and its natural antagonism to HIF-1 alpha. It is worth pointing out that this latter activity has been known since 2007, when the prestigious journal "Cancer Cell" accepted a study in which the following can be read: "Vitamin C has been shown to decrease HIF-1 alpha levels by preventing oxidation of the catalytic ferrous ion" (405).

Overall, vitamin C can act both as a cofactor and as an antioxidant, a dual role that highlights its fundamental importance in regulating HIF-1 alpha.

The dynamics just described help illustrate one of the antitumor mechanisms of vitamin C. While cancer tends to destabilize all the components, oxygen, iron and ascorbic acid, through which prolyl hydroxylase can normally regulate HIF-1 alpha levels, vitamin C commendably attempts to counteract this disruption by restoring at least two of these components: iron and, of course, itself.

However, it may also be useful to restore oxygen levels. In fact, there is a growing research focus aimed at reactivating prolyl hydroxylase through oxygen-based strategies with potent antioxidant action. One example is ozone therapy, which is receiving growing attention (566). This research direction is broad and promising, especially when considering, on one hand, the damage that the hypoxia-ROS duo can inflict during cancer, and on the other, the fact that ascorbate is not the only antioxidant capable of improving the challenging hydroxylation of HIF-1 alpha under hypoxic conditions. Other antioxidants, particularly NAC (N-acetylcysteine), have shown similar properties (405), opening up an intriguing scientific competition in which, however, vitamin C remains in pole position. This stems from substantial evidence suggesting that vitamin C exerts antitumor mechanisms beyond the modulation of HIF-1 alpha.

The multidimensional role of vitamin C in the immune system

The immune system is a complex network of organs, tissues, cells, and proteins specialized in protecting the body from all forms of chemical, traumatic, tumor-related, or infectious disturbances. It consists of epithelial barriers as well as the cellular and humoral components of both innate (nonspecific) and adaptive (specific) immunity. These components are integrated into an extensive network of interactions that serves the essential function of identifying and eliminating a wide range of pathogens, aided by an extraordinary feature: the ability to distinguish between structures that pose no real threat and must therefore be preserved (self), and those that are genuinely harmful and must be eliminated (non-self).

In other words, the immune system acts as a sophisticated surveillance network governed by delicate, and still not fully understood, balances. Within this complex framework, there is substantial scientific evidence supporting a fundamental role for vitamin C. In the following sections, this crucial and multidimensional role will be examined from multiple perspectives (98).

The first line of immune defense is provided by the skin, which acts as a powerful barrier against all forms of external aggression. This barrier is rich in vitamin C thanks to the presence of the SVCT2 transporter, which allows the accumulation of high local concentrations. These concentrations stimulate collagen synthesis via enzymatic pathways (hydroxylation of lysine and proline (67)), and also through an independent mechanism that promotes collagen gene expression in the characteristic cells of connective tissue, fibroblasts (99). This is particularly interesting because it highlights an autonomous pathway in collagen synthesis, in which AA, unlike its role as a necessary cofactor for lysine and proline hydroxylation, acts directly at the level of gene transcription.

Equally important is the robust antioxidant protection provided by AA, which shields the skin from oxidative stress caused by pollutants or radiation. This serves as a fitting introduction to the subsequent discussion of the dermatological roles played by AA.

Let us now return to the immunological implications. It has been shown that supplementation with AA strengthens the epithelial barrier by promoting the formation of the so-called barrier lipids (100). Considering that epithelial barrier dysfunction is a common consequence of many infections, this promotion is clinically relevant. Some authors even hypothesize that maintaining a robust and efficient epithelial barrier could help counteract a broad spectrum of infectious diseases (101).

Vitamin C has several dermatological effects, playing a fundamental role that can be directly related to symptoms observed in scurvy. It plays a crucial role in wound healing, in which, in addition to modulating the expression of pro-inflammatory mediators, it stimulates the healing process by optimizing collagen synthesis (378). Interestingly, this property is particularly valuable in postoperative care, where treatment with ascorbic acid has been shown to offer multiple benefits, including improved healing of surgical wounds.

Wound healing requires the intervention of the body's main weapon of defence, namely leukocytes, cells that are the ideal vector for describing the many immune mechanisms in which vitamin C plays a crucial role. Let us start with the large subgroup that accounts for 40-70% of the total leukocytes, namely the neutrophils, cells specialised in protecting against fungal and bacterial infections. Neutrophils come into action in the initial phase of any event that produces inflammation, such as a surgical injury or the entry of a pathogen. In the early phases of an inflammation, specific signals promptly direct the neutrophils to the infected area to "disinfect" it by releasing ROS, the reactive oxygen species. In essence, the neutrophils harness the full oxidative power of ROS to "burn" the invader; among other things, this provides a demonstration of the importance of ROS, identifying their excess as the cause of oxidative stress.

Following ROS-mediated sterilisation, neutrophils undergo a process aimed at their elimination, called apoptosis or programmed cell death.

Vitamin C is involved in all phases of neutrophil activity: chemotaxis, phagocytosis, and apoptosis, as we will see in more detail shortly. This involvement is truly deep, as heuristically demonstrated by the fact that neutrophils, or leukocytes more generally, are among the favourite sites for vitamin C accumulation.

It is now essential to highlight a clear distinction: while under physiological conditions small amounts of ascorbic acid are generally sufficient to saturate leukocytes, a significant change occurs following an infectious or inflammatory insult. In such cases, leukocytes (particularly neutrophils), in addition to multiplying, increase their uptake of ascorbate by capturing circulating DHA via GLUT transporters. In other words, during infectious stress, neutrophils are ready to store vitamin C not only through the transporter that predominates under normal conditions, SVCT2, but also through the GLUT-DHA system, which is typically upregulated in response to infectious triggers. The upregulation of the GLUT-DHA pathway is due to the fact that the ROS cascade generated by infectious or inflammatory stress tends to increase DHA levels. This happens because ascorbic acid is preferentially oxidized when countering the high levels of ROS. Moreover, GLUT transporters themselves appear to be upregulated following an infectious episode (125), making the GLUT-DHA system a valuable additional source of ascorbate under infectious or inflammatory stress conditions.

The upregulation of the GLUT-DHA system is thought to occur predominantly in neutrophils and infected cells (125), and is considered crucial for neutrophil ascorbic acid concentration, as it can profoundly amplify the contribution of GLUTs. In particular, it is estimated that an infection can increase the capacity of neutrophils to absorb vitamin C by up to tenfold, from the typical concentrations of 1-2 millimoles observed under healthy conditions to a potential 10-12 millimoles during illness (67), (102), (378).

This places neutrophil function at the top of the list of examples demonstrating that the pharmacokinetics of AA is not a static entity, but rather a dynamic one, ready to adapt during transitions when health gives way to disease (remember the oft-repeated point about pharmacokinetic models being based on assumptions of full health, no stress, and no deficiencies?). But there's more: the remarkable flexibility with which neutrophils can increase their vitamin C uptake during infection stands as compelling evidence of its central role in the immune system, perhaps the most striking proof of all.

The great variability of ascorbate in neutrophils, therefore, seems to justify massive administration during an infectious disease, an eventuality in which the metabolic requirement for ascorbate tends to increase for various reasons, including the response to neutrophil demands. To summarise, during an infection, particularly of bacterial origin, two key changes occur, both of which significantly increase the body's demand for ascorbate, rendering the usual 200-400 mg required to saturate leukocytes under normal conditions insufficient: first, an increase in the number of neutrophils (a typical immune response to infection); and second, an enhanced capacity of these neutrophils to accumulate and store ascorbate (70).

Why do neutrophils increase their ability to store vitamin C so much?

The most widely accepted hypothesis holds that the high concentrations of AA in neutrophils enhance antioxidant protection during the critical phase in which neutrophils release reactive oxygen species to attack pathogens (67). This release, in fact, represents a double-edged sword: on one hand, it creates a powerful oxidative burst aimed at destroying the invader; on the other, it requires the body to defend bystander components that could be unintentionally damaged during the oxidative storm.

An alternative explanation suggests that the increase in AA concentration within neutrophils primarily serves to enhance ROS generation, thereby enabling a more aggressive attack against pathogens (67). These two hypotheses are not necessarily mutually exclusive: it is plausible that AA first supports ROS production during the initial antimicrobial assault, and later shifts to a protective antioxidant role to limit collateral damage to host tissues.

There is no doubt, however, about the mechanisms that support the regeneration of vitamin E, a fundamental process mediated by vitamin C. Clear evidence indicates that this process provides significant indirect antioxidant protection, particularly for the plasma membranes of neutrophils, which are well protected by vitamin E (378).

How do neutrophils act?

The infiltration of neutrophils into infected tissue occurs in response to specific signals emitted by the pathogen. These signals rapidly mobilize neutrophils toward the site of inflammation, creating a rapid and coordinated migration. This process is known as neutrophil chemotaxis and is extremely important, because it represents one of the earliest responses of the innate immune system. Innate immunity, also referred to as non-specific immunity, is the type of immunity present from birth and does not need to be acquired through exposure to pathogens.

Interestingly, several studies conducted on guinea pigs with scurvy have shown a markedly impaired chemotactic response compared to those properly supplemented with vitamin C (378), suggesting that vitamin C deficiency can have a substantial immunological impact on chemotaxis (103). Over time, multiple studies have confirmed this relationship, identifying immunosuppressive mediators and vitamin C depletion as two key factors contributing to impaired chemotaxis. Furthermore, they have shown that appropriate vitamin C supplementation can restore normal chemotactic function (104), (105).

Let us pause for a moment: we have just observed the typical pattern of vitamin C's behaviour. While its deficiency can disrupt various processes (such as chemotaxis in this case), its repletion can restore those functions that were dysregulated by the deficiency. This is a relevant principle whose meaning is clear: inadequate AA levels generally lead to reversible damage, provided the deficiency is properly recognized and treated.

So far, a lot of theory and not much practice. We'll try to remedy that by presenting some interesting studies.

Let us start with a study published in 1990 in the "Journal of Perinatology" (106) and focusing on 20 infants, 10 healthy and 10 with a suspected diagnosis of sepsis. This study, which aimed to analyse the effect of oral AA supplementation on neutrophil chemotaxis, is significant both for the good results obtained and for the treatment protocol chosen, a real gem in the ascorbic literature. In fact, the researchers opted for a total dosage of 400 mg, divided into 4 intakes, equivalent to a body-weight adjusted dose of about 8 g for an adult. This is a well-conceived scheme in pharmacokinetic terms, close to Klenner's ideology and far removed from the principles of modern clinical research on oral vitamin C. Chemotaxis significantly improved following vitamin C therapy, indicating the strong impact vitamin C may have on chemotaxis in diseased conditions. "The significant improvement in chemotaxis and random migration may justify the inclusion of vitamin C as an adjunct to the therapy of neonatal sepsis", the authors jointly wrote (106).

We now present an example involving a rare genetic disorder known as chronic granulomatous disease, an immunodeficiency characterized by defective leukocyte function resulting in impaired production of reactive oxygen species. This defect predisposes individuals to recurrent bacterial infections. Interestingly, ascorbate therapy appears to confer clinical benefits in this context, potentially reducing both the incidence of infections and enhancing the host response during the acute phase. In essence, both prevention and therapy. Particularly noteworthy is the case of three brothers affected by chronic granulomatous disease (107). When oral vitamin C supplementation (1 g per day for two years) was added to their antibiotic prophylaxis regimen, the results were remarkable: the children experienced no infectious episodes throughout the treatment period, an outcome not previously achieved with antibiotic prophylaxis alone (107).

The potential benefit that adequate vitamin C supplementation might offer to chemotaxis is a widely described topic in the literature, where one also finds the intriguing hypothesis that the antihistamine function of vitamin C is related to the efficiency of neutrophil chemotaxis. This was supported by a clinical investigation (359), which reported a surprising inverse association between plasma histamine levels and neutrophil chemotaxis, thereby proposing that vitamin C may improve chemotaxis via its established ability to lower circulating histamine concentrations: "Vitamin C may indirectly enhance chemotaxis by detoxifying histamine in vivo" (359).

Once they reach the site of infection through the process of chemotaxis, neutrophils carry out phagocytosis, an essential mechanism by which they engulf and neutralize pathogens. This process is characteristic of a broad class of cells known as phagocytes, with neutrophils representing the primary component. Phagocytosis occurs in two stages: first, the cell engulfs the foreign material, then it destroys it through the action of reactive oxygen species. Simply put, phagocytes, including neutrophils, "eat" the invaders and then destroy them using oxidants. Numerous studies have highlighted the crucial role of vitamin C in this process: inadequate levels of ascorbic acid have been associated with reduced phagocytic efficiency, similarly to what has been observed in chemotaxis (108).

Interestingly, some studies (108) have shown very promising results in patients with recurrent infections or primary defects in neutrophil function. In these individuals, vitamin C supplementation has often enhanced neutrophil activity, providing significant antibacterial benefits. Based on the collected data, some authors have put forward the intriguing hypothesis that ascorbic acid may represent a specific therapy for primary phagocytic function defects in patients with recurrent infections (108).

Following phagocytosis, the defensive task of neutrophils comes to an end, and they may then undergo a process of programmed cell death known as apoptosis. This is a physiological and regulated form of cell death, necessary to ensure proper cellular turnover. However, as we know, biological programs do not always proceed as expected. Several studies have shown that neutrophil apoptosis is inhibited in patients with severe infections (109), highlighting the negative impact that serious infectious states can have on this process. Severe infections, therefore, have the potential to disrupt the body's natural regulatory programs. Notably, the suppression of apoptosis appears to be directly correlated with the severity of the infection. In septic patients, for instance, one of the main drivers of tissue damage is believed to be the attenuation of apoptosis, which is generally attributed to the action of pro-inflammatory cytokines (378).

This leads us to an important presentation. Pro-inflammatory cytokines are signaling molecules released by the immune system in response to a stimulus, and their primary role is to promote the activation and proliferation of cells involved in the inflammatory response. The influence of pro-inflammatory cytokines on neutrophil apoptosis has been the subject of increasingly detailed studies, which have led to a key finding: particularly, but not exclusively, in the context of sepsis, the prolonged survival of neutrophils is largely attributed to the persistent stimulation exerted by pro-inflammatory cytokines (378).

Introducing the concept of cytokines allows us to highlight a facet of vitamin C's multifaceted biological profile that deserves to be explored: its immunomodulatory action, namely its ability to restore balance in a dysregulated immune response. Take cancer as an example: some clinical studies have suggested that high-dose intravenous vitamin C may modulate cytokine levels by reducing the expression of pro-inflammatory cytokines (110). This finding is significant, as it indicates that adequate concentrations of vitamin C could help mitigate the chronic inflammatory state associated with cancer, thereby revealing a potentially beneficial antitumor property of the compound.

However, cancer is not the only condition in which vitamin C may regulate immune dysregulation. Clinical data also suggest that its action can attenuate the overexpression of pro-inflammatory cytokines in various inflammatory disorders. Rheumatoid arthritis, a chronic inflammatory disorder of autoimmune origin that primarily affects the joints, is an important example in which high-dose intravenous vitamin C has been shown to reduce levels of pro-inflammatory cytokines and, consequently, the overall inflammatory burden. The results of a small clinical study published in the journal "Modern Research in Inflammation" (389) are very interesting: in this study, the intravenous administration of 7.5-50 g reduced the values of the main biomarker of the inflammatory state (C-reactive protein or CRP) in rheumatoid arthritis patients by 44%. "Based on our pilot study, we hypothesise that high-dose intravenous vitamin C therapy may be a useful strategy in the treatment of rheumatoid arthritis" (389).

The mechanisms by which vitamin C can stem the avalanche of proinflammatory cytokines that hits the body during inflammation are still partly unknown. One of the known aspects concerns the negative influence that ROS can exert on a central element in the regulation of the immune response, the transcription factor NF-kB (457). The nuclear factor kappa-light-chain-enhancer of activated B-cells, or more simply NF-kB, is a crucial transcription factor for the organism. This factor acts as a switch of inflammation, so much so that its activation is believed to considerably promote the gene transcription of several proinflammatory cytokines (378), (389). Considering that oxidative stress is believed to be one of the main activators of NF-kB, it should come as no surprise that vitamin C is considered one of the strongest inhibitors of NF-kB (457), (378).

Let's return to the neutrophils, cells in which the immunomodulatory role of AA appears particularly important: by limiting proinflammatory cytokines, AA can ensure, or possibly restore, the regular apoptosis of neutrophils, thus avoiding the deleterious complications that altered apoptosis could cause. What are these complications?

Neutrophils that fail to undergo apoptosis initiate a delicate "emergency manoeuvre" characterized by inherently unstable mechanisms. This alternative pathway, known as necrotic cell death or necrosis, leads to the release of specific intracellular components, among which neutrophil extracellular traps (NETs) are predominant. NETs are biologically beneficial only when maintained within a precise physiological balance, which depends on their tightly regulated and limited expression. It is well documented that excessive NET formation can result in tissue damage and significant disruptions of the coagulation system. More importantly, and of particular clinical relevance, NET overproduction has been implicated in the development of multiple organ dysfunction syndrome, a very serious systemic condition characterized by the sudden and simultaneous impairment of multiple organ systems (111).

Therefore, necrotic cell death is an alternative pathway that is often harmful. This only strengthens the position of vitamin C, whose adequate levels could also modulate such a crucial process as neutrophil apoptosis.

The topic of neutrophils also reveals an interesting connection with HIFs, further evidence of the extensive role of vitamin C in immune functions. Here, it is necessary to introduce a result in which it was shown that HIF-1 alpha can facilitate the survival of neutrophils in hypoxic areas, which clearly indicates that overexpression of HIF-1 alpha can delay neutrophil apoptosis (112). Several studies have confirmed this finding: in GULO knockout mice (mice with genetically modified GULO, thus tending to be deficient in vitamin C), for example, a strong overexpression of HIF-1 alpha was observed, with consequent attenuation of neutrophil apoptosis (378). Put simply, high levels of HIF-1 alpha induce neutrophils to remain at the infectious site even during the resolution phase of inflammation, when they should instead migrate elsewhere (112).

What has just been described is not merely a reaffirmation. Infectious or inflammatory states are not the only conditions capable of altering neutrophil apoptosis; this process can also be disrupted by any vitamin C deficiency, regardless of the underlying cause. Based on these data, some scientists have proposed HIF-1 alpha as an efficient modulator of neutrophil-dependent NET generation (113), proposing the hypothesis that AA may act upstream, downregulating NET generation through the degradation of HIF-1 alpha (114); such activity is crucial because it could avert the potentially serious effects associated with excess NETs, including multiple organ dysfunction syndrome.

Overall, vitamin C may provide two key contributions to ensuring or restoring proper neutrophil apoptosis: the reduction of pro-inflammatory cytokines and the downregulation of HIF-1 alpha expression.

In summary, neutrophil chemotaxis, phagocytosis and apoptosis are immune processes that depend on a constant and adequate supply of vitamin C.

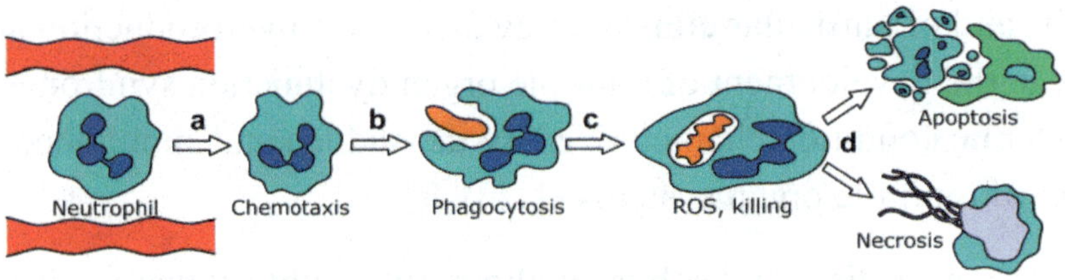

graph adapted from (378)

Shifting our focus from neutrophils to lymphocytes, we encounter a class of white blood cells involved in what is known as adaptive, or specific, immunity. This term refers to the immune system's ability to learn, adapt and remember. This is a capacity acquired over time as it encounters external pathogens.

In addition to antioxidant protection, various lines of evidence suggest that vitamin C can promote lymphocyte proliferation and enhance the generation of antibodies, i.e. proteins produced by B-lymphocytes to neutralize pathogens (115).

More broadly, AA contributes to lymphocyte biology in several ways. For instance, studies conducted in healthy individuals, asthma patients, and elderly subjects (378) have shown that AA can positively influence lymphocyte populations, particularly T cells and natural killer (NK) cells, by promoting their differentiation, development and maturation (116).

The descriptions on lymphocytes tie in perfectly with the immunomodulating capacity of ascorbic acid. Notably, a study in genetically modified GULO-deficient mice found that a parenteral administration of 200 mg/kg modulated the immunosuppression of T-regulatory cells (TREGs) during sepsis (117). In this model, vitamin C not only optimized TREGs' proliferation but also reduced the production of pro-inflammatory cytokines.

At this point, it is necessary to pause briefly and provide some clarifications. We begin with a technical limitation inherent to animal experiments, an essential step before moving to clinical trials. The therapeutic impact of vitamin C in animals that maintain its biosynthesis can be difficult to interpret. Any equivalence in outcomes between treated and control groups may mask the true effects of the intervention, precisely because these animals synthesize their own vitamin C. Furthermore, basic principles of pharmacokinetics remind us that its administration in such models may be ineffective, especially at low doses, and could even paradoxically produce opposing effects (69), (363). These concerns justify the widespread use of animals deprived of biosynthesis. By artificially inducing vitamin C deficiency, this strategy mimics human physiology (which lacks endogenous vitamin C synthesis) and therefore provides a unique opportunity to unequivocally evaluate the pharmacological efficacy of vitamin C.

Another concept worth clarifying relates to an area where vitamin C appears to have a natural affinity with potentially profound implications, already hinted at in the previously cited study (117): the promotion of regulatory T cells (TREGs), both in terms of their development and their functional modulation (378). But what exactly are TREGs?

Regulatory T cells (TREGs) are a critical subset of T-lymphocytes with a sophisticated immunosuppressive function, capable of "shutting down" the immune response when appropriate. They are essential for maintaining immune balance, also known as immune homeostasis. TREGs play a central role in suppressing excessive immune reactions, such as those seen in conditions like sepsis.

The importance of TREGs is highlighted by multiple observations: their deficiency is associated with the development of various autoimmune diseases, allergic responses, and even transplant rejection (118). Mechanistically, the link between TREG function and ascorbic acid is mediated by its capacity to enhance and stabilize the expression of Foxp3, the transcription factor regarded as the master regulator and defining marker of TREG identity and function (568).

In this context, an illuminating study published in the journal "International Immunology" in 2017 (118) proposed a compelling hypothesis: vitamin C could serve as a potential immunotherapeutic agent for certain diseases, including autoimmune disorders and graft-versus-host disease (GVHD), a condition in which immune cells from transplanted tissue attack the recipient's body as if it were foreign.

What has been described so far enriches the immunomodulatory profile of vitamin C: beyond modulating cytokine synthesis, vitamin C may support immune equilibrium by promoting the function of the cells responsible for regulating it, namely TREGs.

We now arrive at a crucial point. Unlike cytokine modulation, which primarily depends on the antioxidant properties of AA, the involvement with TREGs appears to be regulated by different mechanisms. Indeed, the pathways through which AA supports TREG development and function are linked to its enzymatic cofactor properties and belong to a completely different domain: epigenetics (378). An increasing body of evidence, in fact, attributes key epigenetic functions to vitamin C. But what does this actually mean?

Without going into unnecessary technical detail, we should point out that AA acts as a cofactor for a large group of dioxygenase enzymes. Among these is a specialized class known as TETs, a family of ten-eleven translocation methylcytosine dioxygenases (119). Although the discovery of TET enzymes is relatively recent, they are gaining increasing importance in the field of epigenetics, challenging several long-standing assumptions. TET enzymes are involved in a process known as DNA demethylation, a specific type of epigenetic modification that removes methyl groups from DNA. A methyl group is one of the most common structural units found in organic compounds within the body.

While DNA demethylation removes these groups and can reactivate certain genes, allowing them to be expressed again, DNA methylation does the opposite: it adds methyl groups at specific sites on the DNA, preventing the expression of certain genes, effectively "silencing" them. These two opposing mechanisms, methylation and demethylation, do not change the DNA sequence itself, but rather influence how the cell uses the genetic information encoded in the DNA (119).

Although DNA methylation might sound harmful, it's actually a beneficial process when properly regulated. Contrary to older views that saw methylation as static and permanent, we now know it is dynamic and reversible. This flexibility is essential because it allows demethylation to correct excessive or abnormal methylation triggered by various stressors, such as environmental insults, a phenomenon increasingly referred to as hypermethylation. By reactivating genes that have been mistakenly silenced, DNA demethylation can help counteract the negative effects of hypermethylation, which include accelerated aging and, more importantly, the onset and progression of various diseases (119).

In this way, DNA demethylation acts as a modulator of DNA methylation, a capacity that not only supports overall health but may also help correct dysfunctions. There is growing evidence supporting this idea: multiple studies have shown that DNA demethylation plays a key role in both physiological transitions (such as embryogenesis, gametogenesis, learning, and pain perception) and in pathophysiological conditions, including cancer, making it a process with significant therapeutic potential.

Therefore, the discovery that TETs require AA as a cofactor has opened up extraordinary horizons: AA, as a cofactor of TET enzymes, actively participates in DNA demethylation. This allows it to modify gene expression without altering the DNA sequence (the definition of epigenetics), which can ensure optimal adaptation to environmental conditions. In essence, AA appears to possess the characteristics of an efficient mediator at the genome-environment interface. In fact, according to some scientists, it is considered a key mediator, a quality that could open exceptional perspectives. "Ascorbate is a key mediator of the interface between the genome and environment", Young, Zuchner and Wang state in the "Annual Review of Nutrition" (119).

It is therefore no exaggeration to say that vitamin C can offer epigenetics a kind of liberation, enabling the "sentence" imposed by genetics to be reconsidered. In short: while we cannot alter our genes, we can influence their expression by harnessing one of vitamin C's many remarkable properties.

From scurvy to epigenetics, a colossal leap that should prompt reflection among those who still consider vitamin C solely as a nutrient. This conceptual leap challenges the notion of genetic determinism, underscoring that our destiny is not entirely inscribed in our DNA. As Jung observed: "Until you make the unconscious conscious, it will direct your life and you will call it fate". Mathematics, psychoanalysis, physics, chemistry, and medicine appear deeply intertwined, echoing certain quantum theories that envision the universe as a hologram, in which each part contains the whole.

Let us return to the immune system with some studies that revealed a further epigenetic pathway in which the AA-TETs pair seems to be able to enhance the maturation of the entire subpopulation of T cells (116), (120). What are T cells?

T cells, or T-lymphocytes, constitute the subpopulation of lymphocytes that play a central role in so-called cell-mediated immunity, a type of immune response primarily aimed at eliminating microbes that survive phagocytosis. Their involvement with AA has become increasingly broader and more evident in recent years, thus demonstrating that AA's influence on TREGs is only one specific aspect (455). A significant example concerns the subgroup of T cells called gamma-delta T cells, cells that can be significantly enhanced by vitamin C. This paves the way for a promising research project: building a bridge that connects the qualities of AA with the therapeutic intelligence of immunotherapy in order to control the vast ocean called cancer (455).

On the basis of so much evidence, the immunomodulatory role of ascorbic acid appears increasingly important and not exclusively related to antioxidant properties.

One note: the AA-TETs-DNA demethylation triangle will later be reinterpreted in a new space, where it seems to be able to calm the vast ocean mentioned above.

It is now useful to elaborate on the relationship between ascorbate and cytokines. As already mentioned, cytokines represent an important group of molecules with a cell signalling function, usually secreted in response to inflammatory or infectious stimuli. They are able to modulate cellular responses and can express both pro-inflammatory and anti-inflammatory activities; the cytokines with the greatest biological value include the chemokine, interleukin, interferon, and TNF alpha families.

A necessary reminder: there are many studies suggesting that AA can modulate cytokine production by decreasing the synthesis of proinflammatory cytokines (we have already documented a study on inflammation caused by cancer (110) and a study on rheumatoid arthritis (389)) and also by increasing the production of anti-inflammatory cytokines. This evidence is varied and some of it reflects findings that differ from the studies on cancer and rheumatoid arthritis, where efficacy is associated with high-dose intravenous administrations. We will shortly note the independent role, probably less strong than that of intravenous vitamin C, of oral vitamin C as an anti-inflammatory agent.

An interesting study (121) examined the effects of ascorbate on 29 athletes who participated in an intense source of oxidative stress and inflammation such as a 90 km marathon. This study, aimed at testing immunomodulating abilities in a borderline context, divided the athletes into three supplementation groups: 0-500-1500 mg, doses that were administered orally for 10 consecutive days starting 7 days before the marathon. The measurement of plasma concentrations of the main cytokines indicated that only the 1500 mg supplementation was able to significantly attenuate the increase in proinflammatory cytokines resulting from great physical exertion; in addition to cytokines, the "1500 mg group" was the only one in which a reduction in cortisol levels was noted, which once again confirms the effectiveness of adequate AA administration in modulating cortisol under stressful conditions.

But there is one further noteworthy finding: no significant differences were observed between the two weak groups, i.e. the "0 mg group" (the control group), and the "500 mg group".

Overall, this study highlighted AA's ability to reduce proinflammatory cytokine synthesis even through the secondary route of oral supplementation, provided it is used at sufficiently adequate dosages.

It is time for some questions. The first: what would have emerged if the researchers had used only two supplementation groups (0 mg, 500 mg)?

Furthermore, what would have emerged with four supplementation groups (0 mg, 500 mg, 1500 mg, 3 g every 4 hours)?

Let us now proceed by modifying the basic conditions. Although there is no substantial uniformity, even during disease states oral vitamin C supplementation has often demonstrated the ability to reduce proinflammatory cytokines and key inflammatory biomarkers, reaffirming an anti-inflammatory identity in many clinical scenarios. This is the case with diabetes, hypertension and the so-called Barrett's esophagus, a precancerous condition affecting the esophagus. These three diseases have been the subject of a number of studies in which oral ascorbic therapy produced anti-inflammatory benefits expressed through a reduction in proinflammatory cytokines and key biomarkers of inflammation (459), (460). What Babar and co-workers stated in (459) is pioneering. These researchers were among the first to clinically analyse the downregulation of NF-kB exerted by AA, a finding that until then had only been verified in laboratories (the study dates back to 2010). The results in humans appeared consistent: vitamin C inhibited NF-kB in a significant percentage of patients (459).

We conclude with a systematic review and meta-analysis of randomized clinical trials (122) focused on a biologically crucial cytokine: IL-6, or interleukin-6. This cytokine is a multifunctional protein with significant roles in both pro-inflammatory and anti-inflammatory processes. Under normal physiological conditions, IL-6 is essential for various cellular functions. However, during infection, trauma, or intense physical exertion, IL-6 becomes equally important by rapidly stimulating the immune response. Secreted primarily by T-lymphocytes, it is one of the main mediators of the so-called acute-phase response, a complex mechanism aimed at eliminating the cause of tissue damage while simultaneously initiating tissue repair (569).

The fact that many chronic diseases, including diabetes, rheumatoid arthritis, inflammatory bowel disease and cancer, are associated with elevated IL-6 levels has prompted scientists to develop IL-6 antagonists. Could vitamin C be one of these agents?

The analysis of the 24 articles included in the meta-analysis provides encouraging results: despite the low doses administered in clinical trials, vitamin C has been shown to effectively reduce IL-6 levels (122).

Overall, although it is plausible that the reduction of proinflammatory cytokines is plasma concentration-dependent (as Mikirova, Riordan and Casciari suggest: "The effects of ascorbate on inflammatory cytokines are concentration-dependent" (110)), the above illustrations show that vitamin C is often effective, even when forced to travel on secondary roads or at very low speeds.

The topic of cytokines now allows us to introduce a function that made Klenner famous in the long history of vitamin C. Its immunomodulatory properties, in fact, seem to be deeply intertwined with its antiviral properties. It would not have been wrong to write a whole chapter on the antiviral properties of vitamin C, a preliminary insight of which has already been given with paediatric viral myocarditis (41). Especially the figure of the immense Klenner, author of a scientific feat during the polio epidemic, would have deserved it. However, the role of vitamin C in physiology is so extensive that it is necessary to optimise descriptive space.

Many studies have helped clarify the role of ascorbic acid against viral infections. One interesting study (378) concerns an experiment on genetically modified GULO mice infected with the influenza virus. The data showed that these mice had an increase in proinflammatory cytokines (TNF alpha and some interleukins) in the lungs and also a decrease in antiviral cytokines alpha and beta (i.e. interferons: IFN alpha and IFN beta), which suggests that the combination of AA deficiency and influenza may be doubly negative.

Another study (378) on septic mice with genetically modified GULO showed that parenteral administration of 200 mg/kg considerably stimulated the synthesis of the two main types of interferons, IFN alpha and IFN beta. What are interferons?

Interferons constitute a versatile and powerful family of cytokines, produced by white blood cells and tissue cells in response to the presence of viral or tumour agents. They possess strong antiviral and potentially even anticancer properties. It would therefore not be surprising if there were a correlation between the antiviral properties of vitamin C and interferon synthesis.

The antiviral action of vitamin C was analysed in detail in an interesting study that confirmed the theoretical assumptions outlined above (123). In this study, mice were genetically deprived of biosynthesis and subjected to intranasal inoculation of the influenza virus. The mice were grouped into two categories: the first consisted of mice without supplementation, the second category of mice subjected to constant AA supplementation. The first observation concerned the death of mice not treated with supplements, which occurred within a week of viral inoculation. The mice that had received AA, on the other hand, survived. In addition, the "rescue" administration, carried out the day after inoculation to some of the deficient mice, was ineffective in saving most of them, probably due to insufficient dosage or delayed therapy. These results suggest that a therapeutic response requires adequate dosages, without neglecting the time element: indeed, it is likely that the damage produced by influenza virus replication can be neutralised as long as the concentration of vitamin C is sufficiently high in the early phase of viral infection. I repeat, a high concentration in the early phase of viral infection.

This is an appropriate moment to support orthomolecular ideology, because the empirical approaches of the great vitamin C pioneers, such as Pauling and Cathcart, are increasingly supported by scientific evidence. Remember that Pauling and Cathcart recommended massive and frequent intakes of vitamin C from the first signs of infection. The data from the aforementioned study (123), therefore, seem to justify many of the failures of vitamin C in the treatment of the common cold, because inadequate therapy (i.e. not immediate or massive) may have been insufficient, thus obscuring the antiviral potential of vitamin C.

Let's return to the study mentioned above (123). Measurement of the levels of IFN alpha, IFN beta and other cytokines in the bronchoalveolar fluid and plasma of mice after intranasal inoculation was crucial because it identified a twofold difference: in vitamin C-deficient mice there was a decrease in the concentration of interferons (both in plasma and lungs) and an increase in proinflammatory cytokines. This indicates that vitamin C deficiency subverted the physiological expression of cytokines during viral infection, considerably altering the balance between proinflammatory and antiviral cytokines.

Overall, what has been examined is very important because it shows that vitamin C is an essential factor in the production of an adequate antiviral immune response during the initial phase of a viral infection. This factor acts by stimulating the synthesis of molecules with antiviral propensity, i.e. interferons, and also by modulating the inflammatory response through the reduction of proinflammatory cytokines.

It is now time to formulate a personal hypothesis. It is conceivable that the dosage required to achieve a strong antiviral response depends on the timing of the therapy, as it is reasonable to assume that a delayed intervention may require higher doses to compensate for the harmful effects of late treatment. Indeed, it is plausible that delayed ascorbic therapy could amplify the depletion of vitamin C in proportion to the time elapsed between the onset of damage and the start of treatment. This dynamic, in addition to being consistent with orthomolecular ideology, will be revisited later in different and clinically much more challenging contexts than influenza.

We conclude this aside by emphasising the great importance of the time factor, which can be responsible for incorrect clinical interpretations: any delayed therapy may require very high doses, which, however, have rarely been used in clinical studies on oral vitamin C.

Let us return to the literature, which contains further evidence on the antiviral properties of AA. A study published in the journal "Expert Review of Anti-infective Therapy" (124), for instance, found that pretreatment of human foreskin and endothelial cells, carried out prior to cytomegalovirus infection, significantly reduced viral antigen expression and cellular viral load. Interestingly, this result was not obtained when AA was administered exclusively after viral contamination. This difference could be explained by the fact that AA is more of an immunomodulator than a direct antiviral agent (as the authors claim), without however neglecting the alternative hypothesis: the dosage used after viral contamination was inadequate.

In another study (124), mice subjected to confinement stress and suffering from H1N1 virus-induced pneumonia showed a dose-dependent reduction in mortality following ascorbic treatment. This discovery has been attributed to improved mitochondrial function and strong immunomodulatory properties of AA.

Interestingly, the antiviral properties of vitamin C have been described in the literature for over 70 years. Poliovirus, encephalitis, HIV, parvovirus and the rabies virus are viruses that have appeared sensitive to vitamin C in many studies

(124), (378), something that was extraordinarily intuited by the brilliant Klenner in the 1940s.

We're not done with viruses yet. A double-blind study (124) involving 41 patients with herpes zoster evaluated the efficacy of a moderate dose of intravenous ascorbic acid (50 mg/kg administered on alternate days, specifically on days 1, 3 and 5) in reducing herpetic pain and postherpetic neuralgia, two debilitating complications of the disease. The results were noteworthy, despite what could be considered a "suboptimal" administration schedule in light of the pharmacokinetics of vitamin C, as its short half-life may not align well with alternate-day dosing. Furthermore, the mechanisms underlying the observed effects remain unclear. Although patients treated with ascorbic acid experienced a significant reduction in pain scores, it is still uncertain whether this outcome is due to direct analgesic effects, immunomodulatory activity, or antiviral properties of the compound.

Still on the topic of herpes zoster, some authors (124) attempted to quantify the depletion of ascorbic acid caused by this infection and reported alarming findings: compared to healthy volunteers, patients with herpes zoster showed plasma concentrations that were three times lower. This is a significant observation, particularly when considered alongside the consequences of a "neglected rescue". Put simply: since the early phase of a viral infection tends to deplete vitamin C levels, and low levels of vitamin C impair the antiviral response, it becomes evident that high-dose ascorbic acid supplementation is necessary to achieve clinically meaningful outcomes. We will explore this further in light of additional insights shortly.

All this reinforces the logic of the criticism of the scientific research on ascorbic acid, in this case aimed at the days 1-3-5 schedule used in the previous study. I believe that a more rational approach would have given vitamin C the support it needs to unleash its full therapeutic potential. For example, imitating the schemes used experimentally in intensive care units, where moderate intravenous doses (50 mg/kg) are usually administered every 6 hours to ensure that plasma concentrations are in a steady state, essential for maintaining proper vitamin C physiology. And I stress physiology, not pharmacology.

At this point, it is necessary to focus on another key observation. The so-called incubation period of a viral agent, that is, the interval between its entry into the body and the appearance of the first symptoms, is generally long for most viruses, in some cases lasting more than a week. What does this imply?

If we combine this factor with two well-established facts, a critical picture emerges: an effective antiviral response requires adequate levels of ascorbate; viruses begin depleting AA from the very first moments of their establishment in the host. Taken together, these data suggest a personal hypothesis: the body's initial vitamin C reserves may serve only as a temporary buffer, since they are rapidly exhausted during viral establishment. Therefore, an effective antiviral response likely requires not only sufficient baseline levels, but also continuous replenishment to counteract acute ascorbate depletion and sustain therapeutic concentrations throughout the early and critical stages of infection. Such supportive action appears essential to halt the infection at its onset, yet it is rarely feasible within the narrow time window necessary for ascorbate therapy to be truly effective. The reason lies in the ambiguity of the incubation period, which can mask the earliest stages of viral establishment (sometimes for several days), allowing the infection to progress unchecked.

As a result, it is nearly impossible to determine the precise optimal moment for intervention, since the perception of the first signs of illness (symptoms) generally occurs too late to enable an effective therapeutic strategy. In short, the situation becomes highly complex. This is precisely where the power of dynamic flow could come into play, that is, the continuous and massive supply of ascorbate that enabled Klenner to win many battles against the most formidable viruses.

One note: this personal working hypothesis, which can be called "Antiviral Flow Conjecture" or "Partipilo's Conjecture", appears consistent with the dynamics observed in previous studies (123), (124).

We return to the clinical evidence to illustrate a pioneering retrospective study (479) from 2018 (retrospective means a study based on data collected in the past, comparing it with the results obtained from the current trial). The results of that study are among the first to propose oral vitamin C therapy as a valid prophylaxis for recurrences of an insidious infection called herpes simplex keratitis, an infection that affects the cornea and is caused by the herpes simplex virus. "To our knowledge, this is the first study to show that oral ascorbic acid treatment may prevent herpes simplex keratitis recurrence" (479).

A general overview reveals that low ascorbic acid levels weaken antiviral immune responses, highlighting the need to rapidly restore plasma concentrations to physiological levels in order to effectively counter viral progression.

But what would happen if supraphysiological concentrations were considered by administering vitamin C intravenously?

One answer comes from a study on patients with Epstein-Barr virus (EBV), conducted by the well-known Riordan Clinic. This study analysed the impact of high-dose intravenous administrations (7.5 to 50 g) over the period 1997-2006 (125). Not surprisingly, high-dose intravenous vitamin C therapy favourably influenced both disease duration and EBV-specific antibody titers. Furthermore, it was found that patients with high AA concentrations had low antigen levels during the acute phase of infection, a finding that suggests an inverse correlation between plasma ascorbate and antigen burden in this stage of the disease.

According to scientists at the Riordan Clinic, the antiviral efficacy of vitamin C at supraphysiological concentrations can be attributed to the overexpression of GLUTs triggered by infection, an overexpression capable of promoting the entry of DHA into infected cells. This hypothesis, therefore, proposes a mechanism of action other than the stimulation of interferon synthesis. The conceptual clouds could clear thanks to an appropriate distinction: while physiological concentrations stimulate interferons, supraphysiological ones seem to promote an oxidant attack mediated by DHA. This attack is greatly facilitated by the overexpression of GLUTs, whose selectivity would also guarantee the absence of toxicity.

One note: what has just been described is a similar dynamic to what is considered to be the most powerful anticancer dynamic, in which the main actor is hydrogen peroxide, excellently supported by the pharmacological vitamin C in very high doses.

Overall, the Riordan Clinic's promising results seem to be due to the use of very high dosages, which are unfortunately seldom explored in conventional trials.

Thus, we return to the problem of dosages, the fear of dosages. This conservative approach may be unjustified, given the well-established safety profile of vitamin C. What rationale has prompted scientists to generally use low dosages?

It is not easy to provide a clear answer, because vitamin C is not subject to the typical requirements of conventional drugs, for which even slightly more intensive use could dangerously compromise the risk-benefit ratio. Let's take oral dynamic flow as a model, an approach that has never been used in non-orthomolecular scientific research. It is reasonable to assume that its use would have produced better results compared to commonly used supplementation doses (500-1000 mg per day). Even in studies exploring intravenous administration, the pattern is similar: aside from cancer therapy, the use of low doses (1-10 g) is the norm. What might have emerged with higher dosages?

The highly dose-dependent nature of AA, especially with regard to intravenous administrations, whose pharmacokinetics are vertical rather than sigmoidal, suggests the reality of therapeutic improvements.

In addition to the low dosages, many clinical studies are characterised by a deficit that can compromise interpretations: the absence of plasma concentration measurement. This is a fundamental point. Suppose we have a patient with a severe viral infection, for whom intravenous ascorbic therapy is used at a total dose of 1 g per day, wisely divided into 4 solutions of 250 mg. At the end of the therapy, however, there is no obvious improvement. This is a disappointment for the antiviral capabilities of AA, which may, however, have been misrepresented by the fact that the clinicians may have overlooked the importance of monitoring plasma ascorbate levels. It is plausible, in fact, that this therapy (1 g per day), having been set in a clinical context in which physiological reconstitution of ascorbate concentrations (clearly depleted by the infection) usually requires at least 3 g intravenously (34), did not sufficiently increase circulating levels, thus keeping the patient ascorbate-deficient. Add to this the fact that an ascorbate deficiency can significantly weaken antiviral responses, and the picture becomes clear: monitoring plasma concentrations would have provided a more analytical picture of the situation, allowing, for example, verification of recovery from the underlying deficiency. In short, it would have been a crucial confirmation, since it is indisputable that the ascorbic acid therapeutic response requires that its deficiency be remedied.

Without plasma measurements of ascorbate, considerable confusion may arise, an unacceptable condition in scientific discourse. The use of low dosages may involve significant risks, especially in the absence of plasma monitoring, as it can lead to distorted and misleading representations that underestimate the therapeutic impact of vitamin C.

In other words, the application of inadequate dosages and timing may obscure the pharmacological potential of vitamin C, leading to interpretations that do not reflect reality and giving rise to irrational scientific conclusions (let us recall Jungeblut, Sabin, and the case of poliomyelitis). This provides sufficiently strong reasons to identify dynamic flow as the gold standard for oral administration, the only experimental approach based on achieving the molecule's maximum oral expression (i.e., the highest possible orally administered dose). It is not difficult to see how this method could be decisive. In fact, if such a therapeutic strategy were to yield no clinical benefit in managing a given disease X, one could legitimately state: "Oral vitamin C is not effective in treating disease X". And I emphasize: oral vitamin C, not vitamin C in absolute terms!

Conversely, the clinical use of 500-1000 mg cannot provide any definitive verdict, and should therefore not be used, as has sometimes happened, to draw definitive conclusions that have, in some cases, evolved into even more entrenched beliefs.

Definitive, and I emphasize this for the third time, is an adjective that only mathematicians can use with true certainty, because all other sciences, including medicine, are inherently characterized by a degree of uncertainty. In mathematics, on the other hand, we can be completely certain about statements: the famous Pythagorean theorem, whose origins likely trace back to the Babylonians but which has, in essence, always existed (and here we could go on...), will never be disproven in the future. At most, and this is fundamentally what mathematicians do, it can be embedded within a broader theoretical framework. And indeed, this has already happened: consider its extension to much more general spaces than the traditional geometric plane we are familiar with, the so-called Hilbert spaces, immensely abstract spaces in which the Pythagorean theorem continues, quite astonishingly, to hold true.

Putting aside considerations on the quality of the studies, we can conclude that physiological levels of ascorbic acid may counter viral infections by exerting immunomodulatory effects, particularly through the stimulation of interferon synthesis.

What about antimicrobial properties in general?

This question will be addressed only after illustrating one last crucial role in the immune system, which is closely linked to interferons. Specifically, this involves natural killer (NK) cells, a type of lymphocyte with potent antiviral activity. These cells act in tight coordination with cytokines, both during the activation phase, when cytokines signal the presence of viral infection and activate NK cells, and during the so called effector phase, in which NK cells themselves secrete "destructive" cytokines such as IFN-gamma and TNF alpha. It is worth noting that, among all cytokines, interferons are the most efficient at alerting NK cells to viral presence. This concept is now widely accepted. In fact, some researchers have described the relationship between type I interferons (namely IFN-alpha and IFN-beta) and NK cells as a true "alliance": "Evidence from both murine models and in vitro studies supports the existence of an alliance between type 1 IFNs and NK cells to provide effective protection against viral infections", wrote Paolini, Bernardini, Molfetta and Santoni in an article published in the journal "Cytokine & Growth Factor Reviews" (466).

Virus → IFN-α/β → NK cells → IFN-γ + TNF-α → Enhanced antiviral defense

We therefore have the basis to show the great influence that vitamin C can have on NK cells. Clear evidence can be found in an interesting study published in 1997 in the journal "Immunopharmacology and Immunotoxicology" (416). This study evaluated the impact of AA on NK lymphocytes in 55 patients exposed to toxic substances, a factor that can significantly debilitate immune cell function. Remarkable results were found: a single oral dose of 60 mg/kg (equivalent to 4.2 g on an average weight of 70 kg) was able to correct the immune dysfunction due to intoxication in 78% of the participants. AA treatment increased NK-cell activity up to tenfold and also revitalised B and T-lymphocytes. This is a great success, as authors Heuser and Vojdani stated: "We conclude that immune functional abnormalities can be restored after toxic chemical exposure by oral usage of vitamin C" (416).

However, attention should be paid to a detail found in this study in (416), on which a rational criticism can be built, suggesting an underestimation of the results. Analyses of NK and T cells functionality were carried out on a blood sample taken approximately 24 hours after the administration of vitamin C, a timing which, as we know, is incompatible with the pharmacokinetics of high oral doses (24 hours is generally more than sufficient for the complete excretion of a high dose of vitamin C). Why was the sample taken so late? And furthermore, what effects would a sample taken 150 minutes after administration, i.e. close to the plasma peak, have revealed?

It is reasonable to hypothesise that the immune restoration produced by vitamin C, although having an important impact on the immune profile, was nevertheless limited because it was confined to a very few hours (due to the short-stay law), in contrast to the persistent damage generated by toxic substances. In fact, the authors argued that: "After exposure to many toxic chemicals, NK cells function can decrease significantly. Weeks or months later, NK cells function may return to normal levels in some patients and may be suppressed for prolonged periods in others" (416).

Therefore, a 24-hour analysis would have been more realistic had the only therapeutic approach capable of fully covering the entire 24-hour period been selected, namely, the protocol based on 4 to 6 administrations throughout the day. Such an approach would have maximized the value of vitamin C, allowing for a fair comparison between it and toxic substances.

In any case, this study is important because it has clinically demonstrated that vitamin C can substantially enhance NK cell activity (416).

As promised, we now turn our attention to the antimicrobial qualities of vitamin C. The article "Immunomodulatory and Antimicrobial Effects of Vitamin C" (126), published in the authoritative "European Journal of Microbiology and Immunology", is one of the most representative in providing in-depth data on the immunomodulatory and antimicrobial properties, highlighting its great antimicrobial potential: "Vitamin C supplementation is well tolerated and safe, given a virtual absent risk of intoxication upon uncompromised renal function. The biological role of vitamin C is related to its reversibly oxidized form and is involved in a multitude of both enzymatic and non-enzymatic processes. Additionally, vitamin C is a powerful antioxidant compound directed against free radicals and ROS. Leukocytes including lymphocytes can actively accumulate vitamin C against a concentration gradient, which underlines not only vitamin C dependent functional but also developmental immune cell features. In fact, vitamin C has a pivotal impact on both innate and adaptive immune responses. Vitamin C is also involved in bacterial metabolism. It is known that several bacteria can ferment vitamin C, whereas the presence of this vitamin exposes others to oxidative stress, which may result in bacterial growth inhibition. The potent antibacterial effects of vitamin C are, at least in part, due to its low pH and thus milieu-modifying properties. Notably, vitamin C is able to inhibit the growth of S. aureus and streptococci even under neutral pH conditions. Potent growth-inhibitory effects against multi-drug resistant (MDR) bacteria such as MRSA and proven synergistic effects with natural or synthetic antibiotic compounds open novel avenues for the combat of infections with emerging MDR bacterial species. However, both in vitro and in vivo (experimental and clinical) studies are needed to better understand the molecular mechanism of antimicrobial synergies. This applies not only to bacterial, but also to viral, parasitic, and fungal infections" (126).

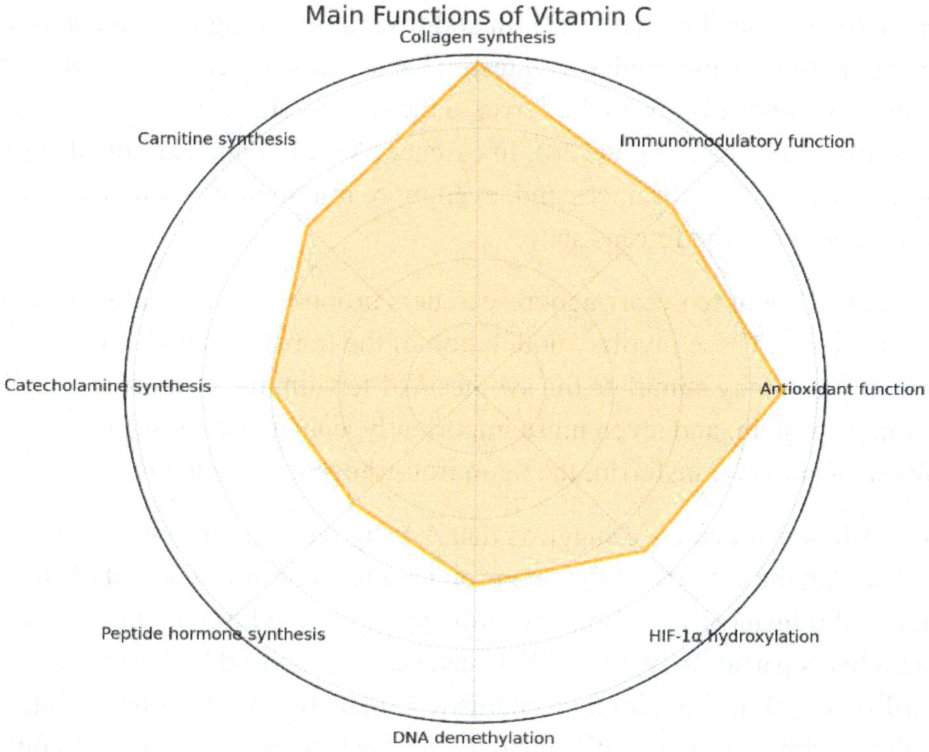

Further physiological roles

It has long been known that vitamin C plays a fundamental role in the mechanisms of iron absorption. Iron is a biologically valuable mineral, necessary for many biological functions, most notably the synthesis of hemoglobin. Furthermore, iron requires the essential support of vitamin C in the form of an enzymatic cofactor to activate certain enzymes involved in important metabolic processes.

Iron is found in food in the form of "heme iron" or inorganic iron, also known as "non-heme" iron. The latter exists in two different chemical states depending on its oxidation state: the ferric state and the ferrous state. While heme iron is virtually absent in plant-based foods (whereas meat is very rich in it) and its absorption is not affected by other foods, non-heme iron is abundantly present in plant-based foods and its absorption is influenced by the foods it is consumed with.

These premises help introduce the close relationship with AA, recognized for several decades, whereby the intestinal absorption of non-heme iron can be significantly enhanced by AA (127). In addition to inhibiting certain compounds that can bind to iron and hinder its intestinal absorption (such as tannins), AA has the ability to reduce iron from the ferric to the ferrous state, the form considered ideal for intestinal absorption (128). In essence, AA can enhance iron absorption by inhibiting harmful substances and, even more importantly, by maintaining iron in its reduced form, the ferrous state.

However, about ten years ago, researchers proposed additional mechanisms mediated by AA. These involve modulation of the transferrin pathway. Specifically, AA may stimulate the synthesis of ferritin, the primary intracellular iron-storage protein, and, even more importantly, enhance the transport of iron in the bloodstream via transferrin, the main iron-transport protein (129).

Overall, much evidence suggests that AA, by reducing iron to its ferrous state and enhancing the activity of the two proteins involved in iron metabolism (ferritin and transferrin), can improve iron absorption in both the intestine and tissues. This is particularly interesting because, as proposed by Lane and Richardson (129), it provides a mechanistic explanation for the onset of anemia in individuals with vitamin C deficiency. In fact, insufficient levels of AA could trigger dysregulation in the iron-transferrin system, leading to a reduction in hemoglobin levels and, consequently, to anemia (129).

The question therefore seems obvious: can adequate AA supplementation counteract anemia?

It is well known that the ability of ascorbic acid to promote iron absorption can be particularly beneficial for individuals affected by a specific type of anemia: iron deficiency anemia, also known as sideropenic anemia. This condition is often resistant to what should be the rational therapeutic approach, iron supplementation, whose effectiveness, however, is often limited to the duration of the treatment period. Therefore, stimulating iron absorption, an area in which vitamin C is unmatched, appears more advantageous than repeated administration of iron, the excess of which could also be harmful. In short, enhancing absorption is preferable to forcing it.

Unfortunately, practice and theory do not always go hand in hand: the few clinical studies on the subject are unsatisfactory. This was observed in a recent randomized study (130) in which ascorbic acid supplementation did not significantly improve the outcomes of iron therapy. Nonetheless, this study is valuable because it offers several insights, including the interpretation that links the inconclusive results to a non-functional use of vitamin C. In fact, the study was based on oral supplementation of 200 mg every 8 hours, a dosage that would likely have been met with sarcasm from the pioneers of vitamin C. This raises a question: do diseases require a decisive pharmacological approach or a gentle therapy?

There are many reasons for a more robust therapy. One of these is that anaemic patients often have an AA deficiency (399), (570). This suggests that the dosage used in the study (130) was unable to correct the probable underlying deficiency. It is therefore plausible that ascorbic therapy was ineffective due to an unsatisfactory restoration of plasma concentrations, which could not reestablish vitamin C-related physiological processes (clearly impaired by the underlying deficiency), including, of course, improved iron absorption. Importantly, the lack of plasma vitamin C measurements before and after treatment significantly undermines the reliability of the study's findings.

In simple words, how could we relaunch a company in difficulty without knowing the extent of the accumulated losses? And how could we evaluate the corrective measures undertaken without having an idea of their economic impact?

Supporting this point of view is one of the few authoritative clinical studies, published in the prestigious journal "The American Journal of Clinical Nutrition", in which vitamin C was used at doses exceeding one gram (514). Eleven volunteers underwent a therapy involving dietary iron restriction combined with either a placebo or supplementation with 1500 mg of AA, skillfully divided into three doses throughout the day. This therapy proved effective: the women treated with AA showed a significant increase in both iron and hemoglobin levels (514).

To conclude the discussion, it is important to address the safety of vitamin C in relation to the risks of iron accumulation. There is strong evidence to suggest that its supplementation, even at relatively high doses, is generally safe for the entire population, including individuals with iron overload, and possibly even for those affected by hemochromatosis, a hereditary disease that causes excessive iron absorption, leading to dangerous tissue accumulation and organ damage (131). "Extensive studies have shown that overall the uptake and storage of iron in humans is efficiently controlled by a network of regulatory mechanisms. Even high vitamin C intakes do not cause iron imbalance in healthy persons and probably in persons who are heterozygous for hemochromatosis", stated Gerster in the "International Journal for Vitamin and Nutrition Research" (131).

Regarding hemochromatosis, Brissot and co-workers found in a 1978 study (132) severe ascorbic deficiencies in untreated patients: "These results affirm an important vitamin C deficiency in the untreated disease". This is a clinically relevant finding and supports considering vitamin C supplementation even in individuals at risk of iron overload.

Doubts about excessive iron accumulation due to vitamin C were further dispelled by an interesting 2018 study (360). The findings suggested a dual potential therapeutic benefit against iron deficiency anaemia: in addition to enhancing iron absorption, vitamin C may offer substantial hepatoprotection in situations where inadvertent iron overload occurs during iron therapy (360).

Therefore, ascorbic acid therapy appears to be truly safe, as it can modulate iron absorption and may also protect the liver, which is considered the organ most affected by any excess iron resulting from overly aggressive therapy.

Let us now move from iron to another fundamental substance: cholesterol. It is physiologically produced by the body, is a key component of cell membranes, and serves as the precursor of vitamin D and steroid hormones.

It has long been known that vitamin C is involved in cholesterol metabolism, an involvement that broadens the cardiovascular health benefits attributed to vitamin C. One of the first articles on this topic was published in the prestigious journal "Science" (133), back in 1973. This study showed that cholesterol tends to accumulate more intensely in the blood and liver of animals with altered GULO activity. This is due to a kinetic defect in the transformation of cholesterol into so-called bile acids, the "detergents" that aid digestion by emulsifying dietary fats. This abnormality appears to be most prominent in the livers of animals deficient in vitamin C (or deprived of its biosynthesis), and it tends to slow down the normal process of converting cholesterol into bile acids. Overall, this indicates a direct correlation between hepatic/plasma concentrations of vitamin C and the body's ability to physiologically convert cholesterol into bile acids (133).

It should be noted that the conversion of cholesterol into bile acids is a biologically essential process, as elevated cholesterol levels are widely recognized as a significant risk factor for cardiovascular disease.

How does vitamin C affect cholesterol metabolism?

There is ample evidence showing that ascorbic acid acts as a cofactor for the enzyme CYP7A1, also known as cholesterol 7-alpha monooxygenase, the enzyme involved in the conversion of cholesterol into bile acids (134).

From a practical standpoint, numerous studies have observed a reduction in cholesterol levels associated with the use of vitamin C (134), highlighting its cholesterol-lowering potential: "High doses of ascorbic acid significantly stimulate the transformation of cholesterol into bile acids in guinea pigs and reduce plasma cholesterol concentrations in humans". This was stated in an important article published in the journal "Annals of the New York Academy of Sciences" in 1975 (134).

In a study published in 1980 in the "British Journal of Nutrition" (135), Jenkins showed that the liver of guinea pigs treated with low doses of AA contained more cholesterol than animals given higher doses of AA, which suggested an inverse correlation between AA and cholesterol levels. This correlation was confirmed clinically: a 2006 review based on 51 studies showed an inverse correlation between plasma ascorbate concentrations and cholesterol levels (136), preceding a 2008 meta-analysis (137) in which 13 randomized controlled trials reconfirmed the hypocholesterolaemic abilities of vitamin C despite the low dosages used. This meta-analysis showed that even an oral supplementation of 500 mg can significantly reduce LDL-cholesterol and triglyceride levels (137).

However, similar to iron deficiency anemia, there are disappointing studies that may reflect certain important inconsistencies. Some of these inconsistencies relate to the issue of appropriate dosing, as suggested by an animal study (138) which showed that a high dose of ascorbic acid (30 mg/100 g/day) was very effective in reducing LDL cholesterol, triglycerides and total lipids, while simultaneously increasing HDL cholesterol. However, these benefits were not observed when AA was administered at a much lower dose, 30 times lower, specifically 1 mg/100 g/day (138). This provides further rationale for the inconclusive results seen in studies where vitamin C was used at extremely low doses.

These findings suggest the need for a paradigm shift in the clinical use of vitamin C, whereby dietary-level doses (300 mg, 400 mg) should be replaced by more consistent pharmacological approaches. This could offer several advantages, beginning with the development of clinical trials focused on the pharmacological value of vitamin C, not merely its nutritional value.

From cholesterol we move on to another compound that the body can synthesise, uric acid. It is an endogenous antioxidant that is formed as a byproduct of normal metabolism. However, when present in excess, uric acid can become harmful. Elevated levels in the blood, a condition known as hyperuricemia, can trigger a pro-inflammatory state and represent a significant risk factor for gout. Gout is a complex metabolic disease marked by recurrent episodes of inflammatory arthritis, often causing intense pain and swelling in the joints.

The versatility of vitamin C is so broad that its uric acid-lowering effect (hypouricemic action) should come as no surprise. Multiple in vitro, animal, and clinical studies have supported this hypothesis, which gained further strength in 2011 thanks to a paradigmatic meta-analysis of randomized controlled trials published in "Arthritis Care and Research" (139). What makes this meta-analysis paradigmatic is the fact that vitamin C exhibited hypouricemic properties despite the modest therapeutic dosing commonly used, the average dose being just 500 mg per day.

Thus, ascorbic acid appears capable of modulating uric acid levels. This finding has been reinforced by various observational studies, which have shown an inverse correlation between plasma vitamin C levels and serum uric acid concentrations (139), (542). But that's not all: more recently, it has been noted that a modest dose of intravenous ascorbate (500 mg) produced a significant reduction in serum uric acid in patients with acute ischaemic stroke (518).

Interestingly, the hypouricemic abilities have been known since the 1970s, as suggested by a clinical study (140) in which the use of high oral dosages (4-8 g) significantly reduced excessive uric acid levels. These results, obtained by Stein, Hasan and Fox in 1976, seem valuable because vitamin C was used in the form of "vitamin megatherapy": "These observations show a pharmacological effect of megadoses of a simple vitamin" (140).

How can the inverse correlation between AA and uric acid be explained mechanistically?

Some in vivo studies have suggested a renal mechanism behind the hypouricemic effect of vitamin C. Specifically, this effect appears to be linked to an increase in the renal clearance of uric acid, that is the volume of plasma from which uric acid is completely removed per unit of time. This enhanced clearance is thought to be stimulated by competition between uric acid transporters and SVCTs in the renal proximal tubule. In simpler terms, it is believed that high levels of ascorbic acid may act directly at the sites of uric acid reabsorption in the proximal tubule, competitively inhibiting uric acid reuptake (139).

However, some scientists have put forward an alternative hypothesis: technically, AA's antioxidant power could increase glomerular filtration speed by acting on the reduction of glomerular microvascular ischaemia (139), (141),

(513). The question remains open, reflecting the vast sea of uncertainties that still surrounds the science of vitamin C; speaking of the sea, it is interesting to note that in a placebo-controlled study a single oral dose of 2 g was found to be effective in managing motion sickness (406).

One of the most recent reviews on the subject, dating back to 2021 (142), offers solid grounds to encourage more careful studies: the promising animal and clinical studies, combined with epidemiological data indicating an inverse correlation between AA and uric acid, constitute robust evidence for further investigation with large clinical studies.

The paragraph concludes with the role of ascorbic acid in bone health, which has been investigated in many animal models and epidemiological studies (366). In addition to the well-known enzymatic role in bone formation, recent discoveries have revealed new epigenetic mechanisms that allow ascorbic acid to participate in skeletal development and maintenance (366). In recent years, therefore, more and more evidence has shown the importance of AA in bone health, both in terms of prevention and therapy, especially in osteoporosis. Its powerful antioxidant functions, along with its role as an enzymatic cofactor in collagen synthesis and in the gene regulation of bone regeneration, are the main properties that make it a promising therapeutic candidate for various bone diseases, as highlighted in a comprehensive systematic review published in 2018 (403).

Chapter 5
Vitamin C In The Prevention And Treatment Of Cardiovascular Diseases

General premises

Prevention and treatment of diseases: these will be the topics covered in the following chapters. This reflects a perspective in which vitamin C is considered a potential pharmacological therapy, a concept first promoted by Klenner over 70 years ago but which still fails to gain meaningful scientific acceptance today.

It will soon become apparent that scientific research on vitamin C is characterized by a series of interpretative inconsistencies, mostly attributable to the pharmacological framing of vitamin C, which can be effective across a wide spectrum of applications, ranging from oral doses of 500 mg to intravenous doses of 100 g. The goal, therefore, is to provide some essential clarifications in order to safeguard and uphold the scientific credibility of vitamin C, focusing in particular on the following factors:

1- The lower ascorbic requirement that distinguishes a healthy person from an unhealthy one;

2- The difference between a prophylactic and a therapeutic approach.

Consider the example of hypertension, in which AA plays a potential preventive role. It is clear that a preventive model for hypertension would require a higher AA intake if another disease, such as diabetes, is also present. This is due to the fact that diabetes tends to reduce plasma and intracellular concentrations of AA in a clinically meaningful manner.

Moreover, higher doses may be required to achieve a therapeutic effect compared to a prophylactic one, not only because the presence of disease increases the metabolic demand for AA. In fact, in certain circumstances, the pharmacological efficacy of AA seems to necessarily require supraphysiological concentrations, as suggested by many studies on its pro-oxidant action against cancer cells.

Regarding the heart, many studies have examined the relationship between vitamin C and cardiovascular diseases such as heart failure, coronary heart disease and hypertension, with inconsistent results. Some cohort studies and several randomized trials have shown no significant association between vitamin C intake and the risk of heart disease, while other studies have suggested varying degrees of benefit. However, it is important to note that in most of these studies, the dosages used were quite low, typically between 500-1000 mg per day.

In contrast, other studies have demonstrated notable benefits, showing that vitamin C may have a dual role in both prevention and therapy. For example, a meta-analysis suggested interesting biological impacts, indicating that AA is effective in controlling blood pressure and maintaining endothelial function (143).

As for heart failure, one of the most dangerous cardiovascular diseases, two large-scale studies (EPIC-Norfolk, European Prospective Investigation into Cancer and Nutrition) provided very promising data (501), (143), (334). These studies, conducted on around 20000 individuals, showed that plasma ascorbate was inversely associated with the risk of heart failure, ischemic heart disease, and even all-cause mortality.

Interestingly, the average range in which plasma concentrations were most strongly associated with disease risk was well above the critical threshold of 11 micromoles/L. This is a particularly important finding, as it suggests the potential usefulness of AA supplementation even in the absence of deficiency, supporting the idea that higher concentrations may enhance coenzymatic and antioxidant actions. Furthermore, the fact that cardiac absorption of AA appears to differ from that of favourite sites, as observed in other studies (69), (363), makes this hypothesis even more plausible.

In summary: the important EPIC-Norfolk studies have suggested that a level below the plasma saturation level may provide much less cardiovascular protection than the saturation level (70-80 micromoles/L). This is a reasonable concept, but it does not seem sufficiently clear to those who think that vitamin C supplementation is only useful when the reservoir is empty. If Stone had intervened, he probably would have convinced the sceptics that the gap between an empty reservoir (frank scurvy) and a plasma level of 20-30 micromoles/L (subclinical scurvy) is much smaller than it seems.

It is interesting to note that other epidemiological studies have also found benefits of vitamin C in relation to the risk of heart failure, thus reinforcing a protective model that is not always replicated by other nutrients, primarily vitamin E, as will be seen below (500).

Before concluding, it is worth mentioning an important piece of evidence in favour of the therapeutic role of vitamin C. A meta-analysis (502) published in 2022 in the specialist journal "Frontiers in Cardiovascular Medicine" highlighted its ability to increase the left ventricular ejection fraction, a key parameter for measuring the severity of heart failure. This parameter measures the effectiveness of the heart's pumping function and is therefore a good indicator of myocardial contractility. Based on the data collected in the meta-analysis (502), vitamin C may also have a therapeutic effect in heart failure, helping to improve the efficiency of a heart affected by this serious condition.

These findings reinforce the dual preventive and therapeutic role of ascorbic acid. Consider its antioxidant, immunomodulatory and cholesterol-lowering properties; its ability to enhance nitric oxide synthesis by protecting BH4; and its function as a cofactor in the synthesis of collagen and carnitine, which has been shown to improve the management of heart failure and hypertension (541). These data provide strong biological plausibility for vitamin C's role in the management of cardiovascular disorders, both from a preventive and a therapeutic standpoint.

Atrial fibrillation

Atrial fibrillation (AF) is the most common form of cardiac arrhythmia. It occurs when the heart's electrical activity becomes disorganized, causing the two upper chambers, the atria, to contract in an uncoordinated manner. The result is a rapid and irregular heartbeat, which significantly increases the risk of thromboembolic events.

Among the many factors that contribute to the onset of AF, surgical procedures, especially cardiac surgeries, play a significant role. This has been extensively documented in numerous studies (144), (561), which report a very high incidence of postoperative AF following cardiac surgery, ranging from 25%

to 60%, depending on the specific type of procedure performed. Postoperative AF after cardiac surgery, therefore, represents not only a frequent occurrence but also a clinically challenging complication, as it can lead to severe adverse events such as ischaemic stroke, thromboembolism, myocardial infarction, and acute kidney injury (144), (561).

In recent years, the pathophysiological relevance of oxidative stress and inflammation in AF has become increasingly recognised (144). Several animal studies have demonstrated a strong association between the development of AF and elevated levels of inflammatory markers (e.g., leukocyte count, IL-6, CRP) as well as oxidative damage (e.g., malondialdehyde), thus suggesting a potential antiarrhythmic role for vitamin C (144). This hypothesis has been further supported by several meta-analyses. For instance, a 2016 meta-analysis (144) associated ascorbic acid supplementation with a significant reduction in the incidence of postoperative AF following cardiac surgery, as well as a shortening of hospitalisation times. Of note, the meta-analysis includes a variety of administration protocols: oral supplementation with 1 g/day, oral administration of 2 g on the day of surgery followed by a maintenance dosage in subsequent days, and intravenous administration with low doses (144). This reflects a considerable heterogeneity in study design, as well as the limitation of a 2 g daily dose, which was the maximum dosage used in all the studies. This context emphasises the therapeutic potential of AA: despite a debatably low "speed" (2 g/day representing a speed that is far too low compared to those that could, and I emphasise could, cause adverse effects), AA has often proven effective.

In synthesis, the meta-analysis (144) supports the prophylactic efficacy of vitamin C in the prevention of postoperative AF following cardiac surgery, prompting the authors to conclude: "In conclusion, vitamin C as prophylaxis for postoperative AF after cardiac surgery is effective. Due to the safe and relatively inexpensive nature of vitamin C, supplementation with vitamin C may be considered in all patients undergoing cardiac surgery" (144).

Even more compelling findings have emerged from studies employing intravenous administration. A noteworthy example involves a cohort of 170 patients, in which 2 g of intravenous vitamin C administered three hours prior to cardiac surgery was associated with a reduced incidence of postoperative AF, a shorter duration of hospitalisation, and a faster restoration of normal cardiac rhythm (145).

Additional evidence is provided by the meta-analysis "Efficacy and safety of vitamin C for atrial fibrillation after cardiac surgery: A meta-analysis with trial sequential analysis of randomized controlled trials" (348), published in "International Journal of Surgery" in 2017. This analysis reviewed eight randomized controlled trials involving a total of 1060 patients, confirming both the safety and the prophylactic efficacy of vitamin C in the context of postoperative AF following cardiac surgery. Similar findings were reported by Hemilä in 2017, whose meta-analysis, based on data from 2050 high-risk individuals undergoing cardiac surgery, demonstrated that vitamin C therapy could reduce the incidence of postoperative AF and decrease length of stay in intensive care units (562).

Conversely, certain clinical trials have failed to demonstrate benefit. This outcome appears more frequently in studies utilising solely oral administration, such as a randomized trial involving 105 patients undergoing coronary artery bypass surgery, in which a daily oral dose of 2 g did not reduce the incidence of postoperative AF (563).

Given the high incidence of postoperative AF after cardiac surgery and the relevant role of oxidative stress in its pathogenesis, I believe that the above-mentioned studies deserve close attention and justify the design of more rigorous clinical investigations.

Moreover, an important general principle appears to be emerging with increasing consistency: regardless of its potential antiarrhythmic effect, the administration of vitamin C may be indicated in surgical patients both for its strong antioxidant and anti-inflammatory properties, and for its ability to compensate for cardiac surgery-induced depletion, which, as will be noted later, is so profound that it frequently leads to an actual deficiency (levels < 11 micromoles/L) (383), (499).

Therefore, it is plausible that the negative results observed in studies exploring the oral route are due to a very restrictive experimental model, probably incompatible with the complex physiological mechanisms and pharmacokinetics of vitamin C. In simple terms, the extent of surgical stress appears to necessarily require the use of intravenous vitamin C to promptly restore reduced plasma levels. In such a complex clinical context, where it must also be taken into account that the need for surgical intervention may reflect an underlying condition already associated with further depletion, oral administration of 1-2 g appears clearly insufficient, metaphorically comparable to going into battle armed only with knives.

Regarding combination therapies in AF management, several studies have highlighted a consistent and compelling theme throughout the literature: the remarkable synergistic potential of vitamin C. A representative example is a randomized double-blind study (146) in which intravenous AA complemented a specific therapeutic approach to AF, namely, catheter ablation. In addition to reaffirming the safety of intravenous vitamin C, this trial suggested that its anti-inflammatory properties may mitigate ablation-related complications (146). Even more striking results were observed in the context of electrical cardioversion, another non-pharmacological intervention for AF. A 2005 clinical trial reported that oral vitamin C supplementation significantly reduced the recurrence of AF after cardioversion, again highlighting its anti-inflammatory efficacy (558).

Positive results have also been reported in combination with pharmacological agents. Notably, a double-blind clinical study evaluated the prophylactic value of AA in combination with amiodarone, a well-known antiarrhythmic agent (147). The study compared two groups of 42 patients each: one treated with amiodarone monotherapy (300 mg intravenously) and the other with amiodarone (150 mg intravenously) plus AA (2 g intravenously). The second group showed a lower incidence of postoperative arrhythmias, including AF (147). This result clearly highlights the potential of AA in enhancing certain pharmacological agents.

However, some methodological inconsistencies deserve to be taken into account. For instance, the AA group received a halved dose of amiodarone, raising the question of how the results would have been interpreted if they had not been favourable. Despite this uneven comparison, however, the outcomes were very positive. Intravenous AA not only reduced the incidence of arrhythmias but also suggested the possibility of lowering the pharmacological dose of amiodarone (from 300 mg to 150 mg), improving its safety profile. These findings indicate that AA, when appropriately used, may reduce the required dose of antiarrhythmic drugs, thereby lowering the risk of adverse effects, which are particularly significant in the case of amiodarone (571), while simultaneously enhancing therapeutic efficacy.

Combination therapy has been the subject of some meta-analyses which have reported very promising results. A particularly illustrative example is the systematic review and meta-analysis of RCTs published in 2018 in "Clinical Cardiology" (454). The authors stated: "This further systematic review and meta-analysis of RCTs evaluating the efficacy of vitamin C on prevention of POAF in patients undergoing cardiac surgery suggested that vitamin C itself and combined vitamin C could prevent POAF, and that vitamin C as an adjunct to routine therapy (e.g., statins, beta-blockers) exerts a stronger preventive effect than vitamin C alone. Additionally, vitamin C supplementation was associated with a markedly shorter ICU length of stay and HLOS and reduced risk of adverse events" (454).

Finally, a 2011 meta-analysis of RCTs concluded that vitamin C, either alone or in combination with vitamin E, can significantly reduce both the incidence of postoperative arrhythmias and the length of hospital stay in both intensive care and non-intensive care units (452).

Endothelial dysfunction

There is substantial evidence supporting the crucial role that oxidative stress plays in the pathophysiology of endothelial dysfunction, a condition characterized by impaired endothelial function, leading to vasoconstriction, increased vascular permeability and inflammation. The endothelium is a large and dynamic tissue that lines the inner surface of blood vessels, lymphatic vessels and the heart. It plays a crucial role in maintaining vascular tone by releasing vasoactive mediators involved in both vasodilation and vasoconstriction.

Vitamin C may exert both preventive and therapeutic effects on endothelial dysfunction through two molecular mechanisms: its strong antioxidant capacity and its regulatory action on the synthesis of nitric oxide (NO), a key mediator of endothelial function. Specifically, vitamin C has the ability to preserve and recycle tetrahydrobiopterin (BH4), a crucial cofactor for the activity of endothelial nitric oxide synthase (eNOS). This role becomes especially important considering that inadequate antioxidant protection, particularly the lack of effective BH4 recycling, can lead to BH4 oxidation. Moreover, it's worth noting that no other antioxidant has been shown to recycle BH4 as efficiently as vitamin C (149), (565).

In the absence of adequate protection, BH4 loses its efficiency, leading to eNOS uncoupling. As a result, the activity of the eNOS enzyme shifts from its physiological function of synthesizing NO to the production of superoxide, thereby contributing to oxidative stress and vascular damage (149), (527). This uncoupling of eNOS disrupts the physiological NO biosynthetic pathway, decreasing NO bioavailability and enhancing superoxide production. Superoxide may then react with NO to form peroxynitrite, a highly reactive nitrogen species (149), (565). Peroxynitrite can cause extensive damage to lipids, proteins and nucleic acids, and is involved in the onset of nitrosative stress, further exacerbating endothelial damage. As such, peroxynitrite represents a serious threat to cellular integrity (565).

In this context, AA can be viewed as a critical regulator of vascular homeostasis. When present in sufficient concentrations, it can preserve BH4 activity, supporting and enhancing the physiological synthesis of NO. Conversely, its deficiency may lead to reduced NO bioavailability and consequent endothelial dysfunction.

Some studies have reported a more pronounced protective effect on BH4 when AA is administered intravenously, likely due to improved tissue concentration. This has led to the potential formulation of a functional equivalence: maximum BH4 protection = endothelial ascorbate saturation (149), (527). This is corroborated by findings from a pivotal study published in the "Journal of Biological Chemistry", which stated: "The present study suggests that saturated ascorbic acid levels in endothelial cells are necessary to protect tetrahydrobiopterin from oxidation and to provide optimal conditions for cellular NO synthesis" (527). These data suggest the importance of achieving ascorbic saturation in all tissues to optimise the numerous physiological modulations, including NO biosynthesis.

Why is the interaction between vitamin C and nitric oxide so important?

Beyond its vasodilatory effects, NO possesses several additional properties of fundamental importance to vascular health. NO deficiency can lead to endothelial dysfunction by impairing arteriolar dilation. Furthermore, NO modulates immune responses and reduces platelet aggregation, thus exerting antithrombotic effects. It also promotes mitochondrial biogenesis, and inhibits leukocyte adhesion to the endothelium, a key inflammatory trigger (149).

Notably, some studies suggest that vitamin C may act synergistically with NO in counteracting leukocyte adhesion, outlining a promising interaction (148). It has also been hypothesised that vitamin C may stimulate NO production via pathways independent of the classical arginine-eNOS axis (148). Additionally, AA contributes to endothelial cell proliferation by promoting collagen synthesis. Taken together, these findings provide strong mechanistic support for the vasoprotective role of vitamin C.

What do clinical studies reveal?

A 2021 clinical trial (361) demonstrated that oral administration of 2 g of AA effectively reversed endothelial dysfunction induced by a pharmacologically triggered inflammatory state. This finding is particularly noteworthy as it supports the therapeutic efficacy of oral AA, an outcome not consistently observed in the literature, and may be attributed to the use of dosages higher than the conventional 500-1000 mg.

Nonetheless, some studies have shown beneficial effects even at relatively low doses. One example is a double-blind, placebo-controlled randomized trial published in the important journal "Circulation", involving 46 patients with coronary artery disease. Participants received either placebo or a regimen consisting of a single oral loading dose of 2 g of AA followed by 500 mg/day for 30 days. Despite the modest dosing, significant improvements were reported in flow-mediated dilation of the brachial artery, a key marker of endothelial function (534).

More compelling outcomes have been observed with intravenous administration. A 2014 clinical study (385) investigated the effects of high-dose intravenous AA (320 mg/kg and 480 mg/kg) on inflammation induced by lipopolysaccharide (LPS) endotoxin, a potent disruptor of NO signalling and vascular integrity. High-dose intravenous treatment with AA restored endothelium-dependent vasodilation and significantly reduced acute inflammation, once again highlighting its anti-inflammatory efficacy.

Several additional clinical studies have confirmed the vasodilatory effects of intravenous AA, particularly in patients with endothelial dysfunction due to atherosclerosis, hypertension, smoking, or diabetes (149). In some trials, AA was even infused directly into the coronary arteries, potentially representing the most effective route of administration in this context (149).

Much of the aforementioned evidence is summarised in a seminal review article (149) by May and Harrison, published in 2013 in "Antioxidants & Redox Signaling". The authors highlighted a significant shortcoming in the existing clinical literature: the lack of plasma ascorbate measurements, which may account for some of the inconsistent or null findings observed in prior studies. This observation reinforces earlier theoretical arguments. May and Harrison further commented on the clinical community's general unawareness of the need to restore plasma ascorbate levels in deficiency states, stating: "Supplementation to upper normal plasma ascorbate levels is clearly indicated in most diseases and conditions in which ascorbate is depleted. However, it is seldom a priority, because patients, physicians, and health authorities are unaware of the increasing evidence for multiple potentially important functions of ascorbate. With regard to the endothelium, it is worth emphasizing observations made more than 50 years ago that early scurvy generates endothelial disruption in guinea pigs, which resembles atherosclerosis and is fully and rapidly reversible with ascorbate repletion" (149).

The available evidence therefore supports the need for a paradigm shift in the clinical use of vitamin C. Although it is universally recognized as an essential nutrient, current clinical and experimental practice still does not reflect the importance of monitoring plasma levels, which is a prerequisite for any rational therapeutic intervention ("measure and correct"). In the absence of such monitoring, many clinical trials risk becoming unreliable, producing ambiguous or misleading results, like a ship forced to sail without a compass on a cloudy day. While sailors of the past had no alternatives, it seems paradoxical that modern medicine continues to overlook such a fundamental principle.

Indeed, no physician would ever administer a hypoglycemic drug without first checking the patient's blood glucose level. The same logic should apply to vitamin C: any strategy should be based on an objective measurement of ascorbemia. Yet the prevailing scientific narrative treats glucose and ascorbic acid very differently. While blood glucose is clearly a priority, the complex biological role of ascorbic acid is often underestimated, despite growing evidence of its many important physiological functions.

Atherosclerosis

The beneficial influence that vitamin C can have on heart health becomes more evident upon considering that endothelial dysfunction is one of the earliest signs of atherosclerotic disease. Atherosclerosis is a chronic vascular condition that typically manifests in adulthood and can lead to numerous cardiovascular pathologies. It is characterised by chronic inflammation of the innermost layer of the arteries (the so-called tunica intima, which is rich in endothelial cells), due to the accumulation and oxidation of lipoproteins within the arterial wall. This process tends to cause the formation of various multifocal lesions, among which the well-known atherosclerotic plaque is particularly prominent.

Lipoprotein oxidation is widely recognized as a key contributing factor in the development of atherosclerosis. This understanding has prompted researchers to explore vitamin C as a potentially protective agent. Owing to its potent antioxidant capacity, capable of inhibiting LDL oxidation and regenerating vitamin E, along with its immunomodulatory, endothelial-protective and lipid-lowering effects, vitamin C provides compelling biological plausibility for the prevention of atherosclerosis.

Surprisingly, some studies (e.g., (150) and (151)) have not found significant anti-atherosclerotic benefits of vitamin C. Nevertheless, other investigations have yielded more encouraging results. For instance, a study published in the journal "Food & Function" (412) demonstrated that a daily intake of 1250 mg of vitamin C resulted in a marked improvement in the lipoprotein profile and a significant reduction in oxidative stress.

An intriguing new line of research has recently emerged (152), proposing a novel hypothesis: the inhibitory action of vitamin C on one of the most important cardiovascular risk factors, vascular calcification. This hypothesis represents a modern reformulation of Pauling's ideas regarding the inverse correlation between vitamin C and lipoprotein-a (37). What does this entail?

Matthias Rath (one of Pauling's last collaborators), along with other researchers, has conducted a series of studies highlighting a crucial characteristic of ascorbic acid: its support for the extracellular matrix, the acellular component of tissues. Although it may seem surprising, tissues are not composed solely of cells; a substantial portion of their volume consists of an extracellular matrix, composed of a complex network of polysaccharides and proteins, especially collagen, which functions as a structural scaffold. In essence, the extracellular matrix, which is highly collagen-rich, plays a fundamental role in ensuring the structural and functional integrity of tissues, particularly connective tissues where it is especially abundant.

This highlights the biological relevance of AA. An illustrative example comes from an in vitro experiment that observed a reduction in calcium accumulation within the extracellular matrix following the introduction of AA, suggesting its potential benefits in counteracting the arterial wall calcification process (153). "We conclude that ascorbic acid supplementation may actively and beneficially interfere with the process of arterial wall calcification, with potential implications for human health" (153).

The benefits that AA may offer against calcification processes are linked to its critical involvement in the integrity of the extracellular matrix, a relationship that is due to the matrix's high collagen content and is supported by numerous studies (153). There is also an additional potential benefit related to a well-known class of cholesterol-lowering drugs: statins. Although definitive scientific evidence is lacking, some studies suggest that statin therapy may paradoxically promote coronary calcification (564). Notably, this effect was also documented in (153) and, of particular interest, was mitigated by vitamin C. Hence, vitamin C may be beneficial not only for directly lowering cholesterol but also by mitigating the potential side effects associated with conventional lipid-lowering medications.

Together with the antiarrhythmic agent amiodarone, this represents another example of pharmacological synergy involving AA, one of many that will be progressively discussed throughout this book. It is worth noting that the synergy between AA and statins may have an additional clinical significance, as suggested in the context of postoperative atrial fibrillation following cardiac surgery: "Based on our results, combined prophylaxis against post-CABG atrial fibrillation with oral atorvastatin plus vitamin C is significantly more effective than single oral atorvastatin", reads the conclusion of a randomized double-blind study involving 120 participants (436).

Returning to Linus Pauling, we consider a study (154) published in the prestigious "Proceedings of the National Academy of Sciences of the United States of America". In this work, Pauling and Rath demonstrated that a dosage of 40 mg/kg/day of AA, administered to an animal model incapable of synthesising ascorbate endogenously, could prevent the development of atherosclerotic lesions and the accumulation of lipoprotein-a in the arterial wall. "We suggest a similar mechanism in humans, given the similarity between guinea pigs and humans with regard to both the lack of endogenous ascorbate production and the role played by lipoprotein-a in human atherosclerosis", the authors wrote (154).

These studies offer a different scientific perspective on atherosclerosis, one that is increasingly supported by a growing number of researchers. The contributions of Pauling and Rath have been particularly significant, as they were among the first to propose distinct mechanisms in the etiology of atherosclerosis, as effectively outlined in a 2016 article titled "Atherosclerosis and the Cholesterol Theory: A Reappraisal" (155). In this paper, the authors presented evidence that challenges the prevailing theory attributing atherosclerosis to excess cholesterol or lipoproteins. Instead, they propose an alternative hypothesis: the weakening of the vascular extracellular matrix in the coronary arteries (which supply oxygen-rich blood to the myocardium) initiates lipoprotein-a infiltration and subsequent plaque formation. Thus, the vascular deposition of molecules such as lipoprotein-a, and the development of atherosclerosis itself, may represent an endogenous protective mechanism aimed at reinforcing arterial walls.

This alternative framework has been described as the "vascular lesion response hypothesis". According to this view, vascular weakening due to reduced collagen synthesis, resulting from chronically insufficient vitamin C levels typical in humans, triggers a compensatory physiological response. This hypothesis, which is a fundamental component of the broader "Vitamin C–Lp(a)–CHD connection" theory, argues that high cholesterol levels represent a protective adaptation aimed at counteracting arterial fragility, acting as a form of "lipoprotein cement" to prevent cardiovascular damage. The theory gains additional support from several considerations:

1- The role of lipoprotein-a as a cardiovascular risk factor is now well documented (473);

2- Symptoms of scurvy predominantly involve vascular fragility, connective tissue impairment, and haemorrhage;

3- An inverse association has been observed between plasma vitamin C and the risk of stroke, particularly haemorrhagic stroke (217);

4- A provocative question posed by the authors of (155): "Why is atherosclerosis characteristic of humans while it is practically unknown in the animal kingdom, except in a few species that are incapable of synthesising vitamin C endogenously?".

Arterial hypertension

Hypertension represents one of the most prevalent clinical conditions in industrialised nations, affecting more than 30% of the adult population. Vitamin C may also help lower blood pressure. We have already observed this, for example, in a previous study on stress reactivity, where it also showed substantial antihypertensive effects (26).

A 2012 meta-analysis published in the prestigious "American Journal of Clinical Nutrition" (156) linked moderate vitamin C supplementation with the potential to lower blood pressure levels, revealing an antihypertensive effect (with an average dosage of 500 mg across the included studies). In addition to the biological plausibility supporting the efficacy of vitamin C, namely its antioxidant, anti-inflammatory, and endothelium-protective functions, the authors of the meta-analysis also noted an inverse correlation between plasma ascorbate and blood pressure values (156). This suggests that maintaining adequate vitamin C levels may reduce the risk of hypertension, an important consideration given its high global prevalence (156), (536).

A 2020 systematic review and meta-analysis of observational studies (157) further confirmed this inverse association between plasma vitamin C levels and both systolic and diastolic blood pressure. In addition, individuals with hypertension were found to have plasma levels approximately 15 micromoles/L lower than healthy controls.

Beyond epidemiological findings, the antihypertensive effects of AA were also observed in a specific cohort study in which a single intravenous administration of 30 grams of vitamin C produced a significant reduction in blood pressure (351). This study, the first to evaluate the antihypertensive potential of intravenous AA, suggested that intravenous ascorbate could be a viable therapeutic option in managing complex clinical scenarios such as hypertensive crises, given its potent antioxidant properties and its ability to enhance the synthesis of nitric oxide, a powerful vasodilator.

A final consideration may help to broaden the overall perspective. Reference is made to the alarming epidemiological data indicating that over 30% of the global adult population suffers from hypertension (536). This figure becomes even more concerning when considered alongside the growing prevalence of other chronic diseases and the pervasive impact of stress. This highlights the increasingly plausible hypothesis of widespread subclinical vitamin C deficiency, which seems to echo Stone's brilliant description of chronic subclinical scurvy.

Ischaemias

Ischaemia is a serious vascular condition caused by a significant reduction in blood flow to a specific area of the body, leading to a reduced supply of oxygen and nutrients. In the absence of timely intervention, the lack of these essential elements triggers an irreversible process leading to necrosis of the affected tissues.

It is not surprising that numerous studies have highlighted the beneficial role of vitamin C in reducing ischemic risk. One example is an article (158) published in "The Journal of the American College of Nutrition", which demonstrated an association between long-term use of ascorbic acid and a reduced risk of ischemia, particularly among individuals with a high tendency to smoke. In this regard, it is worth noting that smoking, which induces oxidative stress and inflammation, can also lead to a marked depletion of vitamin C (159).

Therefore, smoking reduces vitamin C levels, and vitamin C appears to counteract some of the smoking-induced damage. A large epidemiological study (159) provided clear evidence of an inverse correlation between the number of cigarettes smoked and plasma levels of AA. Notably, this correlation was independent of diet, suggesting that dietary intake alone may be insufficient to restore AA levels in smokers. These findings tend to support the hypothesis of supplementation.

In addition to neutralising oxidative stress and limiting inflammation, some evidence suggests that AA may improve microcirculation compromised by smoking. This was demonstrated in a clinical study (379), in which a single oral dose of 2 g improved microcirculatory flow in the 24 subjects examined. The improvement was evidenced by the finding that AA pretreatment attenuated the vascular damage caused by subsequent smoke exposure.

This study is particularly significant as it underscores the predominant role of vitamin C. Indeed, whereas vitamin C demonstrated an improvement in microcirculation, aspirin, a compound commonly regarded as beneficial for microvascular health, showed no efficacy: "The effect of smoking a single cigarette on nail-fold microcirculation was analyzed in 24 healthy subjects with varying smoking habits. Vital capillary microscopy was used and the blood cell flow velocity in the capillaries was evaluated before and 1-30 min after smoking. Smoking induced a marked decrease in microcirculatory blood flow in 23 of the 24 subjects (40–50% decrease 1-5 min after smoking). This change was reduced by more than 50% in the same subjects after intake of 2 g of vitamin C 2 h before smoking ($P < 0.0001$ by ANOVA test), with smokers responding similarly to nonsmokers in these experiments. Intake of 1 g of vitamin C had no significant effect on the smoking-induced changes in most of the subjects tested ($n = 11$). Pretreatment with aspirin had little or no effect on the response to smoking ($n = 9$). Our results show that treatment with a single high dose of vitamin C can reduce and, in some individuals, even completely abolish the negative acute effect on microcirculation induced by smoking a single cigarette. This effect of vitamin C is not likely to be mediated by the cyclooxygenase system" (379).

Overall, there is no doubt about the benefits that smokers could gain from adequate AA supplementation, just as there is no doubt about the extension of the inverse correlation between AA and ischemic risk to the general population (92), (217).

However, vitamin C is not merely a preventive agent. Its potential therapeutic role in managing ischaemia-reperfusion injury, a severe clinical condition occurring when blood flow is restored after a period of ischaemia, further underscores its significance. The deprivation of oxygen and nutrients during ischemia creates a situation in which the restoration of blood flow paradoxically triggers severe inflammation and a surge in oxidative stress, leading to further tissue damage rather than functional recovery. This condition is known as ischemia-reperfusion injury.

The strong protective effects of vitamin C in this context are well documented and are primarily attributed to its antioxidant and anti-inflammatory properties. Interestingly, these effects are exemplified by a discovery involving marsh turtles, which exhibit a remarkable tolerance to oxygen deprivation during prolonged dives. This tolerance is attributed to the extremely high concentration of vitamin C that accumulates in their brains, affording significant neuroprotection during reoxygenation (160), (551). Unfortunately, unlike turtles, humans have the well-known genetic defect affecting GULO, which increases susceptibility to injury under these conditions, supporting the rationale for considering vitamin C as a potential therapeutic agent.

As noted, reperfusion injury leads to massive reactive oxygen species production, which in turn results in substantial vitamin C depletion. Furthermore, the intense inflammation may impair SVCTs, potentially reducing AA absorption both in plasma and cells.

What role could AA play in this clinical context?

The central mechanism is undoubtedly the neutralization of ROS. AA is, in fact, the first antioxidant to respond to oxidative stress (67), (427), (528), preserving and restoring glutathione and vitamin E. In vitro studies have consistently demonstrated this sequence of depletion: ROS exposure first depletes vitamin C, followed by vitamin E, glutathione, and other endogenous antioxidants (427), (528). In short, vitamin C is the first line of antioxidant defence (first-line ROS sink) (67), (427), (160), (528). Therefore, neutralising the ROS surge generated during reperfusion is the main mechanism of action. However, this process is extremely time-sensitive: the rapid depletion of ascorbic acid that occurs during reperfusion injury or cardiac arrest necessitates early intervention.

Some striking numbers deserve attention: following cardiac arrest, plasma AA concentrations can fall by 50-70% within 24 hours, with most patients becoming deficient within three days (160), (161), (548). These findings are especially relevant when considered alongside another key observation: in patients admitted to intensive care units, vitamin C deficiency is associated with a poorer prognosis. Numerous studies have linked ascorbic acid deficiency to increased use of vasopressors, acute kidney injury and multiple organ dysfunction syndrome, as well as elevated SOFA scores, an important clinical index used in intensive care units. All of these factors are clearly associated with higher mortality rates (450), (160), (161). As reported in the prestigious journal "Critical Care": "Vitamin C deficient patients had an 8-point higher SOFA score, corresponding to two fully failing organs and 6.9 times higher odds of dying" (160).

Could this be a compelling reason to consider pharmacological vitamin C in managing critical illness?

This possibility is reinforced by another important piece of evidence: in critically ill patients, standard oral supplementation (in the absence of data on dynamic flow) fails to restore ascorbate levels. For example, various studies have shown that a daily oral intake of 700 mg does not significantly increase plasma concentrations in these patients (34), (160), (162). "The administration of high-dose vitamin C is often considered as unnecessary or even alternative medicine. This does not do justice to the strong scientific base of the pleiotropic beneficial effects of high i.v. doses (not enteral!) as demonstrated in multiple preclinical and clinical studies. Beyond simply preventing scurvy by the correction of vitamin C deficiency, supraphysiological vitamin C levels can exert very strong multifaceted effects" (160).

Describing it as "unnecessary or alternative", some researchers (160) criticise those in the scientific community who continue to overlook the pharmacological potential of vitamin C. Nevertheless, the evidence in support of its therapeutic role, especially in post-ischaemic or post-cardiac arrest phases, is growing.

In some animal studies, rats were subjected to electrically induced cardiac arrest and treated with intravenous ascorbate at doses of 50-200 mg/kg. These treatments resulted in reduced myocardial and neurological injury and increased survival (163), (165). Other preclinical studies have yielded conflicting but intriguing results: some showed a reduction in cardiac damage only in diabetic animals, while others observed neurological benefits only when vitamin C was administered in the form of DHA. The latter is a very interesting point that will be discussed later (160), (165).

Intravenous AA has also shown efficacy in protecting against reperfusion arrhythmias, including the highly dangerous ventricular fibrillation (164), (165). This protective effect is thought to stem from AA's ability to prevent mitochondrial dysfunction due to glutathione depletion. Mitochondrial dysfunction is a condition that leads to a deficiency in cellular energy production, primarily due to mitochondrial oxidative stress, among other causes. It has been associated with a wide range of diseases, including neurodegenerative disorders, metabolic syndromes and cardiovascular conditions.

Supporting this, an animal study (164) demonstrated that coronary reperfusion leads to mitochondrial glutathione depletion, but that high-dose AA administration prevents this outcome: "These results suggest that coronary reperfusion induces mitochondrial dysfunction and a depletion of mitochondrial glutathione concentration, and that a high dose of ascorbate prevents reperfusion damage".

Other promising results come from studies on primates: intravenous administration of 2 g of AA significantly reduced infarct size following cerebral ischaemia (160), underscoring the neuroprotective role of vitamin C and supporting its use in ischaemic stroke scenarios. In support of this, animal models of focal cerebral ischaemia have shown that neurons respond by increasing SVCT2 expression (355), suggesting the neurophysiological importance of AA and pointing to novel therapeutic opportunities.

From a clinical perspective, unfortunately, the quality of the evidence is suboptimal. A 2010 study (518) involving 60 patients with ischemic stroke showed no clinical benefit following intravenous administration of 500 mg/day for 10 days. However, this dose was well below the 3 g/day generally needed to restore plasma vitamin C levels in critically ill patients (34). Why adopt such a conservative dosage of a compound that does not appear to be toxic even at doses up to 200 times higher (424), (367)?

Why impose such restrictive dosing parameters on vitamin C, as though it were a conventional drug with a narrow therapeutic index?

Such a conservative approach appears unjustified in light of the available evidence.

More encouraging results came from a study (519) in which healthy volunteers were subjected to controlled ischaemia–reperfusion. Intravenous AA administration, which achieved millimolar plasma peaks, increased BH4 levels and markedly reduced oxidative stress, enhancing endothelial function. Similar benefits were observed in patients undergoing percutaneous coronary intervention: 1 g of intravenous AA administered beforehand significantly improved microcirculatory reperfusion, likely due to increased nitric oxide bioavailability (160), (165), (552).

Overall, various preclinical studies, and some clinical studies made possible through the participation of volunteers, suggest that pharmacological vitamin C may enhance antioxidant defenses, support nitric oxide biosynthesis, and mitigate microvascular deterioration, myocardial damage and neurological injury in severe clinical contexts such as the post-ischemic phase (165).

However, the overall evaluation remains uncertain, likely due to variability in dose, frequency and timing. "The huge burst of ROS is generated within minutes after the start of reperfusion. Therefore, a late start of vitamin C infusion may lead to negative results" (160).

In other words, timing is critical: if administered too late, even high-dose AA may be ineffective. We can only hope for a paradigm shift, in which vitamin C is regarded not as a mere dietary supplement, but as a first-line pharmacological agent. A major step in this direction is the upcoming large, double-blind, multicentre, randomized, placebo-controlled clinical trial in the Netherlands (166), designed to evaluate the effect of early vitamin C administration in the post-cardiac arrest setting. This study is especially important for three reasons:

1- It is the first randomized controlled trial assessing vitamin C in post-cardiac arrest organ dysfunction;

2- It employs a rational design, including three arms: placebo, 3 g, and a pharmacological 10 g dose;

3- It includes measurement of plasma concentrations.

I believe that the design of similar studies could mark a turning point in research on vitamin C, which requires particular scientific rigour due to its atypical pharmacokinetics and unparalleled therapeutic window.

This section concludes with some insights into chronic ischaemic heart disease, where oxidative stress-mediated coronary deterioration plays a key role. A 2007 study (358) used intracoronary doppler ultrasound to assess microcirculatory flow in 12 patients with ischaemic cardiomyopathy undergoing coronary intervention. Following the infusion of 3 g of AA, microcirculatory flow, initially impaired by intervention and induced hyperoxia (excessive levels of oxygen), improved significantly. The authors urged clinicians to consider these results (358), and although the 3 g dose was likely the minimum required to restore plasma levels, the findings reinforce the central importance of vitamin C in cardiovascular physiology.

These benefits may reflect the biological importance of correcting acute hypoascorbemia, a condition that Cathcart referred to as anascorbemia. This raises some fundamental questions:

1- Is the mere correction of anascorbemia sufficient to achieve clinical improvements in patients with acute conditions?

2- Can the restoration of physiological levels of ascorbic acid in critically ill patients be considered the optimal therapeutic intervention?

The next chapter will provide some important clarifications.

Chapter 6
Pharmacological Ascorbate In Critically Ill Patients

'In critical care medicine, the therapeutic potential of pharmacological ascorbate remains overshadowed by a persistent nutritional mindset'

Introduction

As mentioned several times, the majority of critically ill patients have extremely low levels of vitamin C in both plasma and tissues, to the extent that it becomes clinically relevant to investigate the discriminating factor that enables a minority of individuals to resist the depleting effects of critical illness. Identifying this factor could open up important clinical perspectives, given the numerous negative implications associated with ascorbic acid deficiency.

Here are some noteworthy data: Carr and other authors (34), (160) have reported a high prevalence of ascorbate deficiency in intensive care units, despite regular administration of standard nutritional support. For instance, a study from Christchurch Hospital's intensive care unit (New Zealand) found that 70% of patients had hypovitaminosis, and 32% had a deficiency (34), suggesting that many critically ill patients are in a subclinical state of scurvy. The situation may be even more severe in certain subgroups, such as critically ill patients undergoing haemodialysis, as indicated by a 2018 retrospective study (167), in which ascorbic acid deficiency (87% of patients) was more prevalent than folic acid deficiency (33% of patients) as well as all other vitamin deficiencies examined.

Overall, the available data indicate that conventional nutritional support is insufficient for these patients. It is worth noting that oral administration of 700 mg/24 h failed to increase plasma concentrations in critically ill individuals (34), (160), (162), thereby reinforcing the need for a paradigm shift from a nutritional to a pharmacological approach. More explicitly: a critical condition appears to require the pharmacological use of vitamin C, even when the goal is simply the normalization of plasma levels (34), (535). This excludes the possibility that the discriminating factor lies in nutritional intake, thus directing scientific research towards a potential genetic dysfunction. My personal impression is that resistance, understood as the ability to limit the profound ascorbic acid depletion typically observed in severe illness, may be genetically mediated, perhaps involving the upregulation of SVCTs. Identifying this factor could enhance our understanding of the metabolic variability observed in critical illnesses, conditions in which ascorbate appears to be the first substance to be depleted, though certainly not the only one (165), (383).

Scientific evidence therefore suggests that the normalization of ascorbemia may need to be regarded as a relevant clinical objective during critical illness. As already mentioned, inadequate vitamin C levels expose critically ill patients to potentially lethal consequences, including acute kidney injury and multiple organ dysfunction syndrome (450), (34), (160), (161), (165). Furthermore, unlike other essential substances such as zinc or vitamin E, which appear to have no significant implications in the progression of critical illness, ascorbic acid plays a unique frontline role in defending against oxidative stress, underscoring its fundamental importance. Indeed, some studies have found no correlation between zinc or vitamin E levels and life-threatening events such as multiple organ dysfunction syndrome (450).

This underscores the growing importance of identifying a therapeutic regimen capable of correcting the depletion of ascorbic acid caused by critical illness, a complex task in which pharmacokinetic differences may play a pivotal role. Oral versus intravenous: it is important to recall the profound pharmacokinetic differences between these two routes of administration. Only intravenous administration allows for the attainment of millimolar plasma concentrations. This considerable advantage, however, poses certain theoretical challenges.

While the oral route is strictly limited to plasma concentrations in the range of 70-80 micromoles/L, generally considered optimal, the ideal value required to achieve the maximum clinical benefit via the intravenous route remains undefined. In other words, 70-80 micromoles/L represents the saturation point for standard oral administration, though levels between 220-250 micromoles/L may be reached through dynamic flow. By contrast, the virtually unrestricted potential of the intravenous route raises a crucial question: What is the optimal plasma concentration for correcting a deficiency and producing clinical benefit?

Why aim for 70 micromoles/L? Why should an intravenous strategy conform to a target that reflects the pharmacokinetic ceiling of oral administration rather than its own therapeutic potential?

Logic suggests that 70-80 micromoles/L is not the optimal therapeutic target.

Among the many uncertainties, one rational certainty emerges: the correction of the deficiency, which can otherwise seriously compromise the biochemical functions of vitamin C.

However, three factors must be carefully considered:

1- The low toxicity of high-dose ascorbic acid;

2- The fact that its biochemical activity is dose-dependent: its ROS-neutralising capacity appears to correlate with plasma levels, which implies that supraphysiological levels can considerably enhance the antioxidant effects;

3- The consistently elevated metabolic demand during critical illness.

Therefore, it is reasonable to propose the concept of limit L, previously introduced as the antioxidant-prooxidant threshold, as a potential, albeit currently theoretical, therapeutic target. In the absence of definitive evidence, the current body of literature forces clinicians to rely on more practical objectives. This is precisely what some researchers have done, producing numerous studies that converge on a key clinical conclusion (34), (535): three grams. This is the minimum intravenous dose required to restore a functional plasma concentration of vitamin C. Specifically, some data suggest that a single infusion of 3 grams leads to plasma concentrations of approximately 68 micromoles/L (34), (535). Although transient, this equivalence is critical, as the profound metabolic imbalance associated with critical illnesses and the short half-life of vitamin C require frequent dosages to maintain sufficient levels. Not surprisingly, most experimental protocols involve intravenous administration every 6 hours.

The equation 3 g = 68 micromoles/L is important both because it provides useful guidance for clinicians and because it illustrates the severity of the metabolic earthquake induced by critical illness, which seriously impairs the accumulation of ascorbic acid through various mechanisms: increased cellular metabolism, massive oxidative stress and alterations in SVCT function. Notably, one of the main causes of SVCT dysfunction in critical illness is the cascade of pro-inflammatory cytokines, a hallmark of all critical conditions, which also explains the ineffectiveness of the oral route. Specifically, dysfunction of the intestinal SVCT1 transporter impairs gastrointestinal absorption, thereby compromising systemic bioavailability (451), (63), (298).

As a side note, this mechanism will be explored in greater depth, particularly the way in which TNF alpha overexpression downregulates SVCT1 in various clinical contexts not limited to critical illness, such as certain inflammatory bowel diseases (298).

Returning to the concept of a metabolic earthquake, let us consider some telling numbers. In healthy volunteers, an intravenous dose of 3 grams of vitamin C has been shown to yield plasma concentrations of 1760 micromoles/L (22). This value, which is approximately 26 times higher than the 68 micromoles/L found in critical illnesses, provides a clear indication of the extremely high metabolic consumption that characterises a critical illness. Moreover, the 1760-68 discrepancy reinforces the inadequacy of oral administration in critically ill patients, and provides irrefutable evidence that critical conditions maximise the oral-intravenous pharmacokinetic gap.

Therefore, the evidence strongly suggests: no to the nutritional approach, yes to the pharmacological one, at least when life is at stake.

Sepsis

Paul Marik described this paragraph as “a comprehensive review”, acknowledging its scientific relevance and connection to his recent studies. While until a few years ago the experimental and clinical use of pharmacological ascorbic acid was mainly focused on cancer treatment, recently there has been a great deal of interest in the treatment of another highly insidious disease: sepsis. It is a particularly severe clinical condition, albeit perhaps less well-known than other major pathologies. Consider that in the United States, 750000 people are hospitalized each year with a diagnosis of sepsis, a frightening figure accompanied by mortality rates ranging from 20% for sepsis to 60% for its most feared complication, septic shock. Although less known than other diseases, sepsis is characterized by high mortality rates, five times higher than that of stroke and ten times higher than myocardial infarction. In addition to short-term mortality, septic patients often develop numerous long-term complications, frequently experiencing reduced quality of life and increased risk of death for up to five years after the acute event. For example, about 50% of sepsis survivors develop post-sepsis syndrome, characterized by the onset of cognitive disorders (168).

Sepsis is an organ dysfunction caused by the body's dysregulated response to infection, and its course depends on a complex network of interactions involving the infecting microorganism, the immune system, inflammatory responses, and coagulation. To appreciate its insidious nature, it suffices to consider that over the past 30 years, numerous phase 2 and phase 3 clinical trials have been conducted to evaluate new therapeutic interventions in the management of patients with sepsis or septic shock. Unfortunately, all these efforts have failed to yield a new pharmacological model that is truly effective in reducing organ failure and, more importantly, in increasing survival rates (169). The treatment of sepsis essentially involves controlling the underlying infection and supporting vital functions. Marik's statement is particularly noteworthy, namely the fact that a factor consistently involved in both the pathogenesis and clinical evolution of sepsis has been systematically overlooked: oxidative stress, "The central role of ROS has been ignored" (170).

It remains unclear why scientific research has failed to assign a meaningful role to oxidative stress, despite a growing body of evidence increasingly pointing to the central harmful impact of ROS (170). Nevertheless, some researchers have pursued this direction, opening a scenario in which vitamin C appears to possess the biological properties necessary to play a significant role against sepsis. So, what is the current state of scientific evidence?

In recent years, Marik and other scientists have conducted a series of studies on the so-called HAT therapy (also known as the Marik protocol), an intravenous treatment combining corticosteroids, vitamin C, and thiamine (vitamin B1). "The premise behind HAT therapy is the use of a combination of readily available, safe and cheap agents that target multiple components of the host's response to an infectious agent such that they synergistically restore the dysregulated host immune response, neutralize damaging oxidants, and restore mitochondrial function", said Marik (170). From this statement, it is evident that the use of AA in the treatment of sepsis is justified by several biological mechanisms, beginning with the correction of a probable deficiency.

Speaking of deficiency states, many studies have found extremely low ascorbic acid levels in septic patients, often compatible with acute scurvy (34), (170), (171). This is a particularly significant finding: some studies report that virtually all septic patients exhibit insufficient plasma concentrations, with "insufficient" conventionally defined as a plasma value < 50 micromoles/L. These data become even more alarming when considering that 40% of septic patients have levels below 11 micromoles/L, and 90% fall below 23 micromoles/L (34), (170). What consequences may arise from these deficiencies?

Failure to restore physiological concentrations may lead to serious complications due to the impairment of numerous AA-dependent physiological functions. The idea that low AA levels can significantly disrupt physiology may seem exaggerated to some; however, the scientific evidence is increasingly clear. Critically ill patients with low AA levels can experience devastating consequences, including increased vasopressor requirements, acute kidney injury, and an exaggerated inflammatory response. AA levels in critically ill patients are believed to be inversely correlated with CRP, the main inflammatory biomarker, and possibly with procalcitonin, the specific biomarker of sepsis (34), (171). Furthermore, low AA levels increase the risk of multiple organ dysfunction syndrome and are associated with higher SOFA scores and mortality rates (450), (34), (160), (161), (165), (170).

There are solid biological reasons underlying these data. The typical deficiency state in septic patients is due to four main factors: massive oxidative stress, increased cellular metabolism, inefficient renal reabsorption, and SVCT downregulation triggered by inflammation and oxidative stress. A fifth factor is the intensive drug therapy commonly administered in critical care, whose effects impose such extreme stress that, in animals, they would trigger a compensatory increase in biosynthesis, a mechanism that humans, unfortunately, lack (29), (30), (31).

What are the specific effects of vitamin C? Is it merely a powerful antioxidant?

The sepsis model is epistemologically and didactically ideal, as it challenges the reductionist view of vitamin C as merely an antioxidant. First, it is important to underscore the notion of a priority antioxidant: AA provides the first line of antioxidant defense against oxidative stress, indirectly preserving key endogenous antioxidants such as glutathione, vitamin E, and even BH4 (critical for endothelial function). This makes AA an ideal candidate for countering the massive oxidative stress characteristic of sepsis.

With respect to oxidative stress, an important implication involves mitochondrial protection, as mitochondrial dysfunction is associated with clinical deterioration. Vitamin C may act specifically through two mechanisms: first, by reducing mitochondrial oxidative damage through DHA, its only form able to penetrate mitochondria (via GLUT1). This is crucial because the mitochondrial respiratory chain is a major source of ROS, and limiting mitochondrial damage could provide clinical benefit (170).

Second, vitamin C participates in the biosynthesis of carnitine, an amino acid derivative essential for the transport of fatty acids into the mitochondrial matrix (172). Carnitine deficiency could result in additional complications, as suggested by studies in which its intravenous administration produced benefits in septic shock (170).

Even in its antioxidant role, vitamin C proves to be unique. Why?

Its administration has often led to a reduction in inflammatory and oxidative biomarkers, an effect not generally observed with NAC or other powerful antioxidants (173).

Vitamin C may support a septic organism in several other ways: through its immunomodulatory activity (regulation of proinflammatory cytokine synthesis), its role as a cofactor in catecholamine and vasopressin biosynthesis, its antimicrobial properties, its endothelial protective capacity, and its antihistamine action. In fact, high histamine levels have been observed to contribute to the progression of sepsis (567).

Overall, vitamin C can be considered a pharmacological tool so versatile as to effectively counteract a complex condition such as sepsis. Consider, for instance, its role in vasopressor synthesis. During sepsis, noradrenaline levels decrease in animals lacking ascorbate, which aligns with its role as a cofactor for dopamine beta-hydroxylase. This suggests that adequate supplementation may enhance catecholamine biosynthesis, especially noradrenaline. Such stimulation is essential in the presence of refractory hypotension, whose improvement often depends on sufficient catecholamine levels. Refractory hypotension is notoriously difficult to manage and is one of the hallmarks of progression toward septic shock (defined as sepsis with hypoperfusion and hypotension refractory to fluid replacement therapy). Against this complication, pharmacological use of catecholamines, particularly noradrenaline, remains the mainstay of treatment; it effectively increases heart rate and cardiac contractility, thereby raising blood pressure.

Another strategy against refractory hypotension is the use of vasopressin (ADH), whose levels, however, decline sharply in the late stages of sepsis (91), (174). It is not surprising that vitamin C could provide further support: as a cofactor of the enzyme responsible for synthesizing ADH (PAM), it can increase ADH levels and thus enhance vasoconstriction, contributing to blood pressure maintenance (91). This mechanism, combined with the synthesis of noradrenaline, also dependent on AA, may offer a dual contribution in managing severe septic hypotension. Interestingly, this dual mechanism suggests a powerful synergy whereby the pharmacological requirements for both noradrenaline and vasopressin could be significantly reduced.

The crucial role of AA in the biosynthesis of noradrenaline and ADH underscores a key pharmacodynamic property: promoting endogenous biosynthesis, which is generally preferable to exogenous pharmacological replacement. As will be discussed later, this is part of a broader "saving system" through which various pharmacological agents may benefit. This is one of the main reasons why vitamin C is considered a potentially valuable adjuvant agent.

Now, consider the following logic: the biosynthesis of ADH and noradrenaline requires AA, which, however, is almost completely depleted by sepsis (recall that 90% of septic patients suffer from hypovitaminosis). In combination with the inefficacy of the oral route, this necessarily implies the use of intravenous ascorbate. In other words, intravenous therapy appears indispensable in sepsis, and the triad refractory hypotension-strong vasoconstrictive capacity of ADH and noradrenaline-AA is the most substantial evidence of this.

Additional clinical benefits may derive from AA's ability to reduce cortisol secretion under stress, a phenomenon well-documented in previously commented research (25), (26). Modulation of cortisol levels has been associated with a more balanced immune profile and a reduced risk of clinical deterioration (175).

But there is more: AA protects the endothelial barrier (highly vulnerable in sepsis) and enhances the function of lymphocytes and neutrophils, attenuating two key contributors to multiple organ dysfunction syndrome, neutrophil necrosis and the formation of neutrophil extracellular traps.

Furthermore, AA effectively regulates NF-kB, a transcription factor central to the immune response to infection. Through its modulation of HIF-1 alpha and its strong antioxidant properties, AA helps prevent NF-kB dysregulation, thereby mitigating the inflammatory cascade (170), (177). In relation to inflammation, it is worth noting that AA supports TREG cells, crucial in modulating immune balance and mitigating the hyperinflammation typical of sepsis (126). This is due to its ability to promote TREG differentiation via DNA demethylation mechanisms.

Taken together, these findings establish the biological plausibility of incorporating pharmacological vitamin C into the therapeutic arsenal against sepsis. What, then, has clinical research shown?

A phase 1 randomized trial involving 24 patients with severe sepsis evaluated different intravenous ascorbate doses (0, 50, or 200 mg/kg/24 h), revealing rapid reductions in SOFA scores and inflammatory biomarkers CRP and procalcitonin (171). The study confirmed the safety of the therapy and demonstrated a dose-dependent effect: patients who received 200 mg/kg/24 h had significantly lower SOFA scores than those receiving 50 mg/kg/24 h.

As for HAT therapy, a 2016 retrospective analysis (176) showed that early use of this metabolic multi-therapy (200 mg hydrocortisone, 400 mg thiamine, and 6 g AA daily intravenously) may effectively prevent organ dysfunction, including acute kidney injury, and reduce mortality in septic shock patients. The numbers are striking: mortality was 8.5% in the HAT group versus 40.4% in the control group (176).

It is important to note that all experimental protocols rely on intermittent use of pharmacological vitamin C, consistent with its short half-life. HAT therapy, for example, involves dividing the 6 g dose into four 1.5 g infusions every 6 hours (170).

A different regimen was tested in a 2016 RCT in which 28 septic shock patients were treated with 25 mg/kg intravenous AA every 6 hours for 3 days. Results were impressive: 28-day mortality was 14.3% in the ascorbate group versus 64.3% in the control group (448), (177). In addition to this significant difference, the study demonstrated that ascorbic therapy enhances noradrenaline synthesis. A subsequent meta-analysis confirmed a significant benefit of intravenous vitamin C in reducing mortality and the need for vasopressors (178).

Clinical research has intensified in recent years. Of particular interest is a large 2019 multicenter, randomized, double-blind study (449), (177). It assessed pharmacological vitamin C as monotherapy in 167 patients with sepsis or acute respiratory distress, a serious condition that causes severe respiratory failure. Participants received either placebo or 50 mg/kg intravenous ascorbate every 6 hours for 4 days. Results showed significantly reduced all-cause mortality at 28 and 60 days (29.8% vs. 46.3%) (449), (177), and decreased mechanical ventilation time in the ascorbate group. However, there were no significant differences in SOFA scores. Notably, the authors did not mention the 46.3%-29.8% mortality reduction in the article abstract (published in "JAMA"), as if it were a trivial finding (449).

A meta-analysis (370) published in December 2021 in "The American Journal of Emergency Medicine" produced a different view on SOFA scores. Analyzing 10 clinical trials and a total of 1400 participants, it concluded that vitamin C (monotherapy) may improve SOFA scores and protect septic patients' organs.

However, as often occurs in the scientific world, the data are conflicting: some studies have not demonstrated significant benefits, offering an opportunity for constructive criticism, specifically regarding the association between disappointing results and the inappropriate use of vitamin C. Among these, a study from 2022 stands out (372). In this study, intravenous vitamin C was evaluated as monotherapy (1 g intravenous bolus followed by 250 mg per hour via continuous infusion for 96 hours, i.e., 7 g per 24 hours) in the treatment of septic shock. Although it reduced all-cause mortality at 28 days, the difference

(26.7% in the vitamin C group versus 40.6% in the placebo group) did not reach statistical significance. In this regard, I would like to offer several observations:

1- A dose of 7 g/24 h may be insufficient, especially considering that septic shock is a more severe condition than sepsis, which appears to benefit from daily doses ranging between 100 and 200 mg/kg (i.e., 7-14 g per 24 hours);

2- Unfortunately, the study presents a recurrent limitation: the absence of plasma vitamin C measurements. "We did not measure serum vitamin C levels, so we are unable to assess the rate of pre-existing hypovitaminosis in the study subjects or the degree of increase in vitamin C levels following supplementation", the authors stated (372). Is this really a negligible limitation? Septic shock, the most severe complication of sepsis, is associated with a significant increase in mortality due to profound circulatory and metabolic abnormalities, which predispose patients to the dreaded multiple organ dysfunction syndrome. Its capacity to deplete AA is maximal, which implies that failure to restore adequate plasma concentrations would result in disrupted ascorbate physiology and, consequently, no pharmacological effect. Therefore, this omission represents a potentially significant methodological limitation. In this context, pre- and post-treatment plasma measurements would have provided objective parameters upon which to base clinical interpretation. Their absence, in my view, renders the study's conclusions unreliable;

3- Based on intravenous pharmacokinetics, mathematical modeling suggests that intermittent infusions (e.g., every 4-6 hours) produce higher average plasma concentrations than continuous infusion, which was the method used in this study. This phenomenon has been observed in various pharmacokinetic analyses, including a 2018 study published in "Chest" (392);

4- Although it did not meet formal statistical significance, vitamin C administration resulted in a 13.9% absolute reduction in mortality (372).

Moreover, the variable of treatment duration has often been underestimated in clinical research. In many studies (such as (372)), AA therapy was administered for only 96 hours, a timeframe likely too short to achieve an effective response. This is a personal consideration, yet it seems to find scientific support. A notable confirmation comes from an impressive cohort study published in "Critical Care" in January 2022 (394). This study analyzed the clinical data of 384282 septic patients admitted to ICUs between 2017 and 2019, demonstrating that intravenous vitamin C monotherapy, when extended to at least five days, can significantly reduce mortality during hospitalization and at 90-day follow-up. Given vitamin C's excellent safety profile, it remains unclear why studies have employed such a short treatment window.

Let me highlight two important points: the rapid and massive depletion of AA during sepsis, and its rapid renal excretion when administered intravenously. These points suggest that, once intravenous administration is stopped, AA plasma levels may quickly fall to scorbutic levels, thereby compromising the patient's condition once again. Therefore, a 96-hour treatment course may be insufficient. Why not extend the therapy until the patient has fully recovered? What disadvantages would a longer treatment duration entail?

Furthermore, what harm would result from a more aggressive strategy, using, for example, a dose never before tested in sepsis, such as 100 mg/kg every 6 hours?

In any case, the most recent meta-analyses (583), (584) are particularly noteworthy as they generally, though not entirely consistently, support the potential pharmacological independence of vitamin C in the treatment of sepsis, especially in its more severe forms. This finding suggests a possible separation from corticosteroids and vitamin B1, which are typically included in the HAT therapy protocol.

Regarding vitamin B1, it is worth noting that it supports fundamental biological processes, including the Krebs cycle. Notably, deficiency of this vitamin is observed in approximately 40% of septic patients, a condition that exacerbates mitochondrial oxidative stress and inflammation, two key mechanisms that reinforce the rationale for its supplementation (170). These findings suggest that HAT therapy aligns with the orthomolecular approach, as it aims to restore compounds that become depleted during severe illness. The concept of replenishing vitamins that are deficient in critically ill patients appears eminently rational. Indeed, restoring physiological levels may provide essential support to an organism experiencing metabolic derangements, potentially enhancing the effectiveness of pharmacological interventions. This reasoning formed the theoretical foundation of megavitamin therapy, as proposed by Hoffer and Cathcart, and could pave the way for promising clinical developments, potentially transforming the management of critical illness.

Historically, vitamin C paved the way in this field, followed, as you may recall, by Hoffer's high-dose vitamin B3 treatments. Today, considerable interest is also focused on vitamin B1 and vitamin D, the latter now recognized as essential for a range of extra-skeletal functions, so much so that it is increasingly compared to a hormone, a term that also reflects the biological role of vitamin C in animals. This evolution challenges the outdated equation "vitamins = nutritional elements" and supports the updated view "high-dose vitamins = pharmacological agents", precisely as the orthomolecular scientists had envisioned.

Returning to the clinical studies on sepsis, we can draw one final and important confirmation: no studies reported significant side effects, not even an increased risk of kidney stones (177), (583). Therefore, vitamin C appears to be cheap, safe, and potentially effective.

Lastly, we must emphasize a fundamental issue: scurvy remains an underrecognized yet real and present threat in septic patients. This concern is strongly underscored by two prominent experts, Marik and Hooper, authors of a paper published in "Critical Care" with the emblematic title: "Doctor, your septic patients have scurvy!" (557).

Burns

A burn is a skin injury caused by intense exposure to heat or other harmful sources. It is a clinical condition that can trigger a severe inflammatory response and the extravasation of fluids and proteins into the interstitial space, the supportive fluid-filled region that surrounds and separates the body's cells. This extravasation often requires the administration of large fluid volumes, thereby increasing the risk of edema, an abnormal accumulation of fluid in the interstitial space that leads to swelling and impaired tissue function (179).

Burns therefore represent a particularly challenging clinical issue. Although certain mathematical models, most notably the Parkland formula, have improved treatment protocols and potentially reduced the risk of edema, the latter remains a significant therapeutic complication. The term "fluid creep", coined to describe the unintentional fluid overload frequently observed in burn patients, is concrete evidence of this issue (184).

Given the risks of edema, the intense oxidative stress and severe inflammation, the use of vitamin C in this clinical context appears highly plausible. Numerous studies have identified it as a doubly beneficial tool, potentially capable of both reducing oxidative stress and decreasing fluid loss into the interstitial space. It is important to emphasize that limiting fluid loss is a critical therapeutic goal, as it reduces the total fluid requirement in burn patients and thereby significantly lowers the risk of edema (180). This highlights a key pharmacodynamic feature of ascorbic acid: its ability to reduce pharmacological requirements, a phenomenon already demonstrated with amiodarone in the prophylaxis of postoperative atrial fibrillation (147), and especially with the vasopressin-noradrenaline combination in the management of sepsis.

Numerous animal studies have produced encouraging data. For example, a 1991 study (180) conducted on guinea pigs with third-degree burns covering 70% of their body surface analyzed three intravenous dosages: 170, 340 and 680 mg/kg. Vitamin C proved effective at all tested doses, reducing fluid requirements while maintaining normal cardiac function (180).

Over time, studies in other animal models (including dogs and sheep (184)) have consistently shown positive outcomes. A pivotal moment came in 2000, when a noteworthy clinical study (181) was conducted on 37 patients with severe burns (> 30% total body surface area) admitted to a Japanese ICU. The patients treated with vitamin C received two distinctive therapeutic features: early intervention and, above all, a novel therapeutic magnitude, continuous infusion at a rate of 66 mg/kg/h for 24 hours, totaling 1584 mg/kg/24 h, equivalent to 110880 mg in a 70 kg adult. This is a dosage typically reserved for oncology settings, although infused here at a much slower rate.

Cardiovascular parameters, such as heart rate, blood pressure and central venous pressure, along with renal and hepatic function, were not adversely affected, confirming once again that even massive, acute administration of vitamin C is safe and does not trigger the much-feared pro-oxidant effects. Conversely, the reduction in serum levels of malondialdehyde, a key marker of oxidative stress, has provided further support for the notion that the potential pro-oxidant effects of millimolar concentrations are likely selective and limited to tumor environments (181). In essence, vitamin C megatherapy was safe, not associated with oxidative stress, and, most importantly, clinically effective: while it did not significantly reduce mortality, early high-dose administration decreased fluid needs, reduced wound edema, and lessened the severity of respiratory failure. The authors noted: "In our small series, there were numerically fewer deaths in the ascorbic acid group at 7 days after injury and fewer fasciotomies as well, which we find encouraging. We believe that this new therapy is also effective in much more serious cases" (181).

At the dawn of the 21st century, the foundations were thus laid for a potentially revolutionary therapy in the treatment of burns. However, it took a full 19 years from that moment to more rigorously examine the impact of vitamin C in the management of severe burns. In 2019, a major cohort study was published in "Critical Care" (182). According to the study, doses of vitamin C ranging from 10 to 24 grams may significantly reduce mortality in patients with severe burns (182). In addition to confirming the importance of timing (already emphasized in other acute conditions such as viral infections, cardiac arrest and sepsis), the study re-proposed the concept of a sigmoidal response, suggesting that there may be a dosage threshold beyond which efficacy plateaus. This appears to partially contradict the principle of dose-dependence. However, the authors caution that this finding may reflect limited statistical power: "It can be assumed that if more patients had been included in the study, we could have reached statistical significance" (182).

The paragraph concludes with a 2021 review (476), which confirmed that both high dosage and early administration are essential for achieving clinical benefits, such as reduced fluid needs and accelerated healing time.

Trauma and haemorrhagic shock

The vibrant life of Irwin Stone included a serious car accident in the early 1960s involving both him and his wife. He was severely injured and attributed his survival to the megadoses of vitamin C he regularly took: "My wife and I were seriously injured, and the only reason we survived is that we had been regularly taking megadoses of ascorbic acid for decades", he stated on several occasions.

Over time, Stone underwent numerous surgeries without complications and attributed his rapid recovery to these megadoses, emphasizing that the massive (or perhaps appropriate?) use of vitamin C had protected him from the potentially fatal risk of hemorrhagic shock during the traumatic incident.

Severe trauma, the leading cause of death between ages 1 and 44, and its major complication, hemorrhagic shock (a condition marked by sudden blood loss and profound hypovolemia) are medical emergencies triggering coagulopathy, inflammation and strong oxidative stress. Hemorrhagic shock is associated with profound vitamin C depletion, providing a clear rationale for its prompt replenishment. Such replenishment may help limit oxidative damage and related complications. It is no coincidence that vitamin C has been explored for hemorrhagic shock management since the 1940s, recognized for its regulatory effects on inflammation, oxidative cascades, and coagulation pathways. This hypothesis was first proposed by De Pasqualini in a groundbreaking 1946 report (183), a paper of considerable historical importance. At the time, vitamin C was still regarded purely as a micronutrient, and the scientific community was primarily focused on its role in preventing scurvy. In contrast, De Pasqualini outlined a pharmacological use of vitamin C in emergency medicine, an approach that paralleled the pioneering work of Frederick Klenner, who, around the same period, advocated high-dose vitamin C therapy for poliomyelitis.

Returning to the present, several studies have evaluated ascorbic acid in models of hemorrhagic shock. One such model (184) randomized animals to receive either intravenous saline, low-dose intravenous AA (50 mg/kg), or high-dose intravenous AA (200 mg/kg). The saline group (control) exhibited the worst outcomes in terms of cellular damage, oxidative stress, and inflammation (184).

Another animal model demonstrated a notable nephroprotective effect of vitamin C, consistently with the previously discussed studies that have linked low ascorbate levels to acute kidney injury (160), (165). In this model, the protective effect was attributed not only to its antioxidant activity but also to the activation of SIRT-1, a protein critically involved in cellular defense through epigenetic mechanisms (184), (185). SIRT-1, a member of the sirtuin family, is thought to counteract oxidative stress and inflammation, thereby providing potent antioxidant protection and substantial mitochondrial support to cells. Recent evidence suggests that elevated concentrations of ascorbic acid may markedly enhance SIRT-1 activity, thereby broadening the spectrum of cellular antioxidant defenses (184), (185).

Hemorrhagic shock models have also demonstrated that AA increases expression of heme oxygenase-1 (HO-1), an inducible stress-response enzyme primarily expressed in the liver and kidneys in response to cellular stress. AA-induced overexpression of HO-1 appears to act as a powerful compensatory mechanism, protecting tissues from typical hemorrhagic shock complications (184). Therefore, high doses of AA seem to activate both SIRT-1 and HO-1, thus considerably improving cellular defence mechanisms.

Pretreatment with ascorbic acid has shown organ-protective effects in several studies. In models of hemorrhagic shock, the intestine and stomach exhibited a significant reduction in inflammation and bleeding when pretreated with AA (184). These findings support Stone's claim: the elevated AA levels in his tissues could indeed have made his body more resistant to trauma and bleeding.

As often happens in research, conflicting results do exist, often due to methodological inconsistencies. For example, in one murine model, pre-shock intravenous AA at 10 mg/kg showed no significant benefit (184), (517). The dosage issue is evident: 10 mg/kg translates to 700 mg in a 70 kg human, far too low to restore deficient plasma levels. "Although an effect of oxygen free radicals on liver tissue could be found during and after hemorrhagic shock, treatment with ascorbic acid alone, in our model, failed to ameliorate the recovery of the animals upon resuscitation", reported the authors of a 1996 study (517). How could such a low dose counteract such a massive injury (60 minutes of hemorrhagic shock can be biologically devastating)?

And more importantly, why use such a low dose given AA's extremely low toxicity? What risk would have been posed by dosages commonly used in animal models, typically 100 to 1000 mg/kg?

A 2018 study partially challenged the idea of strict dose-dependence (185). Researchers concluded that both 100 mg/kg and 500 mg/kg dosages provided similar nephroprotective benefits via SIRT-1 activation, confirming the mechanism, even though both doses were 10-50 times higher than the ineffective 10 mg/kg dose used in the 1996 study (517).

With regard to traumatic brain injury (TBI), ascorbic acid appears to be a highly promising therapeutic agent. TBI is characterized by intense inflammation and oxidative stress, two factors that rapidly deplete vitamin C stores and may contribute to a worse prognosis (362). A study published in "Stroke" demonstrated that plasma levels of vitamin C decrease in proportion to the size of the lesion, whereas levels of other antioxidant vitamins remain largely unchanged (526). This reveals a significant, proportional, and selective depletion, underscoring the key role of AA in managing oxidative stress (362).

Overall, the preliminary data are very promising: numerous preclinical studies suggest that high-dose intravenous administration of ascorbic acid may mitigate oxidative damage and cerebral edema. "Based on its mechanisms of action, animal data, and clinical results in critical illness, high-dose AA has exceptional potential to be an effective treatment strategy in the acute phase of TBI. It may be able to mitigate secondary brain injury due to its antioxidant, anti-inflammatory, and cell membrane-stabilizing properties, while the low adverse effect and cost profile of AA make it well suited for clinical studies in patients with TBI. A key challenge will be to identify the ideal TBI patient population that is most likely to benefit from this treatment strategy. Based on the existing data from related fields, patients with moderate to severe TBI, significant brain edema with elevated intracranial pressure, and the older adult population may represent ideal patient groups for high-dose intravenous AA in the acute setting" (362).

Surgery and analgesia

'In the perioperative phase, overlooking vitamin C borders on omission rather than caution'

Based on what has been observed so far, we can reasonably state that vitamin C may be a valuable adjunct in the context of surgery and the delicate postoperative period. As mentioned, surgery is a procedure that induces intense and multifaceted stress, leading to the depletion of numerous essential compounds. It has already been noted (383) that some studies associate severe vitamin deficiencies (particularly of vitamins C, D, and B1) with cardiovascular and orthopedic surgery. Among these compounds, vitamin C appears to be the most vulnerable to depletion caused by pathological conditions or intense stress such as that induced by surgery.

A 2022 meta-analysis (186) is particularly noteworthy for its evaluation of the postoperative decrease in plasma ascorbic acid concentrations. The findings revealed a drop of 18 micromoles/L within the first postoperative week and, more concerningly, a persistence of this depletion over the following 2-3 months. It would be extremely useful to evaluate this dynamic over longer periods (6-12 months) to address critical questions: does postoperative depletion remain stable over time? Can a sequence of stressful events progressively deplete vitamin C stores beyond what diet alone can replenish, thereby leading to a deficiency state?

Given this, monitoring the balance between vitamin C intake and loss seems rational, particularly under conditions that may jeopardize physiological equilibrium. This balance has been analyzed in detail in relation to surgical events. In uncomplicated procedures, for example, data suggest that 500 mg of vitamin C may be sufficient to increase plasma levels; however, in the presence of complications or during complex surgical procedures, much higher doses may be necessary to normalise plasma concentrations (34). A salient example is cardiac surgery, where vitamin C reductions of up to 80% have been observed, making repletion essential (383), (499), (165). These are significant numbers, suggesting that the oxidative stress associated with cardiac surgery produces such a marked increase in ROS that it underscores the critical role of vitamin C, particularly given its function as a “first-line ROS sink”.

An important observation: many studies have shown that other antioxidant vitamins are not depleted by surgery, a phenomenon observed in both surgical and non-surgical conditions, as previously discussed in relation to traumatic brain injury (526). This provides strong evidence for the predominant antioxidant role of vitamin C (499).

Restoring ascorbic acid levels could be particularly useful in major procedures such as cardiac surgery, especially when considering that its vigorous administration (e.g., 250 mg/kg in a 1994 clinical trial (547)) has often led to improved cardiac performance, shorter ICU stays and reduced mechanical ventilation time (165). Even lower doses have shown effectiveness: 2 g administered intravenously before cardiac surgery, followed by 1 g orally per day for four days, was associated with reduced complications and shorter hospital stays (498). In general, more and more studies support the importance of vitamin C supplementation in the context of cardiac surgery. Consider the very recent review published in the journal “Annals of Medicine and Surgery” (591), in which the authors stated the following: “There seems to be a beneficial effect of vitamin C supplementation in arrhythmias such as in postoperative atrial fibrillation, reduction of ICU length of stay, and hospital length of stay, reduction in postoperative ventilation time, in inotropic demand, and in postoperative fatigue. Vitamin C can act as a scavenger of free radicals to decrease lipid peroxidation in cell membranes, and to protect the myocardium postoperatively from ischemia/reperfusion injury, thus attenuating oxidative stress and inflammation" (591).

In addition to alleviating the severe oxidative stress associated with surgical procedures, vitamin C actively promotes surgical wound healing and may have substantial effects in containing intraoperative bleeding. This has been evaluated in several clinical studies, including a randomized placebo-controlled trial (402) in which a modest intravenous dose (1 g the evening before and 1 g during a total abdominal hysterectomy) resulted in a significant reduction in intraoperative blood loss. More generally, a 2022 meta-analysis indicated that its administration may reduce the rate of blood transfusion in gynecological surgery (597).

Specifically regarding surgical wound healing, an interesting study (497), conducted at a university hospital, revealed not only the high incidence of vitamin C deficiency among surgical patients but also very notable improvements in those with critically low levels (4-8 micromoles/L). In these patients, previously stalled wound healing resumed rapidly following supplementation, prompting the authors to report a "rapid and dramatic recovery of extensive and complicated wounds" and to summarize their findings as follows: "Our cases demonstrate that treating patients with ascorbic acid deficiency leads to a rapid improvement in the wound healing process after surgery, thus reducing the costs of elaborate wound care and prolonged hospitalisation" (497).

Vitamin C is also gaining attention for its potential role in pain management. For instance, a 2016 meta-analysis (187) found that preoperative oral AA (2 g/day) could reduce postoperative morphine requirements. This suggested a synergistic interaction between vitamin C and certain drug classes commonly used in postoperative pain management, a property still under-recognized by much of the medical community. The ability of AA to reduce morphine demand is thus added to the other synergies previously discussed, such as those with vasopressors in sepsis and with fluids in burns.

Furthermore, the same meta-analysis (187) provided a "high-level evidence" recommendation for vitamin C in the prophylaxis of complex regional pain syndrome (CRPS), a painful condition that can develop after surgery or injury, and is marked by ongoing, intense pain that is greater than expected for the original cause. Numerous RCTs have investigated AA's role in preventing CRPS, particularly in patients undergoing wrist or ankle surgery (189). If we were to summarize the results of these studies in a single word, it would be "remarkable": despite the use of very low doses (0.2-1.5 g/day orally for 48 days), significant prophylactic efficacy against CRPS has been demonstrated. It is reasonable to speculate that higher doses might have yielded even greater benefits. This hypothesis is supported by subgroup analyses, which found the risk reduction to be dose-dependent, with better outcomes observed in patients receiving more than 500 mg/day (189).

Very recently, a meta-analysis published in "The International Journal of Orthopaedic and Trauma Nursing" has strengthened the scientific evidence supporting the protective role of vitamin C against complex regional pain syndrome (590).

From a broader perspective, the body of literature on the analgesic effects of vitamin C is substantial. For instance, other studies have examined its intraoperative intravenous use in two particularly painful procedures: tonsillectomy and uvulopalatopharyngoplasty (a surgical treatment for obstructive sleep apnea). In both cases, the administration of 3 g of intravenous vitamin C during surgery resulted in a significant reduction in postoperative pain (188).

Taken together, the evidence for the analgesic role of vitamin C is compelling and suggests potential applications across various clinical settings. Supporting evidence, including its use in CRPS, acute and post-herpetic neuralgia (possibly linked to its antiviral effects (124)), Paget's disease and oncologic pain, suggests that vitamin C is a safe and effective analgesic, distinct from classic agents but capable of synergizing with them (189).

What are the mechanisms underlying this analgesic effect?

Vitamin C contributes to pain control via several mechanisms. The first involves its role in the synthesis of neurotransmitters essential for pain modulation, namely catecholamines and serotonin. Notably, serotonin-noradrenaline reuptake inhibitors (SNRIs) are among the most effective pharmacological agents for managing pain (190), highlighting the importance of these pathways.

A second mechanism is the reduction of ROS, which are known to disrupt normal pain signaling.

A third, and perhaps most intriguing, mechanism is vitamin C's involvement in the synthesis of opioid-like compounds known as opioid peptides. These include endorphins, enkephalins, and endomorphins, which mimic the structure and function of morphine and trigger powerful endogenous analgesic responses. Vitamin C's role becomes evident through its function as a cofactor for peptidylglycine alpha-amidating monooxygenase (PAM), the enzyme responsible for the synthesis and activation of certain opioid peptides. Through this pathway, vitamin C supports the biosynthesis and activation of natural analgesics, with a particularly notable role in the case of endomorphins (189).

Endomorphin-1 and -2 are opioid neurotransmitters predominantly expressed in the central nervous system. They are generally considered to possess high analgesic potency, with relatively few side effects and a low risk of dependence (189). These features suggest that the AA-PAM axis could represent a particularly refined and "intelligent" analgesic system. This view is supported by observations that tissues synthesizing endomorphins tend to contain the highest concentrations of AA, and that severe infections have been reported to deplete both AA and peptide hormones (471), raising the possibility of a causal link and highlighting the potential importance of the AA-PAM pathway in pain physiology.

Another mechanism relates to the role of vitamin C, via PAM, in the synthesis of calcitonin, a hormone that was once widely employed in the management of bone pain (189).

These mechanisms are backed by clinical findings: vitamin C has consistently reduced morphine requirements across several studies (189). Epidemiological support comes from a large American study involving 4742 individuals, which found an inverse correlation between plasma AA levels and various types of pain (472).

The analgesic properties of AA help clarify its interaction with commonly used drugs. These interactions are typically bimodal, enhancing therapeutic efficacy while reducing the required drug dosage. This is particularly evident with opioids: vitamin C has been shown to reduce opioid requirements and, consequently, their associated side effects. "The results of this meta-analysis demonstrated significant postoperative reductions in the need for opioids, as well as a decrease in the severity of pain in patients who received perioperative vitamin C, suggesting that vitamin C can be incorporated into the multimodal approach to postoperative pain control in surgical patients", concluded a recent meta-analysis, in which intravenous administration showed the most pronounced clinical effects (546).

A noteworthy implication is that, in general, no withdrawal symptoms have been reported in studies investigating the therapeutic association between opioids and vitamin C (189). This finding suggests that vitamin C may facilitate a gradual reduction in opioid use, often a challenging process, while still maintaining effective pain control. Remarkable, isn't it?

Even more surprising is a 2000 clinical study (191) in which oral megadoses of vitamin C at 300 mg/kg (21 g for a 70-kg individual) markedly improved withdrawal symptoms in heroin users. This dosage, unusual yet reported as safe and effective, highlights the therapeutic potential of the orthomolecular use of vitamin C. Notably, despite widespread concerns about the poor gastrointestinal tolerability of such high oral doses, the study found otherwise, with patients tolerating the regimen well throughout the treatment period.

Returning to its analgesic benefits, another study showed that patients with Paget's disease, a chronic disorder of abnormal bone remodeling, experienced significant pain reduction through daily intake of 3 grams (189). In the management of cancer-related pain, intravenous administration has proven to be markedly more effective: several studies have demonstrated that high-dose infusions can reduce both opioid consumption and pain intensity (189).

The multifaceted analgesic properties of vitamin C open up new possibilities in still underexplored areas, such as the treatment of Chikungunya, a mosquito-borne viral infection characterized by prolonged and debilitating joint pain. In one study, 56 infected patients underwent intravenous ascorbic acid infusions (25-50 g) combined with hydrogen peroxide therapy (3%), resulting in significant pain relief in most cases and, in 5 cases, even complete resolution (453).

Taken together, the potential analgesic role of vitamin C is receiving growing support, especially in the fields of oncology and postoperative care. Speaking of surgery, a comparative clinical trial (390) showed that 2 g intravenous AA was slightly more effective than 100 mg of aceclofenac (a well-known non-steroidal anti-inflammatory drug) in third molar surgery. One might wonder: what if 10 g had been used?

Reduction in the need for analgesics, shorter hospital stays, antioxidant and anti-inflammatory effects, prevention of cardiac arrhythmias and other cardiac events, infection prophylaxis, prevention of complex regional pain syndrome, improved postoperative recovery, promotion of surgical wound healing, reduction of intraoperative bleeding, and enhanced stress tolerance: these are all factors that should prompt consideration of vitamin C use, despite the lack of high-quality scientific evidence. From my perspective, the potential benefits that ascorbic acid therapy could offer in a postoperative setting are so numerous and diverse that they outweigh the uncertainty stemming from the absence of so-called high-quality evidence, which unfortunately is rarely pursued. In short, while awaiting large-scale studies, the accumulation of numerous small studies demonstrating multiple clinical benefits can form a solid logical basis, especially given the low toxicity of vitamin C. This logical foundation could temporarily stand in for traditional high-quality trials, which, regrettably, require substantial funding, funding that is difficult to secure for a low-cost substance like vitamin C.

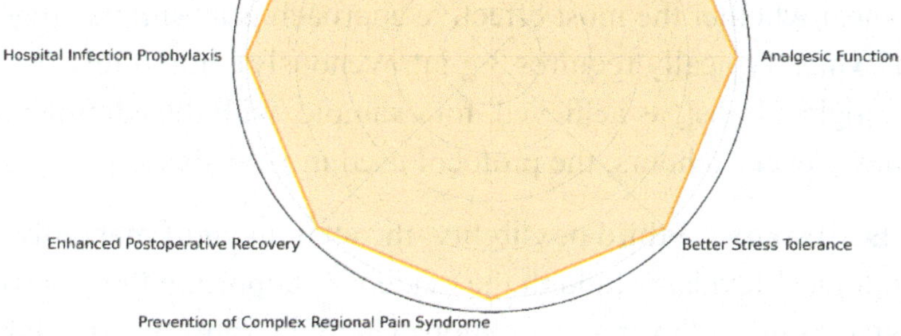

The final point in this section relates to a randomized, double-blind, controlled trial (192) in which 3 g intravenous AA reduced pulmonary complications following cardiac surgery, a common issue (10-25% incidence) often due to reperfusion injury. The protocol divided the 3 g dose into three 1 g administrations (10 minutes post-induction of anesthesia, 10 minutes pre-cardiac resuscitation, and post-sternal closure), highlighting the importance of dose fractionation. Regarding anaesthetic drugs, another clinical study showed that 67 mg/kg intravenous AA during surgery reduced the need for propofol, a widely used anesthetic with potentially significant side effects. This finding reinforces earlier preclinical results and further broadens ascorbic acid's range of pharmacological partnerships (461).

Returning to study (192), the dose-splitting approach aligns with AA's pharmacokinetics, underscoring a vital concept: scientific rigor is essential in vitamin C research. Neglecting any component of the critical tetrad of dose, mode, timing, and frequency can lead to misleading interpretations and unreliable conclusions.

The dire case of Allan Smith

The sensitivity that vitamin C exhibits toward a wide range of clinical conditions should no longer be surprising. It is a form of adaptive sensitivity, capable of intensifying under critical conditions, potentially pushing the affected individual toward scurvy. At the same time, this sensitivity highlights the inadequacy of the oral route for acute administration, thus opening favorable scenarios for the intravenous use of vitamin C.

As previously discussed, this context raises several clinically important questions. Among them is the question of the optimal administration protocol. It remains unclear whether the most effective approach is a "simple" physiological restoration (which typically requires 3 g intravenously) or a mildly supraphysiological boost, as achieved, for example, with the administration of 1.5 g intravenously every 6 hours, the protocol used in HAT therapy.

There is, of course, a third possibility: the attainment of markedly supraphysiological levels. Although the evidence supporting this approach is not yet conclusive, some authoritative opinions lend it credibility: "In addition to simply preventing scurvy by correcting vitamin C deficiency, supraphysiological levels of vitamin C can exert very strong multifaceted effects", wrote Spoelstra-de Man, Elbers and Oudemans-van Straaten in "Critical Care" in 2018 (160).

Until further research is conducted, we will have to rely on logical reasoning. Personally, I believe that the most reasonable approach involves careful and continuous monitoring of clinical responses according to the chosen therapeutic protocol. Such a dynamic strategy would allow the intensity of treatment to be escalated when required by the patient's condition, thereby leveraging all the qualities that make vitamin C a powerful and safe pharmacological agent. This echoes the classic advice of Linus Pauling, who once said: "If you are taking vitamin C and are not getting results, you should increase the dosage because it is likely that the amount administered has been insufficient to obtain the desired effect".

The emblematic case of New Zealand farmer Allan Smith fits perfectly into this framework and has even been featured on major television networks (540), (339). Smith had developed a severe form of pneumonia following the worsening of swine flu contracted during a vacation in Fiji. After several weeks in intensive care, his chances of survival were deemed virtually nonexistent.

High-dose intravenous vitamin C: this was the unconventional request made by Smith's family in response to the failure of conventional treatment. Initially dismissed by the medical team as a waste of time ("Vitamin C is a waste of time"), the request was reluctantly accepted. The response to 50 g of intravenous vitamin C profoundly redefined the concept of "waste of time", as Smith showed remarkable improvement in respiratory function.

Despite the progressive improvement in his condition with the daily 50 g regimen, the ascorbic therapy was inexplicably interrupted a few days later, at the request of a new physician who had taken over the case. A heated therapeutic controversy arose concerning Allan's survival: vitamin C was eventually resumed, but only at a very low dose of 1-2 g per day, which led to a worsening of his condition. It was only after legal intervention that the original high-dose therapy was reinstated, an action that ultimately led to his unexpected recovery.

This story raises a fundamental and pressing question: why does persistent skepticism still surround the pharmacological potential of a molecule as safe, inexpensive, and biologically versatile as vitamin C?

Chapter 7
Vitamin C In The Nervous System

Main functions in the nervous system

It has been shown that the central nervous system is the preferential site for vitamin C accumulation. This is mainly due to its remarkable capacity for local absorption and retention, two properties supported by specific homeostatic mechanisms capable of preserving vitamin C levels even in critical conditions, such as profound deficiency or severe brain disorders (78). Although our understanding of these mechanisms remains limited, it is known that the brain employs two major strategies to ensure adequate ascorbic acid levels in response to critical situations: the functional redistribution of tissue concentrations and the upregulation of SVCT2. This transporter, for instance, appears to be upregulated in neurons in response to cerebral ischemia (355).

In this context, the brain appears to respond to deficiency with remarkable resilience, provided that the deficiency remains reversible. For example, neurotransmitter levels remain unchanged during short-term deficits. However, prolonged deficiency tends to cause a significant reduction in dopamine and noradrenaline levels, and also exposes catecholamines to intense oxidative stress (193).

This remarkable conservation system allows us to underscore a sophisticated interconnection between vitamin C and glucose. In addition to their similar chemical structures and the metabolic dependence of vitamin C on glucose in the biosynthetic pathway of ascorbic acid, both molecules express homeostatic mechanisms aimed at ensuring a constant cerebral supply. The brain, in fact, consistently prioritizes the delivery of both glucose and ascorbic acid, especially under metabolic stress.

Importantly, brain physiology not only requires the sustained availability of both molecules, but also entails extremely high oxygen consumption, which inherently increases the risk of reactive oxygen species overproduction. While

ROS play physiological roles in neuromodulation and neurotransmission, they can also cause significant oxidative damage. The defense against ROS is one of the most crucial functions of vitamin C in the nervous system.

Vitamin C is the most abundant antioxidant in neurons and is often referred to as the "primary antioxidant". Several studies (550) have estimated that its neuronal concentration, approximately 10-12 millimoles, is significantly higher than that of other antioxidants, including glutathione, the most important endogenous intracellular antioxidant, whose neuronal concentration ranges from 2 to 3 millimoles. For this reason, vitamin C plays a multifaceted and highly effective antioxidant role, acting as a central defender of neuronal redox homeostasis. This is further supported by the recycling of ascorbate, which becomes particularly valuable in the brain due to its role in maintaining exceptionally high local concentrations. In fact, if there is one location where dehydroascorbic acid (DHA) becomes critically important, it is the central nervous system: this is demonstrated by the fact that certain cell populations rely exclusively on the oxidized form of vitamin C for uptake; more notably, DHA has the unique ability to rapidly cross the blood-brain barrier (BBB). The blood-brain barrier is a specialized endothelial interface between the bloodstream and brain tissue that tightly regulates the passage of substances, thereby protecting the brain from harmful compounds while allowing the entry of essential nutrients.

It is important to note that, unlike DHA, the penetration of ascorbic acid across the BBB appears to be significantly limited and slowed. This phenomenon, observed in numerous studies (61), (78), (213) and attributable to the lack of SVCT2 expression in the endothelial cells of the blood-brain barrier, tends to centralise the position of GLUT1 and GLUT3, the main transporters of DHA.

Returning to the topic of oxidative stress, vitamin C also plays a key role in supporting and protecting mitochondria, which are highly active in neuronal cells and serve as major sources of ROS. One notable example is superoxide, a highly reactive species generated by mitochondrial metabolism. The substantial accumulation of ascorbate in neurons enables the efficient neutralization of superoxide (78), a capacity that is notably reduced in tissues with lower vitamin C concentrations, as will be discussed later (438).

Additional antioxidant benefits of vitamin C are observed in aqueous compartments, where it participates in the regeneration of vitamin E, an essential factor in lipid protection. Given the high lipid content of brain tissue, this interaction plays a key role in maintaining membrane stability and overall neural integrity.

Vitamin C has also been implicated in neural development. Studies in rats have shown that cerebral ascorbate levels double during late pregnancy, suggesting its involvement in brain maturation. Furthermore, AA has been shown to enhance the differentiation of embryonic stem cells (78), (194). Interestingly, no other antioxidant has replicated this effect, which suggests that the process may not be solely dependent on general redox activity, or perhaps that ascorbate's antioxidant properties are uniquely effective.

Among its numerous roles, one often overlooked function of vitamin C in the nervous system is its involvement in the biosynthesis of carnitine. Carnitine, an amino acid derivative fundamental for the transport of fatty acids into mitochondria, can considerably impact neural function. Several animal studies have revisited its role, showing that supplementation can reduce hypoxia-induced oxidative stress, cognitive decline and even the overexpression of HIF-1 alpha (335). Further evidence comes from research on acetyl-L-carnitine, a more bioavailable form of carnitine with recognized neuroprotective properties, which has demonstrated, among other effects, neuroprotective actions including the enhancement of cognitive performance and the promotion of recovery following traumatic brain injury (335).

Ascorbic acid also plays a crucial role in neurotransmission, as it is deeply involved in the biosynthesis of catecholamines and serotonin in nervous tissue. This underscores a broader perspective, previously mentioned, suggesting that catecholamines, produced not only in the adrenal glands but also by neurons, serve functions that extend beyond their classical role in the stress response. Dopamine, for instance, is essential for motor control and reward mechanisms.

Despite growing evidence supporting these functions, many aspects of vitamin C's role in brain physiology remain poorly understood, some even enigmatic. Recent progress has been made in understanding its neuromodulatory function, particularly in relation to the interaction between vitamin C and glutamate, the brain's primary excitatory neurotransmitter. It has been under scientific scrutiny for quite some time due to a suspected association between its sodium salt (commonly known as monosodium glutamate, or MSG, widely used in the food industry as a flavor enhancer) and the onset of certain pathologies. What we currently know is that high levels of glutamate can indeed be harmful: several studies have reported that exposure to elevated concentrations of glutamate can trigger a phenomenon of severe neuronal toxicity, known as excitotoxicity.

Remarkably, vitamin C has shown the ability to counteract this toxicity, mainly due to its antioxidant properties and its capacity to modulate NMDA receptors, a key class of glutamate receptors. Experimental data suggest that vitamin C may inhibit the binding of glutamate to NMDA receptors (491), (492). While the underlying mechanisms are not fully clear, experiments confirm that ascorbate protects neurons from excitotoxicity triggered by NMDA receptor activation. This neuroprotective effect appears to involve a specific process known as the glutamate-ascorbate hetero-exchange, which may reduce excessive intracellular glutamate accumulation and, consequently, mitigate oxidative stress (78), (491), (492). Therefore, this strongly suggests that extracellular ascorbate concentrations are dynamically regulated by glutamate release. But how?

It appears that an increase in extracellular glutamate concentration triggers a substantial shift of AA into the extracellular fluid, likely as a compensatory mechanism to manage glutamate excess. For instance, in certain conditions or brain regions, ascorbate accumulation may inhibit intracellular glutamate uptake, thereby maintaining elevated glutamate concentrations in the extracellular space (78), (491), (493). One such region is the retina, as highlighted by an intriguing 2018 study published in the "Journal of Neurochemistry" (491).

It is important to note that reciprocal dynamics have also been documented, cases in which ascorbate is the first to accumulate in the extracellular space, such as in response to local injury. This was demonstrated in a compelling animal model (493), where glutamate was shown to functionally respond to an extracellular AA load, modulating its levels according to behavioral context. More specifically, exposure to varying light intensities (lights on vs. lights off) combined with AA supplementation at low and high levels revealed two key findings: in darkness, extracellular glutamate levels increased regardless of AA levels, while under light conditions, only high-dose AA led to a rise in extracellular glutamate (493).

These findings were further clarified in a 2022 study (494), which identified new mechanisms by which AA modulates glutamate levels. Specifically, AA appears capable of regulating the expression of GLT-1, the principal glutamate transporter in the brain.

Taken together, the ascorbate-glutamate hetero-exchange provides strong evidence for ascorbate's neuromodulatory role, with broad implications across various clinical contexts. One such context is cerebral edema, a serious condition characterized by excessive fluid accumulation in the brain. Some experimental models (357), based on the hypothesis that oxidative stress and glutamate NMDA receptor overactivation contribute to the disorder, have investigated the potential protective effects of vitamin C, proposing it as an effective neuroprotective agent. Notably, Brahma, Forman, Stewart, Nicholson and Rice, writing in the "Journal of Neurochemistry" (357) concluded: "These data demonstrate that brain edema, linked to glutamate-receptor activation, can result from intracellular oxidative stress and that this can be prevented by ascorbate".

This neuromodulatory role also highlights a crucial distinction between ascorbate's intracellular and extracellular activities. Inside the cell, AA primarily serves as a potent antioxidant; outside the cell, however, it seems to function as a neuromodulator (78). This duality illustrates the fundamental role of vitamin C in the nervous system, a role still not fully understood. For instance, although advanced imaging techniques have recently allowed for detailed mapping of ascorbate distribution in the brain, this has not yet clarified its neuromodulatory dynamics. The forebrain, a region with high AA concentrations and dense catecholaminergic innervation, has not shown a consistent correlation between extracellular AA and neurotransmitter levels. This continues to complicate efforts to understand the full scope of vitamin C's neuromodulatory functions (78).

Fortunately, in other areas, our understanding has received a significant boost in recent years through important scientific clarifications. Recent discoveries have highlighted that vitamin C is an essential factor for Schwann cells, the peripheral nervous system cells responsible for wrapping neuronal axons in an insulating layer known as myelin. Simply put, axons, the characteristic cellular extensions that allow neurons to transmit signals, are wrapped in a myelin sheath, forming the nerve fiber. In the peripheral nervous system, this sheath is produced by Schwann cells.

Vitamin C plays a crucial role in supporting the activity of Schwann cells, thus enabling axon myelination during development and remyelination following injury (195). This ability appears to depend largely on the epigenetic properties of vitamin C, which, as is well known, can promote DNA demethylation through the activation of TET enzymes. This epigenetic function, distinct from previously discussed immunological roles, is directed toward the regulation of genes associated with the insulating, protective structure known as myelin. Several studies support this hypothesis. One particularly striking observation involved hypomyelination of peripheral nerves caused by AA deficiency, which was rapidly reversed through correction of the deficiency. This intervention led to significant improvements in myelin-related gene transcription and in the expression of key myelin components, including myelin basic protein (195).

Taken together, these findings provide compelling evidence of vitamin C's critical role in myelination. This view is further strengthened by considering a well-known structural partner in myelin formation: collagen. In fact, it was collagen that initially suggested a potential role for AA in myelination processes, as early as the 1980s (205). The link lies in the extracellular matrix, rich in collagen, that makes up the basal lamina, a specialized extracellular structure adjacent to Schwann cells and considered essential for proper myelination (195), (205).

Thus, at least two vitamin C-mediated mechanisms appear to actively contribute to myelin formation, with potential therapeutic implications for diseases such as multiple sclerosis (196).

At this point, it is valuable to return to the topic of DNA demethylation, as recent findings are shedding extraordinary light on the world of vitamin C, an epigenetic radiance that may influence the treatment of a wide array of diseases, including cancer. This emerging perspective supports the growing field of nutrigenomics, the scientific discipline that explores the interaction between nutrients and gene expression. One illustrative example?

Consider how genetic variations in SVCT transporters can impair ascorbate uptake. This is a critical issue in nutrigenomics and simultaneously reinforces significant doubts about the ability of diet alone to ensure adequate tissue levels of vitamin C throughout the body. "Vitamin C may be more than simply a micronutrient in the central nervous system, since it is present in millimolar concentrations in neuron-rich areas", wrote Harrison and May in a seminal paper entitled "Vitamin C Function in the Brain: Vital role of the ascorbate transporter (SVCT2)" (78). This is both a scientifically authoritative and symbolically significant statement. It helps challenge the traditional, purely dietary conception of vitamin C and echoes the visionary thinking of Irwin Stone.

Alzheimer's disease

There are numerous neurodegenerative diseases. The most well-known are Alzheimer's disease, Parkinson's disease, multiple sclerosis and amyotrophic lateral sclerosis. Although pathophysiologically distinct, these conditions share several key features, including glutamate-mediated excitotoxicity and mitochondrial dysfunction (196). The presence of glutamate-mediated excitotoxicity is therefore the first element that supports a potential role for ascorbic acid in the treatment of neurodegenerative diseases. This is not the only relevant aspect: some animal studies have reported very promising experimental data regarding treatments with high doses of vitamin C, particularly in relation to the reduction of one of the hallmarks of Alzheimer's disease, namely, amyloid plaques.

There are also other theoretical considerations that seem to support the potential anti-Alzheimer's role of vitamin C: the neuronal tendency to absorb large amounts of it and its ability to modulate neuroinflammation are additional favorable factors (196).

Alzheimer's disease is considered to be the most common form of neurodegenerative dementia. It is a multifactorial condition characterized by cognitive deficits and neuronal loss, with an onset that depends on genetic, environmental and dietary factors. Given the biologically multifunctional nature of vitamin C, it is not surprising that numerous animal models have yielded encouraging data. For instance, an important study (549) evaluated the effects of vitamin C on neurodegeneration and memory impairment in a pharmacologically induced mouse model of Alzheimer's disease, via administration of the drug colchicine. Intraperitoneal administration of 200 and 400 mg/kg reduced memory impairment, presumably by mitigating neuroinflammation, and normalized several inflammatory biomarkers. However, the study revealed an unusual finding that appears to warrant caution with the use of high doses. Mice that received the

600 mg/kg dose showed moderate memory deterioration and signs of neuroinflammation in the hippocampus. This represents one of the very few experiments to report high doses of ascorbate as potentially "harmful", a phenomenon attributed by the researchers to a negative interaction with colchicine: "The results showed that vitamin C at lower doses had an antioxidant effect and at higher doses produced prooxidant effects in the context of Alzheimer's disease with colchicine-induced neurodegeneration" (549).

The anti-Alzheimer's role of ascorbic acid could be even broader. This is based on the fact that the disease's pathogenesis involves three key factors that vitamin C may help address: the presence of amyloid plaques, the breakdown of the blood-brain barrier, and mitochondrial dysfunction (197). In this regard, a study published in the prestigious journal "Nature" (197) investigated the effects of two different oral dosages (low and high) in mice lacking biosynthetic capacity and carrying familial Alzheimer's mutations. It was found that high-dose vitamin C administration reduced amyloid plaques by 50%, also helping to alleviate mitochondrial dysfunction. This effect is attributed to DHA, which, by entering the mitochondria via GLUT1, is able to protect them by effectively neutralizing mitochondrial ROS. Moreover, the high dose of vitamin C also reduced the breakdown of the blood-brain barrier (197).

In addition to confirming the effectiveness of vitamin C, these positive results also support the dose-dependent effect hypothesis, which suggests that the effects of ascorbate administration are proportional to the dose given, or, more precisely, to the plasma concentration. "These results suggest that vitamin C supplementation could be an important pharmacological avenue for the treatment of Alzheimer's disease and the optimal vitamin C dose is necessary for the prevention of Alzheimer's disease pathogenesis", the authors concluded (197). Therefore, the researchers refer to the "optimal dose", which may be the only one truly capable of reducing the risk of Alzheimer's disease. This further supports the value of the preventive strategy based on constant vitamin C supplementation.

Overall, this study appears highly relevant, offering both clinical and theoretical insights, including the recognition of the biological importance of DHA, the only form of vitamin C capable of acting within the mitochondria.

Unfortunately, there is a significant limitation regarding clinical data. It is not surprising that some authors (198) have found low levels of ascorbic acid in patients with Alzheimer's disease, levels that tended to be proportional to the degree of cognitive decline. These data support the main theorem about vitamin C, which states that its depletion is directly proportional to the severity of the underlying disease. The findings reported by Riviere, Birlouez-Aragon, Nourhashemi, and Vellas are particularly noteworthy (198): "In Alzheimer's patients living at home, plasma vitamin C levels decreased in proportion to the severity of cognitive impairment despite a constant dietary intake of vitamin C, while this was not observed with vitamin E, which remained substantially stable". These observations underscore the asymmetrical behaviour of the two antioxidant vitamins, highlighting the marked sensitivity of vitamin C to pathological conditions. But that's not all: the statement "Plasma vitamin C levels decreased in proportion to the severity of cognitive impairment despite constant intake" reopens the nutritional debate. These findings, in fact, raise further doubts about the adequacy of current nutritional recommendations (70-100 mg per day), at least in individuals affected by disease. As already noted, and as will be explored further, it is highly likely that the full restoration of ascorbic acid levels in a pathological state requires amounts well above the recommended daily allowance (RDA), sometimes making the use of pharmacological doses necessary, as in severe diseases.

From an epidemiological perspective, a large study conducted on 5000 participants demonstrated an inverse correlation: a high intake of ascorbic acid was associated with a reduced risk of Alzheimer's disease (196). The long follow-up period (six years) and the large sample size lend substantial credibility to these findings, making the inverse correlation particularly compelling (196). This research was followed by other studies with similar results: vitamin C supplementation (alone or in combination with vitamin E) reduced the risk of cognitive decline and Alzheimer's disease over extended observation periods (196). In contrast, a smaller study failed to demonstrate this inverse correlation (196).

Altogether, these findings call for a reevaluation of vitamin C's role not only as a nutrient, but as a targeted neuroprotective agent, especially in neurodegenerative contexts like Alzheimer's disease, where conventional treatments remain limited.

Parkinson's disease

Parkinson's disease is a neurodegenerative disorder that primarily affects motor control and balance. Its hallmark symptoms stem from the degeneration of dopamine-producing cells, particularly dopaminergic neurons, which makes it strongly associated with dopamine deficiency. However, the lack of dopamine, although critical, is not the sole determining factor. A potential link with vitamin C has emerged, related to a specific protein called alpha-synuclein, which plays a key biological role in regulating neurotransmitter trafficking at synapses. It is known that, when structurally altered or present in excessive amounts, alpha-synuclein can induce neurodegeneration via the formation of abnormal protein aggregates known as Lewy bodies. This feature supports the hypothesis that alpha-synuclein is closely associated with the pathogenesis and progression of certain neurodegenerative disorders such as Parkinson's disease.

Interestingly, alpha-synuclein appears to be responsive to vitamin C to some extent. One of the most significant processes involves mitochondrial dysfunction: it is hypothesized that the overexpression of alpha-synuclein increases the vulnerability of dopaminergic neurons to oxidative damage, thereby raising the risk of mitochondrial dysfunction. However, this condition may be alleviated by vitamin C (196), (199), (200).

Beyond these theoretical considerations, an intriguing 2021 animal study (469) revealed a novel potential role for vitamin C. The study focused on inflammasomes, multiprotein complexes that function as intracellular sensors of inflammation. First identified in 2002, inflammasomes respond to diverse stimuli by initiating pro-inflammatory cascades through the activation of specific cytokines. Among the various known inflammasomes, NLRP3 is the best-characterized and is most strongly implicated in inflammatory, autoimmune, metabolic, cardiovascular and neurodegenerative diseases (598).

At first glance, the connection between NLRP3 and vitamin C may appear tenuous. However, in the aforementioned study (469), its administration notably reduced neuroinflammation associated with Parkinson's disease. The authors attributed this effect to a decrease in NLRP3 inflammasome activity, revealing a relevant immunological mechanism through which vitamin C may attenuate the pro-inflammatory response driven by this potent inflammasome in specific pathological contexts.

From a clinical and epidemiological perspective, the picture appears more blurred compared to other areas, providing an opportunity to identify apparent inconsistencies in the theoretical foundations of vitamin C. One of the most striking inconsistencies comes from a study that contradicts prevailing theories on vitamin C, reporting unexpectedly normal plasma levels in Parkinson's disease patients (201). This is an atypical and scientifically intriguing finding, and it is not an isolated one. Other studies have confirmed this anomaly, reporting normal plasma concentrations but significantly reduced levels in lymphocytes, leading some scientists to propose lymphocyte AA concentration as a potential biomarker for Parkinson's disease (202). Is there a convincing explanation for this unusual phenomenon?

These asymmetries can be interpreted in at least three ways:

1- Parkinson's disease is one of the rare diseases that does not deplete ascorbic acid stores (which seems unlikely);

2- Plasma is not a reliable compartment for assessing systemic vitamin C status in Parkinson's patients;

3- The results may be due to computational or methodological errors in the studies (also unlikely).

The most plausible hypothesis is that the findings from (201) and (202) reflect a compensatory dynamic resulting from practical constraints. What does this mean?

It is reasonable to consider that patients with Parkinson's disease might exhibit normal plasma levels of vitamin C alongside reduced concentrations within lymphocytes. This observation raises several important questions, beginning with a critical reassessment of the convenient assumption (and it is indeed convenient, because measuring vitamin C levels in tissues is a complex procedure) that plasma concentration serves as a reliable indicator of systemic ascorbate status. Furthermore, one might ask: are there other diseases that display a similar discrepancy between plasma and intracellular ascorbate levels? And more provocatively: could Parkinson's disease involve a specific, possibly genetic, defect that impairs vitamin C transport into lymphocytes? If so, might this open a novel and precisely targeted avenue of investigation?

If it were confirmed that Parkinson's disease causes this unusual combination of normal plasma levels and low lymphocyte levels, we could be witnessing an atypical pattern of vitamin C distribution, where lymphocytes fail to retain it. In short, the portion of vitamin C not retained by lymphocytes might be redirected to the plasma. This would explain the paradoxical finding of normal plasma levels and suggest that the unassimilated fraction is not entirely lost. Therefore, it is plausible that the disease acts at the lymphocytic level, causing a defect in local uptake.

Recent studies seem to support this defective-filling hypothesis, highlighting a direct involvement of lymphocytes in the pathophysiology of Parkinson's, particularly a frequent reduction in T cell subpopulations (456), (382). This may represent a critical point for at least two reasons:

1- The strong immunological connection between AA and T cells (455), (116);

2- The association between abnormal lymphocyte profiles and greater vulnerability to Parkinson's disease (382).

Taken together, these elements provide a rational basis for the unusual finding of low lymphocyte ascorbate levels alongside normal plasma concentrations, suggesting, in a transversal way, a potential immune impairment. Parkinson's disease thus seems to form a biologically relevant triangular relationship involving:

1- Reduced lymphocyte vitamin C concentration;

2- Decreased lymphocyte count, especially T cells;

3- Reduced levels of TREGs, which modulate neuroinflammation.

In this context, intracellular vitamin C in lymphocytes may play a leading role. Adequate levels of lymphocytic ascorbate could help alleviate the neuroinflammatory state associated with Parkinson's disease through various mechanisms, most notably by promoting the function of TREGs. This anti-inflammatory role would complement the other contributions of vitamin C previously discussed, such as the neutralization of oxidative stress and the mitigation of mitochondrial dysfunction. Thus, a new perspective emerges: lymphocytic concentration, already proposed by some researchers as a potential biomarker, may indeed have clear pathophysiological and clinical significance (202).

At this point, a highly plausible question arises: is it possible to restore lymphocytic ascorbate levels even in the presence of an altered lymphocyte count?

In other words, could an intensive supplementation of AA, for example through intravenous administration, help restore the ascorbic levels of the entire lymphocytic architecture in patients with Parkinson's disease?

A possible answer to this question carries a fascinating implication: that normalizing lymphocyte ascorbate levels may require elevated plasma concentrations, suggesting that supraphysiological systemic levels might be necessary to effectively counteract the neuroinflammation associated with Parkinson's disease. It would also be essential to determine whether lymphocytes are the only cell type exhibiting vitamin C deficiency in this condition.

The above considerations are intended to stimulate further scientific research aimed at clarifying some of the dynamics of vitamin C that may have broader relevance, extending beyond Parkinson's disease. For instance, the well-known retention mechanism that preserves vitamin C in the brain during systemic deficiency might behave differently in the context of neurological disorders, possibly remodelling tissue distribution to prioritise brain function, while subtly but substantially weakening extracerebral compartments and rendering them more susceptible to secondary dysfunction.

As far as the therapeutic aspect is concerned, the literature remains very limited and thus far from conclusive. However, a pivotal 1992 study offered a very promising perspective (203). Conducted by Stanley Fahn, one of the world's leading Parkinson's researchers, it demonstrated that a high-dose combination of vitamin C and vitamin E enabled patients with early-stage disease to delay the initiation of levodopa therapy, the gold standard treatment, by up to 2.5 years. These findings strongly suggest that an early and intensive antioxidant regimen may slow disease progression. As emphasized in the text, the terms early and intensive refer to two critical parameters: timing and dosage, which have often been underestimated in scientific research, potentially leading to misleading conclusions. "Results of this pilot study suggest that the progression of Parkinson's disease may be slowed by administration of these antioxidants. Controlled clinical trials using double-blind randomization techniques are required to confirm these results", Fahn concluded in "Annals of Neurology" (203), a request that, to this day, unfortunately remains unmet, due to the lack of specific clinical trials.

A 2004 study (204) sparked renewed hope by investigating the bioavailability of levodopa, which is known to be compromised by various factors, including the advanced age common among Parkinson's patients. Remarkably, the study demonstrated that even a very modest dose of 200 mg of vitamin C could significantly enhance levodopa absorption. The authors concluded that "levodopa therapy in combination with ascorbic acid may be one of the strategies for the treatment of Parkinson's disease" (204). Nearly two decades later, one can only speculate on the additional benefits that might have emerged from a more rational use of vitamin C in this context.

Fortunately, this finding did not suffer the scientific neglect encountered by others, such as those reported in (203). A more recent study (468) revisited the topic and provided further evidence supporting vitamin C's notable potential to enhance levodopa bioavailability.

While broader scientific consensus is still pending, these findings already justify including the vitamin C-levodopa synergy among other documented interactions, such as with vasopressors in sepsis therapy and opioids in pain management, which have been shown to reduce pharmacological requirements. This sparing effect, known as therapeutic window expansion, combined with vitamin C's antioxidant and anti-inflammatory properties, may also reduce drug-related toxicity. In conclusion, levodopa may derive notable benefits from this significant pharmacological synergy (470), with positive implications for the clinical management of a disease that remains extremely difficult to treat.

Multiple sclerosis

Multiple sclerosis is a chronic inflammatory disease of the central nervous system. It is an autoimmune condition that causes demyelination, neurodegeneration, and oxidative stress, resulting in a wide spectrum of neurological symptoms.

The crucial role of vitamin C in the synthesis of collagen, a protein associated with myelin formation, establishes an initial potential connection between multiple sclerosis and vitamin C. It is important to note that vitamin C plays a fundamental role in the formation of myelin by Schwann cells (195), (196), (205). This connection is further supported by the findings of a major study published in "Nature" (349), which revealed a surprising link between TREG cells and myelin regeneration, uncovering interconnections that also involve vitamin C. The study demonstrated an unexpected interdependence, showing that TREGs can assist neural cells with functions similar to those of Schwann cells, namely, oligodendrocytes. While Schwann cells are responsible for myelinating peripheral nerves, oligodendrocytes perform a similar role in the central nervous system. The results of this study (349) therefore attribute to TREGs the ability to support central myelination, a process that is persistently impaired in multiple sclerosis, thereby expanding their known functional repertoire.

This interplay enhances the role of vitamin C: beyond stimulating collagen synthesis and epigenetic pathways associated with Schwann cells, it may also support myelination through the promotion of TREG cells (118), which have proven effective in remyelination processes (349).

Another notable aspect derives from the immunomodulatory properties of TREGs, which some researchers have proposed as potential therapeutic tools for autoimmune diseases such as multiple sclerosis (118). This line of reasoning forms a biologically intriguing triangle: ascorbic acid, TREG cells and myelination processes, a geometric model that helps rationalize the use of vitamin C as a therapeutic agent in multiple sclerosis.

In this context, a 2015 study (206) evaluated the effects of AA and the steroid hormone progesterone in mice within a model of multiple sclerosis. Following injections into the hippocampus, a brain region essential for learning and memory, an important observation was made: unlike progesterone or the combined progesterone + AA treatment, AA monotherapy was the only one to improve memory in mice. This suggests a specific pharmacological action of AA and supports the hypothesis that patients with multiple sclerosis might benefit from its ability to protect key brain regions such as the hippocampus (206).

As is often the case in research involving ascorbic acid, interesting connections emerge. One such case concerns progesterone, a hormone crucial to the female reproductive system. Several studies, including one published in "Fertility and Sterility" (364), have shown that vitamin C supports the biosynthesis of progesterone, with potentially significant benefits for fertility. The conclusions reflect recurring themes in ascorbic research: "Ascorbic acid supplementation may not cause improvements in some patients with luteal phase defect because this condition can have many causes. However, ascorbic acid supplementation should be tried in these patients because it is clearly effective for some cases of luteal phase defect, it is affordable and has no side effects" (364).

Returning to multiple sclerosis, further studies (207) have shown that vitamin C may modulate the enzyme acetylcholinesterase, which is responsible for the degradation of acetylcholine, a neurotransmitter that is essential for nerve transmission. Although preliminary, these findings are encouraging, especially considering their possible implications beyond multiple sclerosis. The role of AA in the neuromodulation of various neurotransmission systems suggests broader pharmacological impact, such as anti-aging applications or benefits against cognitive decline.

From an epidemiological standpoint, data on the correlation between AA levels and multiple sclerosis remain limited. Some researchers have linked low plasma concentrations with active disease phases, likely due to lipid peroxidation that characterises exacerbations (208). A 2019 Egyptian study (419) provided a novel stratification: younger patients appeared more deficient than older ones, and individuals with infratentorial lesions showed greater AA depletion than those without such lesions. This is a particularly valuable study, highlighting not only the AA depletion induced by multiple sclerosis but also suggesting that the disease may be more active in younger individuals and those with specific lesion patterns (419).

Further insight comes from a 1998 Canadian study published in "The International Journal of Epidemiology" (209), which revealed a potential protective role of vitamin C.

Unfortunately, clinical data remain scarce. However, this lack of information might benefit vitamin C, as future studies in the context of multiple sclerosis would operate in a relatively unbiased scientific landscape, free from the methodological preconceptions seen in other areas. With this in mind, well-designed clinical trials focused on more rational administration of oral vitamin C could help answer a key question: could oral vitamin C, when used appropriately, provide clinical benefit in the treatment of multiple sclerosis?

It is interesting to note that this issue has been thoroughly addressed in relation to another vitamin: biotin, a B-vitamin that has demonstrated promising preclinical and clinical effects in treating multiple sclerosis, ultimately earning a place in a phase 3 clinical trial (398). Although the latter trial failed to replicate earlier successes, it highlights an asymmetry in scientific focus: why has vitamin C not received comparable attention, despite a strong biological rationale?

Why has biotin advanced to late-stage clinical testing, while vitamin C remains at the starting line?

Depression

There is no doubt that several neurotransmission systems require vitamin C to function properly, and its critical role in the synthesis of serotonin and catecholamines is just one of many demonstrations of this fact. This has led to the consideration of vitamin C as a potential therapeutic agent in depressive disorders, an idea already suggested by previously cited studies showing a positive association between ascorbate levels and elevated mood (90).

Depression is characterized by symptoms such as low mood, psychomotor slowing, anxiety and somatic disturbances. It has long been associated with dysfunctions in neurotransmitter systems involving noradrenaline, dopamine and especially serotonin, all of which are neurotransmitters whose synthesis depends on vitamin C.

However, recent research has refined this etiological framework by highlighting the role of chronic stress as an additional key factor. Chronic stress not only depletes ascorbic acid, but can also induce immune dysregulation and negatively affect the hypothalamic-pituitary-adrenal axis. For instance, cortisol and pro-inflammatory cytokines are known to promote the conversion of tryptophan, a serotonin precursor, into kynurenine, a neuroactive and largely irreversible metabolite, leading to a significant reduction in brain serotonin levels (213). Therefore, vitamin C's ability to modulate immune responses and cortisol secretion under stress, along with its crucial role in neurotransmitter synthesis, positions it as a highly promising antidepressant agent. This hypothesis is supported by numerous animal studies (210), (211), (212), (213).

More recently, researchers have proposed additional mechanisms of action. Vitamin C may modulate monoaminergic systems by activating the serotonin 5-HT1A receptor, similarly to many antidepressant and antipsychotic drugs. It can also stimulate the expression of heme oxygenase-1 (HO-1), an enzyme with mood-supportive implications and, as previously noted, cell-protective effects (184), (213).

Regarding plasma levels, several data strengthen the theoretical assumptions. It has been found that patients with depression consistently present low plasma concentrations of vitamin C. This is particularly evident in a randomized, double-blind, placebo-controlled study published in 2014 in the "International Journal for Vitamin and Nutrition Research" (214). Among 322 elderly participants, 36% were deficient (plasma levels < 11 micromoles/L), and the study also observed that patients with the lowest concentrations had the most severe symptoms and higher inflammation. "A high percentage of elderly patients had suboptimal vitamin C levels, and this was associated with an increase in symptoms of depression", the study concluded (214).

Are there any clinical studies that have explored the therapeutic role of vitamin C in depression?

Yes. Two examples are particularly noteworthy. In the first case, vitamin C was studied in a hospital setting, where its deficiency is presumed to be both widespread and underestimated. This randomized double-blind trial (407), published in "The American Journal of Clinical Nutrition", demonstrated that patients treated orally with 500 mg of AA twice daily experienced significant improvements in mood and psychological distress. These improvements were not observed in patients who received an alternative therapy, vitamin D supplementation (5000 IU/day). These findings suggest that vitamin C may be more effective than vitamin D in terms of antidepressant effect. Furthermore, C-reactive protein (CRP) levels decreased by 32% with vitamin C, but not with vitamin D, further confirming the strong anti-inflammatory action of vitamin C (407). Despite its low dose compared to the high dose of vitamin D, vitamin C proved to be the more effective agent from various perspectives.

The antidepressant properties of vitamin C have also been investigated in paediatric populations. In a randomized, double-blind, placebo-controlled pilot study (533), children were treated either with fluoxetine alone (10-20 mg/day) or with fluoxetine plus 1000 mg/day of vitamin C. The results were straightforward: the combination therapy outperformed fluoxetine monotherapy, highlighting yet another potential synergy. "These preliminary results suggest that vitamin C can be an effective adjuvant agent in the treatment of major depressive disorder in paediatric patients" (533).

The mention of fluoxetine, a well-known antidepressant, raises an intriguing consideration regarding AA's pharmacological synergies. In an animal study (386) published in "Neuropharmacology", the combination of fluoxetine (1 mg/kg) and intraperitoneal vitamin C (100 mg/kg) showed effectiveness in treating spinal cord injury, significantly reducing inflammation and preserving the blood-spinal cord barrier, a physiological barrier analogous to the blood-brain barrier. The authors reported: "These results demonstrate the synergistic effect of the combination of low doses of fluoxetine and vitamin C on blood-spinal cord barrier disruption after spinal cord injury and support the effectiveness of the combination treatment for managing acute spinal cord injury" (386).

Still on the topic of spinal cord injuries, vitamin C appears to act synergistically with natural compounds, such as the amino acid taurine. In an animal study (387), their combined administration produced a notable anti-inflammatory effect. These data raise the question: Could AA monotherapy be effective in the treatment of acute spinal cord injury?

Some preliminary evidence suggests a positive answer. For example, a comparative study in rats (388) showed that high-dose AA (200 mg/kg, administered intraperitoneally) was as effective as high-dose corticosteroids (methylprednisolone, 30 mg/kg).

Returning to the topic of depression, a growing number of clinical studies continue to support the beneficial role of AA (213). For instance, Fritz and colleagues conducted a systematic review of observational studies (215) evaluating the adjuvant efficacy of AA in cancer therapy. In addition to improvements in quality of life, the review reported a potential prevention of common chemotherapy side effects, such as fatigue, nausea, insomnia, anxiety and depression, thus confirming a significant mood-enhancing effect (215).

In conclusion, both the strong biological plausibility and the accumulating preliminary data underscore the urgent need for well-designed, high-quality clinical studies.

This section concludes with a particularly illustrative clinical case (352). A 66-year-old woman was hospitalized due to a deterioration in mental health against a background of longstanding schizophrenia and depression. Alongside severe anemia, clinicians noted the presence of petechiae, small hemorrhagic skin lesions. Although petechiae can result from various causes (e.g., coagulation disorders, infections), scurvy became a plausible diagnosis when routine tests failed to explain her symptoms. Plasma levels of ascorbic acid were subsequently measured and found to be extremely low (< 5 micromoles/L), confirming acute scurvy and requiring immediate, intensive treatment. A natural question arises: what treatment would have been given if vitamin C levels had not been measured?

It is likely that a non-ascorbic intervention would have provided only symptomatic relief rather than addressing the underlying condition. This raises broader concerns: how many similar cases may have gone unnoticed, given that measuring vitamin C levels is not routine?

The authors remarked: "Although it is now a rare condition in developed countries, this case will remind modern medical practitioners that patients with scurvy may present with non-specific symptoms and clinical findings such as depression and anaemia" (352).

Stroke

Stroke is a potentially life-threatening disorder that often leads to permanent physical disability. It occurs when the supply of oxygenated blood to a region of the brain is interrupted or significantly reduced. The discussion of stroke was not included in Chapter 6, which focuses on critical illnesses, for a specific reason related to a particular aspect of ascorbic acid therapy. What is this reason?

To understand it, we must consider the mechanisms that regulate cerebral vitamin C uptake. This process is controlled by two major physiological barriers: the blood-brain barrier (BBB) and the blood-cerebrospinal fluid barrier, both of which restrict the entry of ascorbate into the central nervous system. Also crucial is the role of the SVCT2 transporter, which enables the transfer of ascorbate from the plasma through the choroid plexus to the cerebrospinal fluid. Equally important are GLUT transporters, especially GLUT1 and GLUT3, which allow dehydroascorbic acid, the oxidised form of vitamin C, to rapidly cross the blood-brain barrier, where it is subsequently recycled into ascorbic acid within cells (78), (213).

DHA plays a crucial role in the central nervous system for two main reasons: it crosses the BBB much more rapidly than ascorbic acid, and its uptake by certain cells, such as astrocytes, is highly selective. Astrocytes, star-shaped glial cells that provide structural and metabolic support to neurons, can in fact absorb only DHA, not ascorbic acid, due to the absence of SVCT2. In contrast, neurons express SVCT2 and can accumulate very high levels of vitamin C (up to 10-12 millimoles), using both transport systems (213). These theoretical elements provide a strong biological rationale for considering DHA a potential therapeutic agent for various neurological disorders, including stroke. Several animal studies (160), (165), (216) support this perspective. For example, in an experimentally induced ischemic stroke model, intravenous DHA, administered as a pretreatment or within 3 hours after stroke onset, produced remarkable outcomes, including a significant reduction in infarct volume (216). Similar findings were reported in other models where pre- or post-stroke DHA administration was tested: DHA effectively reduced both infarct size and mortality (160).

These findings can be attributed to the remarkably rapid distribution of DHA throughout the brain, including regions affected by stroke, where large amounts of reactive oxygen species are swiftly released. These results warrant careful consideration, as they are supported by a robust physiological basis:

1- Rapid depletion of vitamin C during stroke, promptly compensated by DHA's entry into the brain;

2- Preservation of glutathione and vitamin E, two essential antioxidants that act synergistically to mitigate oxidative stress;

3- Epigenetic action of vitamin C through its role as a cofactor for TET enzymes, which increases the expression of brain-derived neurotrophic factor (BDNF), a key protein essential for neuronal survival, synaptic plasticity (the process by which synaptic connections strengthen or weaken over time to support learning and memory) and the growth and differentiation of new neurons;

4- Demonstrated safety in animal studies of intravenous DHA.

These considerations are drawn from one of the most representative and influential works on the subject (216), authored by Reynold Spector and published in "Medical Hypotheses" in 2016.

From an epidemiological standpoint, the evidence consistently underscores the protective value of vitamin C. The inverse correlation between plasma levels and stroke risk is supported by both robust statistical analyses and well-defined mechanistic pathways (92), (217). Among the most relevant mechanisms are its documented effects on:

1- Inhibition of lipoprotein oxidation;

2- Protection against lipid peroxidation;

3- Antihypertensive properties;

4- Anti-inflammatory modulation.

Collectively, these mechanisms provide a strong biological rationale for the hypothesis that vitamin C exerts a meaningful protective role in the pathogenesis of stroke (217).

Chapter 8
Vitamin C In The Treatment Of Cancer

'The tragedy of vitamin C does not lie in the absence of data, but in the persistent reluctance to acknowledge them'

Introduction

Cancer, unfortunately, needs no introduction. Pain, suffering, frustration, despair, hope, courage, and trust, these are the emotions increasingly felt by patients, families, and healthcare professionals. Together, they form a powerful emotional landscape that captures the dramatic nature of the disease more vividly than any set of statistics. Still, it is impossible to ignore the troubling trend reflected in the numbers: a clear and steady rise in incidence.

Let us remain with the numbers, the only tool capable of offering a clear and objective view of scientific reality. Although revisiting the link between cancer and reduced ascorbic acid levels may seem redundant, reasserting this connection remains useful, not only to reaffirm the validity of vitamin C's biological principles but also to raise awareness within the scientific community about the importance of plasma monitoring, which has been largely overlooked until now.

A solid body of studies has revealed progressive deficits of vitamin C in cancer patients, showing, as predicted by the theoretical framework of vitamin C, that patients undergoing treatment (or in advanced stages of disease) exhibit even lower concentrations compared to those who are untreated or in earlier stages. A robust confirmation came in 2020 through a comprehensive study published in "Nutrients", which provided several noteworthy data points, including a threefold increase in the risk of hypovitaminosis (levels < 23 micromoles/L) following the initiation of anticancer therapy (33).

Roughly fifteen years earlier, the journal "Palliative Medicine" published a study of great significance: the investigation, conducted on a sample of terminal patients admitted to a large hospice, revealed a state of deficiency (levels < 11 micromoles/L) in 30% of patients, and also reported a strong inverse correlation between plasma ascorbate and the inflammatory biomarker CRP (32).

Overall, a multitude of observational studies have increasingly and clearly described significant reductions in plasma ascorbate levels in cancer patients, documenting a proportional relationship with variables such as disease stage and treatments administered (367). In this context, it seems that Stone was not wrong to link the progression of leukemia to scurvy. One of the many recent confirmations comes from a 2022 study published in the prestigious journal "Frontiers in Oncology", in which numerous researchers examined antioxidant vitamins A, C and E in the context of acute myeloid leukemia (507). The findings offered a twofold validation. On the one hand, the widespread ascorbic deficiency strengthened Stone's hypotheses, as acknowledged by the authors themselves: "This is in agreement with the hypothesis proposed by Stone, who suggested a role of disease burden in individual patients in relation to the metabolic deficiency stemming from humans' inability to synthesize ascorbic acid". On the other hand, it reaffirmed that vitamin C is the primary "target" of complex diseases, since even in this study, plasma levels of vitamins A and E showed no significant differences compared to the control group.

Therefore, in severe pathological conditions such as cancer, vitamin C replenishment should be regarded as a clinically relevant point, since it is particularly prone to depletion due to multiple metabolic factors. These include the same mechanisms observed in sepsis and other severe conditions: a drastic increase in cellular metabolic demand, massive oxidative insult, intense inflammatory response and potential dysregulation of SVCTs, all of which are further exacerbated by the depleting effects of anticancer therapies (33), (367).

Therefore, considering the body of evidence gathered, especially the fact that inadequate levels are associated with the onset of numerous diseases and thus with potential increased mortality, reaffirming the need for supplementation is scientifically well-founded, regardless of any direct effect on the disease itself. Yet theory and practice do not always align, and this mismatch regrettably occurs in science as well. As paradoxical as it may seem, the monitoring of plasma levels and the potential for restorative therapy remain virtually inaccessible to cancer patients. A telling statement from the authors of (33) illustrates this point: "It is noteworthy that the vast majority of people with cancer will never undergo measurement of plasma ascorbate, and this relationship may prompt increased awareness regarding ascorbate status in oncology patients".

Why this indifference?

Why underestimate a deficiency that could cause scurvy or its subclinical forms?

Why overlook a deficiency that could further compromise the physiology of an organism already devastated by cancer?

Therefore, it is reasonable to state that correcting any deficiency, regardless of vitamin C's potential anticancer properties, represents the most immediate and well-justified indication for its therapeutic use. As Mayland, Bennett and Allan (32) succinctly put it: "Patients with low plasma concentrations of vitamin C have shorter survival". These words speak for themselves.

Pauling and Cameron

The first scientist to hypothesize a role for vitamin C in cancer treatment was William J. McCormick, another specialist in the orthomolecular field. In the 1950s, McCormick proposed two potential antitumor mechanisms. The first was related to collagen synthesis: he observed that ascorbate deficiency might facilitate metastatic spread by weakening the structural integrity of connective tissue. The second involved the inhibition of hyaluronidase, an enzyme that degrades hyaluronic acid, another key component of the extracellular matrix (219). These hypotheses, however, remained underexplored for decades and have only been revisited in recent years.

Toward the late 1960s, McCormick's insights were complemented by the illuminating laboratory findings of Benade, which will be discussed shortly. Yet the most impactful development was still to come; these preliminary results would lay the groundwork for the scientific revolution initiated by Linus Pauling and Ewan Cameron. Their clinical studies on cancer patients marked a radical shift, leaving a lasting and profound impact on the history of vitamin C, especially considering that Pauling had been awarded the Nobel Prize twice. At the time, vitamin C was regarded primarily from a nutritional perspective, while Pauling and Cameron revealed its surprising anticancer properties, radically transforming both its scientific and potential clinical framework.

The turning point came in 1976, when Pauling and Cameron published the results of a bold study (220) involving 100 terminal cancer patients. The therapeutic efficacy and lack of toxicity validated the scientists' boldness, astonishing those who had refused to believe that a "mere" vitamin could have a significant pharmacological impact against cancer.

None of the enrolled patients had received any other form of definitive treatment: "100 terminal cancer patients received ascorbate supplements as the sole form of definitive treatment" (220). The treatment protocol involved daily intravenous administration of 10 grams of ascorbate for the first 10 days, followed by indefinite oral maintenance therapy of 10 grams per day. This two-phase approach included an intensive initial phase (intravenous infusions over 10 days) and a maintenance phase (2.5 grams orally every six hours).

The findings were remarkable, even to the investigators themselves: "The results were surprising even to us", Pauling later wrote. The retrospective analysis revealed that patients receiving ascorbate had a mean survival time 4.2 times longer than that of the control group, which consisted of 1000 patients who had not received ascorbate. Furthermore, a specific subgroup of about 10 patients exhibited an extraordinary 20-fold increase in survival compared to controls (see figure).

Essentially, vitamin C markedly extended survival in treated patients, with a subset demonstrating exceptional longevity that defies simple explanation. It could be hypothesized that this subgroup carried a favorable genetic anomaly, perhaps associated with the upregulation of SVCTs or some other determining factor.

These results, particularly striking given the critical condition of the enrolled subjects (all terminal cancer patients), also included additional benefits, such as relief from often unbearable cancer-related pain.

In summary, ascorbate effectively addressed one of oncology's most complex challenges from two perspectives: it significantly prolonged survival while simultaneously improving quality of life.

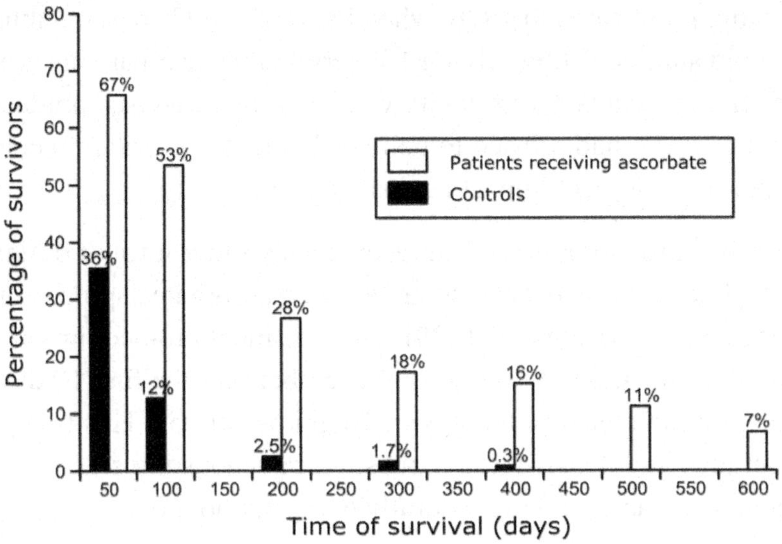

graph adapted from (220)

Encouraged by these promising outcomes, Pauling and Cameron undertook a second clinical study, completed in 1978 (221), involving another cohort of 100 terminally ill patients treated with the same therapeutic regimen. Once again, vitamin C proved beneficial: treated patients showed a 300-day longer survival than controls. This result echoed previous findings and also highlighted a 55-fold improvement in one-year survival rates from the point of declared therapeutic intractability (22% survival in the ascorbate group vs. 0.4% in the control group). "There is no doubt in our minds that treatment with ascorbate in amounts of 10 grams per day, or more, has real value in extending the lives of patients with advanced cancer. Moreover, as previously noted, the quality of life was improved with ascorbate administration. Furthermore, we continue to believe that adding ascorbate earlier in the treatment regimen may have a far more profound effect, potentially extending survival by years", Pauling and Cameron stated in the conclusion of their publication (221). These were bold assertions, supported by compelling yet retrospective data, inherently lacking the robustness of double-blind randomized controlled trials.

It should be noted that Pauling and Cameron's use of a retrospective design was not deliberate but rather a necessity, due to the lack of support from the National Cancer Institute. Their request for adequate patient recruitment and funding to conduct a randomized clinical trial was met with indifference. As

Pauling's wife recounted, having accompanied him to one such meeting, the scientific establishment displayed a stark lack of curiosity, as she later described in the book "How to Live Longer and Feel Better": "I had never seen a group of medical researchers so uninterested in new ideas".

In response to the growing attention drawn by Pauling and Cameron's findings, Creagan, Moertel, and colleagues at the Mayo Clinic, an institution historically tied to cancer research and the earlier work of Szent-Györgyi, undertook their own investigation. In 1979, they published a randomized, double-blind controlled clinical trial involving 123 patients with advanced cancer (222). Sixty patients received 10 grams of oral vitamin C daily, while 63 served as controls. Notably, the intravenous loading phase used by Pauling and Cameron was omitted. Unfortunately, the study yielded no significant survival benefit for the vitamin C group, even though some patients did report improved pain management.

A further study in 1985 replicated the double-blind, placebo-controlled design with a cohort of colorectal cancer patients (223). In this case as well, only oral administration of vitamin C was used, and, although the study partially adhered to Pauling's recommendation to exclude patients previously treated with chemotherapy, no survival benefit was observed.

The results were so disappointing that they had far-reaching implications. These two studies, based on the most rigorous experimental design, effectively halted scientific interest in the anticancer potential of vitamin C for over two decades. Nonetheless, Pauling's perseverance and support from less conventional sources kept the idea alive in less academic circles.

From 1985 until the emergence of Chen's studies in 2005, vitamin C was relegated to the realm of alternative cancer treatments. This position persisted despite other clinical evidence. For instance, Murata's work in Japan in 1982 reproduced results similar to those of Pauling and Cameron, showing increased survival and improved quality of life in cancer patients treated with high doses of vitamin C (408).

Meanwhile, as Creagan's team was planning their 1985 trial, Anthony and Schorah published a groundbreaking study in the "British Journal of Cancer" in 1982 (218). They examined nearly 150 lung cancer patients and discovered alarmingly low vitamin C levels, approaching scurvy in many cases. Furthermore, they noted that cancerous lung tissue showed significantly higher concentrations of vitamin C compared to unaffected regions, suggesting a localized biological response. The study concluded with an appeal: "Given the growing evidence that immune mechanisms play a role in controlling tumor spread and metastasis, the impact of vitamin C supplementation on lung cancer survival should be tested in a clinical trial". This request, however, was ignored, as the Mayo Clinic instead chose to proceed with patients suffering from colorectal cancer, a decision that, in hindsight, appears at the very least questionable.

The influence of the Mayo Clinic was such that it invites a sardonic paraphrase of the Latin phrase: "Ubi Mayo, minor cessat".

It is now crucial to reassess the Mayo Clinic's position with objective clarity.

1- The discrepancies in treatment protocols are evident. Creagan's studies did not include the intravenous loading phase. Given the pharmacokinetic limitations of oral ascorbate, this omission may have been critical;

2- Oral administration alone may have been insufficient to fully restore the depleted vitamin C levels in these patients, who were at very high risk of severe deficiency, thereby preventing any potential pharmacological action;

3- There is a possibility that some participants in the vitamin C or placebo groups self-supplemented, given the publicized findings of Pauling and Cameron and the easy accessibility of vitamin C;

4- The situation is reminiscent of Sabin's flawed replication of Jungeblut's anti-polio work using lower doses and higher viral loads;

5- The 1985 study focused exclusively on colorectal cancer, excluding all other neoplasms, thus presenting a considerable experimental limitation. Nevertheless, both recent high-quality clinical evidence (586) and my father's medical history contribute to challenging the conclusions of the Mayo Clinic;

6- Pauling's request was only partially honored. Although the 1985 trial excluded pretreated patients, both studies allowed substitution of ascorbate with salvage chemotherapy upon signs of disease progression, an approach that significantly diverged from Pauling and Cameron's methods.

There are two key discrepancies. The first stems from the therapeutic substitution applied by Creagan's team, which effectively meant that patients enrolled in Pauling and Cameron's studies received ascorbic therapy for a much longer period than those in the Mayo Clinic trials. The second discrepancy concerns pharmacokinetics. Although pharmacokinetic knowledge of vitamin C was limited at the time, something appears inconsistent upon logical examination. Why did Creagan and colleagues choose to weaken the protocol proposed by Pauling and Cameron?

Although the clear superiority of the intravenous route was not fully understood, Klenner and other scientists, and above all the general foundations of pharmacology, pointed to substantial differences between oral and intravenous administration. In one of the many captivating historical reconstructions dedicated to the topic, one can sense disappointment at the way the scientific debates surrounding Pauling and Cameron's experiments unfolded: "Surprisingly, for years it went unrecognized that the observational studies by Cameron and Pauling used both oral and intravenous administration, while Mayo Clinic studies employed oral dosing only", noted several prominent scientists (429).

Therefore, the Mayo Clinic studies did not provide a reliable or adequate verification of Pauling and Cameron's work. Yet, they were enough to stifle enthusiasm for further research, a missed opportunity for science and, even more tragically, for cancer patients.

What further worsened the situation was that the Mayo Clinic's critical studies were published in the "New England Journal of Medicine", one of the most prestigious medical journals in the world. This leaves much room for reflection. The growing sense of disillusionment echoes the original humility of Pauling and Cameron, who never proposed vitamin C as a standalone cancer cure. Rather, they advocated for its integrative role, supporting both the body and conventional treatments. Their approach aimed to enrich the therapeutic arsenal with a non-toxic, biologically versatile and economically advantageous option.

Despite the humility of Pauling and Cameron, numerous subsequent studies on high-dose vitamin C in animal models have indicated that it may act effectively as a standalone agent against cancer cells. These findings raise critical questions about the previous neglect by the scientific community, which has only recently begun to properly reconsider the pharmacological potential of vitamin C. Yet we are still at the beginning.

The sociological analysis of Evelleen Richards, Honorary Professor of History and Philosophy of Science at the University of Sydney, highlights how much progress is still needed (503). By comparing medical attitudes toward three potential anticancer agents, 5-fluorouracil, interferon and vitamin C, Richards identified a deep-seated bias against the latter. Other researchers have echoed this concern: "Given the poor-quality evidence for many conventional cancer drugs that are allowed to enter the market, the strong negative attitude in mainstream medicine against vitamin C appears particularly concerning. Where do such strong emotions come from that have prevented appropriate investigation of vitamin C for cancer?" (503).

Two prooxidant mechanisms

To provide a technical description of the antitumor properties of ascorbate, we must return to the years during which Stone was arduously engaged in promoting the virtues of the molecule worldwide. Within this context, almost quietly, emerged the scientific work of Benade, an endeavor that would ultimately prove historically invaluable and pioneering from an oncological perspective.

Benade was able to demonstrate in vitro that vitamin C, at least in certain tumors such as the so-called Ehrlich ascites carcinoma, is capable of exerting an intelligent destructive action, that is, one aimed at destroying cancer cells while completely sparing healthy tissues (224). In the late 1960s, he hypothesized that ascorbate's cytotoxic effect was closely linked to the intracellular generation of a byproduct of vitamin C oxidation: hydrogen peroxide (H_2O_2). Yes, you read that correctly, hydrogen peroxide, the well-known active ingredient in common household antiseptic solutions used for wound cleaning.

Benade went on to demonstrate a principle that would later prove central: the cytotoxicity of ascorbate increases in conjunction with the administration of a specific substance (3-amino-1,2,4-triazole or ATA), capable of inhibiting catalase activity in tumor cells. Catalase thus re-emerges as a key player. This is an endogenous antioxidant enzyme capable of degrading hydrogen peroxide (H_2O_2), rapidly decomposing it into oxygen and water. The mechanism thus becomes clear: ATA can suppress a significant portion of the defensive barriers organized by catalase, thus facilitating the entry of H_2O_2, a highly oxidizing compound, into tumor cells. This outlines a scenario in which tumor cells' detoxification capabilities against H_2O_2 are greatly reduced, thus attributing significant antitumor potential to the combination of AA and ATA.

Even more intriguing was a hypothesis by Benade that over time proved accurate: catalase activity within tumor cells is markedly lower than in normal cells. Several subsequent studies have confirmed this finding, identifying reduced levels of catalase and other antioxidant enzymes in malignant cells (426). This historically revealed for the first time an intrinsic weakness of cancer cells, and not just any weakness but a critical defect, as it allowed the hypothesis of a pronounced vulnerability to ascorbate, not necessarily dependent on the influence of ATA (224).

In short, Benade's work marked an increase in interest in the antitumor qualities of vitamin C, culminating in the late 1970s with the turbulent clinical studies by Pauling and Cameron, cornerstone investigations around which a constellation of valuable studies would orbit such as those by Murata, Anthony, and Schorah.

And then? It may seem redundant to repeat that the findings from Creagan's team triggered a sharp shift in the attention paid to vitamin C, initiating a precipitous decline. Some attempts at rebalancing, notably a 1993 study by Leung, Miyashita, Young and Tsao (225), which reconfirmed vitamin C's impressive pharmacological intelligence, proved virtually ineffective.

This collapse continued for at least another decade before being halted in 2005, when Chen's research team, armed with newly acquired pharmacokinetic insights, suddenly reignited scientific enthusiasm. That date marked a new chapter for vitamin C: the dawn of a new day that still seems far from sunset, despite a sky partially overcast.

The path outlined by Chen's team has attracted an entire generation of researchers, leading scientific research in a new direction that has revealed a new application profile: very high doses of intravenous vitamin C.

It all began with a groundbreaking experiment (428) published in 2005 in the journal "Proceedings of the National Academy of Sciences of the United States of America", in which Chen's group incubated both normal and tumor cell types in specific culture media containing varying concentrations of ascorbate, ranging from 0 to 20 millimoles. Something astonishing was observed, albeit formally consistent with Benade's work: healthy cells were unaffected by 20 millimoles of ascorbate, while five cancer cell lines were heavily attacked by it (226), (428). Furthermore, Chen corrected one of Benade's assumptions, proving that it is extracellular ascorbate (not intracellular, as Benade had argued) that destroys tumor cells, thus clarifying several important technical aspects.

The destructive storm results from the formation of H_2O_2 in the extracellular environment, caused by ascorbate oxidation. As previously mentioned, H_2O_2 is generated through the extraordinary ability of AA to reduce metals such as iron and copper, leading to the Fenton reaction. In the extracellular tumor microenvironment, where iron is typically abundant, millimolar concentrations of ascorbate rapidly reduce ferric iron to its ferrous form. This reduction simultaneously leads to the oxidation of AA. In this reactive and effervescent setting, oxygen and iron interact to form superoxide, which then converts, via dismutation, into hydrogen peroxide. This sets the stage for further oxidative reactions that selectively damage cancer cells.

In short, H_2O_2 formation is driven by the extracellular oxidation of ascorbate. This is a crucial point: in a landmark in vivo study (429), Chen's group demonstrated that the extracellular space must be saturated with oxidized vitamin C, specifically, with semidehydroascorbic acid (the intermediate between AA and DHA, formed when vitamin C donates an electron to reduce iron), in order to initiate these pro-oxidant reactions. By "saturated," we mean millimolar plasma concentrations, which, as is well known, can only be achieved through high-dose intravenous administration. Oral supplementation, in contrast, fails to produce detectable levels of oxidized vitamin C. This implies not only that H_2O_2 generation depends on intravenous delivery, but also that oral intake is pharmacologically safe, lacking any pro-oxidative potential (429).

Once this essential point is acknowledged, with an extracellular space abundant in semidehydroascorbic acid, all prerequisites for triggering the Fenton reaction are met. This reaction drives H_2O_2 to oxidize ferrous iron back to ferric, simultaneously generating an extremely reactive free radical: the hydroxyl radical. The high ascorbate flux and recycling of iron to the ferric state tend to restart the sequence, facilitating the cyclic generation of increasingly oxidative compounds (539).

Technical descriptions aside, the crucial point is that Chen paved the way for a wealth of both in vitro and in vivo studies, all of which concur that millimolar concentrations of ascorbate generate H_2O_2 in the extracellular medium, thereby qualifying as an H_2O_2 prodrug. Chen and colleagues further reported that the introduction of catalase into the culture medium quenched the strong antitumor effects (a phenomenon previously observed by Benade), thereby identifying the enzyme as a likely central link in the chain leading to the AA-mediated cytotoxic response (226), (428), (243).

Catalase is in "good" company. Its deficiency, a condition frequently observed in cancer cells (again, originally noted by Benade and subsequently confirmed (426)), is accompanied by additional abnormalities characteristic of malignant cells, which systematically exhibit numerous mitochondrial defects that compromise internal antioxidant enzymes. Induced by tumor degeneration, such alterations can weaken cancer cells, resulting in pronounced endogenous oxidative stress. In short, the malignant cell suffers from an intrinsic and evident antioxidant vulnerability, severe enough to make it a natural target for any pharmacological agent with oxidative action. And what better drug than the canonical prodrug of an excellent oxidant such as hydrogen peroxide could strike at this evident vulnerability?

The understanding of vitamin C's primary cytotoxic mechanism sparked a wide array of studies, many in vitro or in animal models, all of which validated Chen's findings: pharmacological vitamin C generates hydrogen peroxide, against which tumor cells exhibit poor defense. Lacking the enzyme necessary to neutralize hydrogen peroxide, namely, catalase, cancer cells are left defenseless against H_2O_2 attacks resulting from millimolar levels of AA, whereas healthy cells, equipped with sufficient catalase, remain largely protected. As H_2O_2 penetrates deeper into the cancer cells, it ultimately induces cell death, a process facilitated by the weak antioxidant defense system of malignant cells (539).

This is a remarkable mechanistic cascade, with a potential impact extending beyond oncology into other areas of medicine. This is the opinion of clinicians at the Riordan Clinic (125), whose views identify viruses and bacteria as additional targets of the destructive process. Consider, for instance, chikungunya and the promising outcomes from combining high-dose intravenous AA with the adjunctive use of hydrogen peroxide (453).

The second antitumor mechanism is linked to the fact that the presence of H_2O_2 in the extracellular space can dramatically increase levels of DHA. This rise creates a unique oxidative microenvironment that depletes tumor cells of their essential antioxidant reserves. It is a complex dynamic, which will be clarified through several key explanatory digressions. Let us proceed step by step.

First, it is well established that several types of cancer, particularly those belonging to the subgroup characterized by two specific genetic mutations, KRAS and BRAF, tend to overexpress the glucose transporter GLUT1. As we will see later, this overexpression enables DHA, once transported into the malignant cell, to trigger substantial oxidative stress.

Let us now recall a phenomenon first described nearly a century ago by Nobel Laureate Otto Warburg: tumor cells have a high rate of glycolysis, the metabolic process through which glucose is broken down to produce energy. This metabolic reprogramming, known as the Warburg effect, is essential for the survival and proliferation of tumors (227). Why are these two premises important?

It has been observed that the aforementioned mutations KRAS and BRAF contribute to the Warburg effect partly through the overexpression of GLUT1 (228), thus suggesting the possibility of exploiting this selective GLUT1 expression, as well as the associated glycolytic metabolic activity, as a viable therapeutic strategy against cancer. This highly promising hypothesis has recently been supported by several studies demonstrating that high-dose ascorbic acid can exploit these vulnerabilities to selectively kill cancer cells. One such example is colorectal cancer bearing KRAS or BRAF mutations (229), in which the marked overexpression of GLUT1 may facilitate the cytotoxic action of vitamin C. It is also important to note that colorectal tumors with KRAS or BRAF mutations, which represent approximately half of all colorectal cancers, are notoriously resistant to conventional therapies (229).

This is particularly intriguing, and it deserves to be emphasized once again: in colorectal cancer, ascorbate appears to act with even greater efficacy precisely in the large subset of patients who are resistant to standard treatments.

But how does this mechanism actually unfold in practice?

A necessary step back: we know that cancer cells rely on glycolysis to ensure adequate glucose intake, which is transported into the cell primarily via GLUTs, especially GLUT1. We also know that massive AA administration drives semidehydroascorbic acid (a byproduct of iron reduction) to undergo further oxidation, facilitated by an extracellular environment now saturated with H_2O_2 (itself a product of oxygen reacting with reduced ferrous iron). This further oxidation converts semidehydroascorbic acid into DHA. These two points are crucial: due to its structural similarity to glucose, DHA is efficiently and rapidly absorbed, much faster than AA, via GLUT1 in tumor cells with KRAS or BRAF mutations, which are highly glucose-dependent due to GLUT1 overexpression. As a result, tumor cells, particularly those with these mutations, unwittingly offer multiple entry points (GLUT1) for DHA, "fooled" by its chemical resemblance to glucose.

Simply put, they become confused. This confusion within the tumor cell triggers intense competition between glucose and DHA: increased DHA entry and reduced glucose uptake represent a double-edged sword for the tumor cell. In fact, it's a triple blow, because, and this is worth noting, tumor cells tend to retain vitamin C (both AA and DHA) longer than healthy cells, likely mistaking it for their preferred nutrient: glucose (424), (539).

The strategy, therefore, is to saturate glucose transporters with DHA, both to facilitate its entry and to competitively inhibit glucose uptake. If DHA becomes sufficiently abundant to gain preferential access to GLUT1, at the expense of glucose, this would result in a substantial influx of DHA into the tumor cell, followed by its rapid reduction to ascorbate via the well-known ascorbate recycling mechanism. Here lies the crucial point: given the potentially predominant presence of DHA, its recycling would rapidly deplete intracellular antioxidants, particularly glutathione. This depletion would raise intracellular ROS levels, triggering an uncontrollable oxidative cascade that could lead to energy collapse and, ultimately, cell death (539). Naturally, this process is also selective: healthy cells, which express normal levels of GLUTs and are not subjected to excessive oxidative stress, would not experience DHA overload and would therefore recycle it efficiently without incurring irreparable oxidative damage.

Another compelling aspect is the synergy between these molecular mechanisms and targeted therapies, a relationship that is increasingly supported by various researchers: “It is important to emphasize that these antitumor effects have been widely reported as synergistic when vitamin C is combined with targeted therapies” (243).

The matter, in short, appears highly promising, especially considering that the demonstration of these antitumor mechanisms was presented in the article “Vitamin C selectively kills KRAS and BRAF mutant colorectal cancer cells by targeting GAPDH” (229), published in one of the world’s most authoritative scientific journals, “Science”. The article outlines the high cytotoxicity (both in vitro and in animal models) of vitamin C against the same tumor type that was, coincidentally, the subject of the second clinical trial by Creagan and colleagues: colorectal cancer (223). It almost seems like fate: Creagan and Moertel’s team unknowingly selected a tumor against which vitamin C appears particularly effective.

It is also worth noting that the two antitumor mechanisms described above have been observed in vivo in cancer patients, paving the way for extending the therapeutic horizon to other tumors, provided they exhibit high GLUT1 expression and intense glycolytic activity. These two characteristics could help identify a specific tumour profile that is particularly sensitive to pharmacological vitamin C.

Before proceeding, it is useful to mention a historically reported concern regarding high-dose AA cancer therapy: patients with glucose-6-phosphate dehydrogenase (G6PD) deficiency, a condition underlying the well-known favism, might (the conditional is necessary in light of recent findings to be discussed later) develop hemolytic anemia following high-dose intravenous ascorbate therapy (230). The issue lies with the G6PD enzyme, which maintains proper glutathione balance in red blood cells. In G6PD-deficient individuals, massive intravenous vitamin C administration may lead to uncontrolled DHA accumulation in erythrocytes, facilitated by the preferential GLUT1 transporter (note: erythrocytes do not express SVCTs) and by the intrinsic glutathione deficiency of these cells. The resulting oxidative stress could destroy a large number of erythrocytes, leading to anemia. For this reason, researchers recommend that patients intending to undergo intravenous vitamin C therapy first undergo testing to exclude G6PD deficiency.

Thus, we have identified a potential adverse effect of vitamin C, one that is predictable through a simple blood test and appears strictly tied to its pharmacological use. On the topic of harmfulness, however, more should be said. The matter is far more complex than it seems and may give rise to broader reflections. As we will later explore, based on more recent developments, even the mythology surrounding the difficult coexistence of G6PD deficiency and vitamin C has been partially debunked.

A comprehensive and well-defined conceptual framework may even allow for a near-Copernican reversal of the relationship between these two elements, at least under certain objectively defined circumstances. What we shall see underscores a defining trait of scientific research: the healthy culture of doubt must always reign supreme. A critical attitude should be an integral part of the complex process of constructing any scientific truth, especially within the context of Medicine, wisely described by the great Osler as the "Science of uncertainty and the Art of probability". The G6PD case is emblematic in this regard: although the mythology of "red blood cell destruction" has been downsized and the issue redefined with greater accuracy, even identifying a potential protective role for pharmacological vitamin C in the context of G6PD deficiency, a persistent and misleading media narrative continues to suggest otherwise.

Preclinical and clinical studies on high-dose intravenous vitamin C monotherapy

Following the pioneering research initiated by Chen's group in 2005, numerous studies have explored the effects of millimolar concentrations of vitamin C (1-20 millimoles/L) in both preclinical models and, to a lesser extent, clinical settings. These studies have encompassed a variety of cancer types, with a particular focus on leukemia (231), (232), colorectal cancer (233), (234), melanoma (235), (236), pancreatic cancer (237), (238), and prostate cancer (239), (240). Additional investigations have addressed mesothelioma, hepatocellular carcinoma, thyroid cancer, neuroblastoma, and glioblastoma. An extensive bibliography is available in the seminal article "High-dose intravenous vitamin C, a promising multi-targeting agent in the treatment of cancer", published in the renowned "Journal of Experimental & Clinical Cancer Research" (243). What have these studies revealed?

A considerable body of animal studies investigating vitamin C monotherapy has demonstrated that high doses (1-4 g/kg), administered daily by injection, consistently result in significant inhibition of tumor growth (241), (243). Notably, administration frequency appears to be a critical factor. Many researchers support the importance of daily infusions, considered optimal for maintaining adequate intratumoral levels of ascorbic acid (243), (367). This observation, which aligns with fundamental pharmacokinetic principles, suggests a parallel with the dynamic flow model associated with oral administration. In essence, sustaining high plasma and tissue concentrations may support certain physiological and pharmacological mechanisms otherwise unattainable.

In contrast, the clinical domain remains hampered by limited evidence and poor therapeutic efficacy, though one encouraging and consistent finding is the remarkable safety profile of high-dose vitamin C, at least up to 1.5 g/kg, which distinguishes it from all other therapeutic options. Furthermore, as discussed later, this safety may extend beyond mere absence of toxicity to include attenuation of side effects from conventional therapies when vitamin C is used as an adjuvant (424), (242), (243). These properties are of paramount importance: pharmacological vitamin C appears to be non-toxic, may potentially exert antitumor effects, and, when combined with chemotherapy, may reduce its notorious side effects.

However, the number of clinical trials evaluating vitamin C monotherapy is so small that we are far from having definitive answers, creating a stark contrast to the promising preclinical results. This discrepancy may stem from suboptimal study implementation. Clinical studies often employ substantially lower doses and less frequent administration compared to preclinical protocols. As noted in (243), some trials used doses four times lower than those in animal studies, administered only once weekly, an approach that is surprising, considering the short half-life of vitamin C infusions (572), (243), (367). Such asymmetries are as evident as they are difficult to rationalize, especially given the low toxicity of the intervention.

Future research should thus prioritize clinical trials employing more intensive and frequent ascorbic acid regimens, ideally targeting less advanced or unpretreated disease stages, rather than the late-stage or heavily pretreated cohorts currently dominating the literature (243).

Vitamin C as an adjuvant to traditional, innovative and natural therapies

Many preclinical studies exploring the combination of high-dose vitamin C with major approved cancer therapies have demonstrated synergistic effects sufficiently convincing to warrant large-scale clinical trials. Numerous anticancer drugs, from classic chemotherapeutics like platinum compounds to modern targeted therapies, may be potentiated by vitamin C (243). For instance, preclinical data have shown strong synergy between vitamin C and sorafenib, a potent tumor growth inhibitor. Remarkably, this combination led to unexpected disease regression in a patient with metastatic liver cancer (458), (243).

Positive preclinical results have been reported in various aggressive cancer types. The case of small-cell lung cancer is emblematic: in a murine model, the combination of chemotherapy, radiotherapy, and vitamin C at a massive 4 g/kg dose increased survival by 50% (243). Beneficial interactions have also been reported with immunotherapy, whose efficacy, as we will later discuss, appears to be influenced by the efficiency of the immune system.

Preclinical and clinical research has also demonstrated benefits in relation to radiotherapy, indicating that high doses of vitamin C increase its cytotoxic effects and at the same time reduce toxicity, an observation that also supports its radioprotective potential (243), (305).

It is also worth noting vitamin K3 (menadione), a synthetic derivative of vitamin K, since several in vitro studies have demonstrated that it markedly amplifies the pro-oxidant effects of high-dose ascorbate (573), (243). Even more importantly, this synergy has been confirmed in vivo, where combined administration led to reduced growth and metastasis in a lung carcinoma model (243). This is an emerging and particularly interesting area of research, as it suggests the potential for synergy with a wide range of low-toxicity substances. Among the most promising compounds are alpha-lipoic acid, epigallocatechin gallate, curcumin, resveratrol and sulforaphane. These combinations are currently under investigation with the aim of naturally enhancing the cytotoxic activity of vitamin C while preserving excellent safety profiles.

Similarly, a novel therapeutic approach described in "Nature" in 2020, "Synergistic effect of fasting-mimicking diet and vitamin C against KRAS mutated cancers" (435), has been enthusiastically received. In this study, Italian researchers propose clinically testing a strategy combining pharmacological vitamin C with a fasting-mimicking diet, outlining a potentially transformative therapeutic paradigm.

The topic of natural synergisms also allows for an important point to improve clarity in the scientific discussion surrounding vitamin C. Within integrative medicine, an interdisciplinary approach blending traditional and complementary therapies, oncological co-adjuvant treatments often include intravenous combinations of glutathione and vitamin C. However, this association may be counterproductive. Given the mechanistic basis of vitamin C's antitumor activity, glutathione might act antagonistically by compensating for the oxidative vulnerability of cancer cells, for example by neutralizing the hydrogen peroxide generated by high doses of ascorbate. Supporting this hypothesis, several studies have reported significant attenuation of vitamin C's antitumor effects following co-administration of glutathione or its precursor NAC (367). In "Free Radical Biology and Medicine", Ping Chen, Jennifer Stone, Sullivan, Drisko, and Qi Chen explicitly state (553): "There is an antagonism between ascorbate and glutathione in cancer treatment, and therefore intravenous AA and glutathione should not be administered on the same day to cancer patients".

With this necessary premise established, it is now time to evaluate the body of preclinical studies on vitamin C in combination with antineoplastic agents. The outlook is promising: most studies report improved disease control along with reduced toxicity, an ideal combination, especially considering the high toxicity of conventional cancer therapies. Supporting these preclinical successes, some phase 1 and 2 clinical trials have reported encouraging results in terms of disease stabilization and objective response rates (243). However, this body of evidence remains immature, hampered by the small size of the studies and, even more critically, by the lack of standardized treatment protocols. Several researchers, for example, attribute negative outcomes to the high variability in treatment regimens across different studies (243).

Currently, numerous phase 1 and 2 clinical trials, as well as a phase 3 study, are underway to gather more robust evidence on the efficacy of combining vitamin C with standard treatments (243). One particularly encouraging finding is already available: in a very recent phase 2 trial, the addition of high-dose ascorbic acid (75-100 g intravenously, 2-3 times per week) to standard chemotherapy doubled overall survival in patients with metastatic pancreatic cancer, while also improving quality of life (585).

Therefore, although high-quality, large-scale evidence is still lacking, the current scientific outlook suggests that the following three hypotheses are moving in the direction of truth:

1- High-dose intravenous AA is safe and well-tolerated;

2- High-dose intravenous AA can exert selective and substantial cytotoxic effects;

3- AA can enhance the efficacy of conventional therapies while reducing their toxicity.

It is therefore entirely justified to call for large-scale clinical investigations. Such studies could provide robust evidence of vitamin C's antineoplastic potential and help identify the most effective treatment regimens. As stated in (243): "Given that implementing high-dose AA may represent a breakthrough for cancer patients with poor prognosis or limited treatment options, further clinical investigation of this promising and non-toxic oncologic approach is not only desirable but truly imperative".

An even more emblematic and illustrative conclusion comes from Ngo, Van Riper, Cantley, and Yun, who closed their 2019 "Nature" report with the following: "In conclusion, high-dose intravenous ascorbate represents a promising and inexpensive anticancer therapeutic option that should be further explored in clinical trials. Given its low toxicity and low financial cost, ascorbate could become an important weapon in our arsenal against cancer, either acting as a single agent with predictive biomarkers or used in combination as an adjuvant therapy. Although we are still waiting on a definitive answer for the clinical benefits of ascorbate therapy in cancer, current preclinical and early phase I/II clinical trial results suggest that Linus Pauling's claims regarding the therapeutic benefits of vitamin C therapy in cancer may not be so outrageous after all" (539).

Dosage, timing and frequency

In preclinical studies, the concept of dose-dependent response has become central. Doses exceeding 1 g/kg were generally more effective, and just as non-toxic as lower doses (243). Notably, the lack of efficacy in some cases using < 1 g/kg reinforces both the "more is better" paradigm and the long-standing concern that inadequate dosing may obscure vitamin C's true potential (243).

With regard to treatment duration, multiple in vitro models suggest that short exposures lasting 1-2 hours, often referred to as "flash treatments", are most suitable for maximizing pro-oxidative cytotoxic effects.

Regarding frequency, the prevailing consensus is that more frequent administration yields better outcomes, unsurprising given the short half-life of vitamin C. Daily infusions have proven more effective than the typical integrative medicine protocols involving 1-3 weekly infusions (243). For example, a phase 2 trial in prostate cancer patients using a once-weekly 60 g infusion showed no improvement in biomarkers or disease regression after 12 weeks (572). In contrast, high-dose daily administration in prostate cancer mice significantly inhibited primary tumor growth and metastasis (243).

The situation becomes even more complex when considering dosage ranges. Preclinical data have led researchers to propose 1-2 g/kg for monotherapy and 75-100 g when used alongside standard treatments (243). However, these recommendations remain provisional due to a lack of clinical validation and the complex interplay of variables involved.

Importantly, vitamin C's exceptionally wide therapeutic window complicates the effort to define optimal dosing. Even extraordinarily high doses, potentially up to 5 g/kg, could theoretically be non-toxic, which paradoxically makes it difficult to establish clear therapeutic boundaries.

In summary, the assertion that "pharmacological vitamin C monotherapy is clinically ineffective" is one of the most challenging to substantiate. Indeed, the exceptional safety of vitamin C implies that even if a trial using a very high dose (e.g., 5 g/kg/day) fails, one cannot rule out the possibility that a higher dose might succeed. As such, without a clearly defined upper limit of vitamin C's therapeutic window, no definitive negative conclusions can be drawn about its efficacy. This realization underscores the urgent need for intensified research to explore the full potential of a substance that is exceptionally versatile, minimally toxic, and affordable.

Interestingly, the inherent toxicity of standard pharmacological interventions simplifies research by clearly delineating risk-benefit boundaries. In contrast, the near-absence of toxicity in vitamin C makes defining such thresholds inherently difficult.

Looking ahead, several researchers suggest that a promising research direction would be to shift the focus from plasma levels to the direct measurement of intratumoral ascorbate concentrations. Although plasma concentrations around 20 millimoles/L are considered cytotoxic to cancer cells (428), (243), more specific measurements within the tumor microenvironment could provide insights of greater practical relevance.

In conclusion, current evidence outlines the following perspective: higher is better than lower, frequent is better than sporadic, and intravenous is better than oral.

Antitumor role of vitamin C as a cofactor

As insightfully anticipated nearly seventy years ago by McCormick, modulating collagen synthesis may represent a barrier to cancer progression. Rath and other authors revisited this hypothesis, suggesting that extracellular matrix degradation, already implicated in the pathogenesis of atherosclerosis, could play a critical role in tumor formation and, more significantly, metastasis. In line with this perspective, it is worth noting that vitamin C contributes to the stabilization of what are considered the primary components of the extracellular matrix: collagen fibers (244). This function is far from trivial, considering that the extracellular matrix constitutes the main anatomical barrier against the dissemination of cancer cells throughout the body. This reveals one of the key reasons why restoring physiological concentrations of ascorbate can be crucial in oncology patients: the ascorbic deficiency, which commonly characterizes these individuals, leads to a weakened extracellular matrix, making it less reactive to the invasive behavior typical of malignant cells. The breakdown of the extracellular matrix barrier would therefore be highly detrimental, as the extraregional migration of tumor cells, a phenomenon that leads to the formation of metastases, could render cancer progression uncontrollable.

A new research frontier has thus emerged, where various studies have explored the significance of collagen fiber distribution, identifying its distinct role in both cancer progression and therapeutic responsiveness. The reduction in metastasis, and in some cases even complete remission, observed in recent preclinical studies, seems to support the initial theoretical assumptions and expand the general framework of this hypothesis (243). A concrete example: some researchers have proposed that reduced metastatic spread in pancreatic cancer may be closely associated with increased collagen levels, a conceptually sound hypothesis that has found histopathological support (245). This theory is further reinforced by the practical results of a study published in "Nature" (245), which presented a series of positive clinical outcomes, including a marked improvement in a pancreatic cancer patient treated successfully with 70 infusions of intravenous ascorbate (100 g per infusion) in combination with chemotherapy. "These data revealed a multi-target mechanism underlying the antitumor pharmacological action of ascorbate, with minimal toxicity, and provided guidance for the design of larger definitive studies to test the efficacy of high-dose intravenous vitamin C (IVC) in the treatment of advanced pancreatic cancer", states the promising scientific report entitled "High Dose Parenteral Ascorbate Inhibited Pancreatic Cancer Growth and Metastasis: Mechanisms and a Phase I/IIa Study" (245).

Leaving aside, for now, the specific susceptibility of pancreatic cancer to vitamin C (an issue that will be revisited through a representative clinical case later on), it is important not to overlook the findings of a large meta-analysis of observational studies published in 2015 in "Nature" (525), which reported: "Our analysis suggests that higher intake of vitamin C may reduce the risk of pancreatic cancer". This underscores a fundamental principle: although vitamin C is a promising pharmacological agent in oncology and other fields, it is first and foremost an essential prophylactic agent.

Continuing the theoretical discussion, it is essential to revisit the previously mentioned link between vitamin C and hypoxia-inducible factors (HIFs). A considerable body of research has validated the underlying concepts, including the compelling preclinical and clinical studies by Kuiper, which confirmed the inverse correlation between intratumoral ascorbate levels and HIF-1 alpha activity

(246). Other studies on GULO-deficient mice demonstrated that both intraperitoneal and oral administration of vitamin C led to a clear inverse correlation between intratumoral ascorbate levels and key parameters such as HIF-1 alpha activation and tumor growth rate (246). These findings suggest a potential antitumor role for orally administered vitamin C, opening a new and previously underappreciated research avenue.

This perspective, apparently paradoxical and rich in both historical and scientific meaning (as will be discussed later), contrasts with the prevailing view of the past two decades, which has linked vitamin C's antitumor activity almost exclusively to intravenous administration. In fact, similar antineoplastic effects have been observed in other studies where they were attributed to the restoration of physiological plasma and intracellular concentrations. Campbell, Vissers, Bozonet, Dyer, Robinson, and Dachs were among the first to argue that an appropriately dosed oral therapy could effectively suppress HIF-1 alpha activity and its tumor-promoting effects in hypoxic microenvironments (404). "This is the first study to investigate the significance of restoring physiological ascorbate levels in tumor progression. Our data provide evidence, in an animal model, that optimal ascorbate levels may reduce tumor growth and HIF-regulated cancer aggressiveness", stated the authors in a 2015 article accepted by "Cancer Medicine" (404). Their findings open new research horizons where a parallel universe may reveal a constellation of groundbreaking surprises.

Another antitumor mechanism involving vitamin C lies within the multidimensional realm of epigenetics. Owing to its well-known role as a cofactor for the family of dioxygenase enzymes involved in DNA demethylation (the TET enzymes), one might reasonably inquire into the relationship between cancer and DNA demethylation. Despite several unresolved questions, it is believed that many forms of cancer not only cause ascorbate depletion, thereby compromising the coenzymatic functions vital to TET activity, but also exhibit abnormalities in DNA methylation-demethylation dynamics that favor malignant cell progression (247). More specifically, TET enzymes are frequently mutated and thus impaired in various cancers, particularly hematological malignancies. Consequently, epigenetic dysregulation, primarily represented by the repression of TET activity, is increasingly considered a hallmark of oncogenesis. These considerations have paved the way for an ascorbate-based therapeutic approach in some hematological malignancies.

Initial findings in this context warrant deeper investigation: several studies havc shown that vitamin C supplementation can modulate abnormal TET enzyme levels, thereby demonstrating an antitumor effect linked to DNA demethylation (248). This recent and scientifically significant discovery has spurred growing interest in the potential therapeutic role of vitamin C in leukemia, as evidenced by the attention of the late Francesco Lo-Coco, one of the world's foremost hematologists, whose pioneering research revolutionized the treatment of acute promyelocytic leukemia (529), (531), (530).

Further support comes from articles published in "Nature", including "Leukaemia: Vitamin C Regulates Stem Cells and Cancer" (532) and "Ascorbate Regulates Haematopoietic Stem Cell Function and Leukaemogenesis" (249), the latter offering several notable insights. Chief among them is the suggestion that oral supplementation may play an important role, as reflected in the authors' concluding remarks: "Our data suggest that for individuals with clonal hematopoiesis, maintaining adequate dietary ascorbate intake is important to maximize residual TET tumor-suppressor function" (249). This aligns with prior statements by Lo-Coco and collaborators (529), who emphasized the principle of adequacy: "Vitamin C may exhibit antitumor properties even when administered orally, provided the dosage is sufficiently high". Therefore, if used appropriately, oral vitamin C could also exert anti-tumor effects, a point that should absolutely not be underestimated.

The restoration of TET function by vitamin C is also described in four preclinical studies that effectively combined ascorbate with chemotherapy or biological therapy (250), further supporting the compound's strong synergistic potential with anticancer agents.

Alongside TET enzymes, jumonji C domain-containing histone demethylases are another group of important epigenetic regulators whose activity seems to be boosted by vitamin C, with potentially wide therapeutic implications. One important effect of this boost is the suppression of abnormal self-renewal in hematopoietic stem cells, the undifferentiated progenitors of all blood cells, often involved in hematological malignancies. This benefit was highlighted in a 2019 report by Lee Chong, Ahearn and Cimmino, published in "Frontiers in Cell and Developmental Biology" (248).

Given these various epigenetic implications, it is not an overstatement to suggest that vitamin C may promote the re-expression of tumor-suppressor genes, genes that normally inhibit the cell cycle and protect against malignant transformation, which are frequently silenced in cancer. In simple terms, vitamin C can modulate certain epigenetic alterations that cancer leverages to sustain its progression, thereby adding an additional mechanism to its potential antitumor effect. For this reason, its use as an epigenetic agent in cancer treatment represents a scientifically relevant hypothesis, which clearly departs from the traditional nutritional role typically associated with vitamin C.

Yet the antitumor arsenal of vitamin C is not limited to direct mechanisms. An additional, "indirect" mode of action concerns its impact on the immune system. While the antioxidant role of vitamin C within immune architecture is well established, its cofactor activity is increasingly recognized as critical for numerous immune processes (251). These include T cell maturation and activation, neutrophil chemotaxis and apoptosis, antiviral cytokine synthesis, and NK cell-mediated tumor cell cytotoxicity, all of which depend on sufficient plasma and tissue ascorbate levels, especially in high-consumption states such as inflammation and malignancy (251). In this regard, the need to achieve millimolar plasma concentrations, which have been shown to moderate pro-inflammatory cytokine expression (110), further supports the "more is better" philosophy and strengthens the rationale for high-dose therapy in oncology.

From this standpoint, it is reasonable to posit that immune efficiency, which is inherently dependent on optimal vitamin C levels, should be considered both in ascorbate-based strategies and in broader therapeutic contexts. Various animal models support this hypothesis, indicating that immune competence may enhance vitamin C's antitumor effects. For example, several researchers observed that its maximal antitumor effect was achieved in immunocompetent mice, suggesting that its efficacy also relies on its immunomodulatory properties (252). It is also worth recalling vitamin C's relevant role in promoting interferon synthesis and supporting NK cell function.

It is therefore plausible to assert that a well-functioning immune system represents an essential prerequisite for maximizing the antitumor actions of ascorbate, and possibly other antineoplastic agents as well.

This immunological overview concludes with some scientific proposals that point toward an ambitious goal (455): the integration of vitamin C into the increasingly promising field of immunotherapy. “This work provides a rationale for conducting clinical trials that combine immunotherapies with high-dose ascorbate”, as stated by researchers in “Science” (252), the prestigious journal that published their findings.

We now arrive at a critical synthesis. A comprehensive analysis reveals no fewer than seven distinct antineoplastic mechanisms. When combined with the unique pharmacological properties of vitamin C, these constitute a compelling case for the immediate initiation of high-quality clinical trials. The urgency is justified: cancer is not retreating, on the contrary, it appears to be gaining momentum, fueled by modern lifestyles that provide fertile ground for its proliferation. Time is of the essence, particularly in light of vitamin C’s favorable safety profile and low cost. These two features sharply contrast with conventional treatments, highlighting a logical and strategic advantage in favor of ascorbate.

We are talking about a vital molecule, typically deficient in cancer patients, minimally toxic, potentially synergistic with many standard therapies, capable of mitigating side effects, endowed with multiple antitumor mechanisms, and potentially able to improve quality of life. The number seven seems emblematic in the context of vitamin C and cancer: seven known antitumor mechanisms and seven valid reasons to seriously consider its pharmacological use in cancer treatment, initially as an experimental approach, and potentially, in the future, as a clinical mainstay.

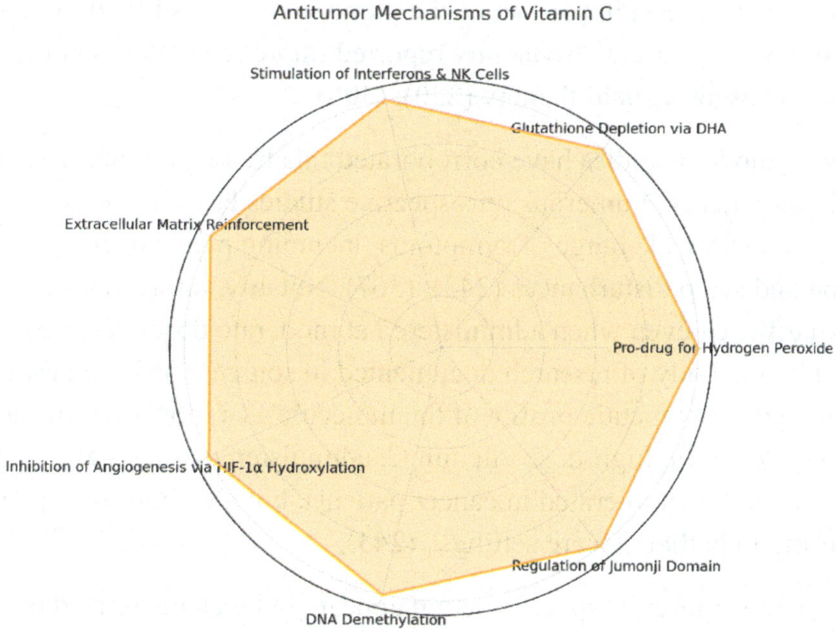

The potential improvements in quality of life

Direct involvement with oncology patients entails navigating a complex array of experiences. Given the countless challenges that characterize the final stages of illness, ensuring dignified days and an acceptable quality of life represents one of the most important, and often extremely difficult, goals to achieve. The understandable psychological frustration, the natural fear of "what comes next," the pain associated with the disease, and the side effects of therapies all contribute to a harmful interplay of forces that can severely destabilize the delicate balance sustaining quality of life. A potential rebalancing force may lie in vitamin C, whose numerous virtues also position it as a promising adjuvant capable of improving quality of life in cancer patients.

One might naturally consider its analgesic properties, which are not only effective but also synergistic with synthetic opioids, drugs that, while potent, are unfortunately not free of toxicity. However, its analgesic effect constitutes just one element within a broader therapeutic arsenal. Consider, for instance, its involvement in carnitine synthesis, supporting physical performance, and, more notably, in the biosynthesis of serotonin and catecholamines, pathways that appear to confer notable antidepressant properties on ascorbic acid. These benefits have been recognized, at least in part, since the pioneering work of Pauling, Cameron and Murata, whose patients frequently reported improvements in vitality and pain control during ascorbic acid therapy (220), (408).

Several modern studies have corroborated this trend, particularly among terminally ill patients. Numerous retrospective studies have reported improvements in a wide range of symptoms, including pain, appetite, fatigue, depression and sleep disturbances (243), (367). Notably, intravenous ascorbic acid has shown efficacy even when administered at moderate doses (2-15 g), as evidenced by the body of research documented in sources (367) and especially (243), where the therapeutic profile of the molecule as a monotherapy can be appreciated: "Overall, high-dose vitamin C, administered as a single agent, was not only safe and well tolerated in cancer patients, but also improved pain and quality of life in palliative care settings" (243).

But there is more: its specific action appears to be characterized by a certain rapidity, with benefits manifesting within a relatively short timeframe. For example, in a prospective study published in 2007 in the "Journal of Korean Medical Science" (253), 39 terminal cancer patients were assessed. Each patient received an intravenous dose of 10 g of vitamin C every three days, along with a daily oral supplement of 4 g, for a duration of just one week. All outcomes were positive: significant improvements in overall quality of life were reported, including reductions in fatigue, nausea and vomiting, as well as increased appetite and better pain control. According to the authors, vitamin C proved to be effective, safe, and fast-acting; their concluding remarks are particularly explicit: "Although there is still controversy regarding the antitumor effects of vitamin C, its use should be considered a safe and effective therapy for improving quality of life in terminal cancer patients" (253).

Overall, the multifaceted support that an intervention with ascorbic acid can provide, combined with the state of hypovitaminosis commonly observed in oncology patients, constitutes a dual rationale for its use in cancer management. It is important not to overlook that this is independent of the mechanisms through which the molecule can act directly on tumor cells, with potential clinical efficacy and high precision.

The extraordinary story of my father Raffaele

My interest in vitamin C began in early 2013, specifically on January 5th, a date that remains etched in my memory and heart. Late that morning, I came across an online discussion forum where a lively and heated debate caught my attention. I was struck by the confidence with which one user praised the therapeutic potential of vitamin C. Driven by curiosity, I embarked on a thorough research journey, whose findings proved to be highly divisive: on one side, a small group of advocates promoted its use even in the treatment of serious conditions like cancer; on the other, a larger and more skeptical majority warned against possible adverse effects, particularly the risk of kidney damage.

What happened to my father in August of that same year, a diagnosis of advanced cancer, would retroactively give that early research an almost "premonitory" quality.

In late spring 2013, Raffaele began to exhibit alarming clinical signs, including a constellation of symptoms suggestive of an evolving intestinal sub-obstruction. These symptoms worsened to the point that specialized evaluation became necessary, ultimately leading to a grim diagnosis: advanced colorectal cancer.

At the time, he was 82 years old and far from a model of perfect health. His medical history was extensive and complex, including ischemic heart disease, arterial hypertension, type 2 diabetes, obesity, atrial fibrillation, obstructive sleep apnea syndrome (one of the main sources of oxidative stress), psoriasis, spinal canal stenosis, and chronic bronchitis. This complex clinical profile required both an elaborate polypharmacy regimen and ventilatory therapy to control nocturnal apnea.

The increasing abdominal pain and severe defecation difficulties indicated a progression from a sub-obstruction to a full intestinal blockage, thereby prompting the medical team to proceed with a high-risk surgical intervention. Performed on October 23rd, 2013, the operation proved extraordinarily complex, highlighting the exceptional skill of the surgical team. The procedure was fraught with technical difficulties, most notably the resection and subsequent reimplantation of the right ureter, and further complicated by Raffaele's compromised physical condition, which forced him to leave the operating room with dangerously low blood pressure.

The surgical intervention, left colectomy and rectal resection, extended to include appendectomy and right pelvic ureter resection with reimplantation, followed by terminal left iliac colostomy, resulted in the diagnosis of "poorly differentiated adenocarcinoma involving the full thickness of the sigmoid-rectum and bladder wall, with focal extension to the cecal appendix, perilymphatic neoplastic invasion, and multiple secondary localizations near the right spermatic vessels".

The staging confirmed an advanced clinical condition, classified as T4N0M1, indicative of a high and widespread tumor burden. The subsequent surgical consultation further highlighted the severity: the biological aggressiveness of the tumor, involvement of the right kidney, depth of invasion, advanced age, and multiple comorbidities all contributed to making the prognosis even more unfavorable.

The family's response was swift and constructive. An open and constructive discussion, partly inspired by my recent interest in vitamin C, led to three measures:

1- The decision to rule out initiating potential chemotherapy;

2- The initiation of high-dose vitamin C supplementation, both orally and in liposomal form (an innovative delivery method to be discussed later), supported by additional compounds such as liposomal curcumin, epigallocatechin gallate, the amino acids lysine and proline, and vitamin D;

3- The adoption of a plant-based diet, combined with a substantial reduction in carbohydrate intake.

The results observed over time were remarkable. One year later, oncological assessments revealed no detectable signs of disease. Moreover, the effects of the polytherapy led to the discontinuation of medications for diabetes and hypertension, which were no longer deemed necessary. This important secondary outcome, namely, the improvement in blood glucose and blood pressure control without the need for previously essential medication, led me to realize that vitamin C can offer "collateral benefits". In fact, this hypothesis aligns well with the holistic nature of the molecule: for example, taking it to strengthen immune function may also yield a range of concurrent benefits, such as increased physical endurance, enhanced mental clarity and improved skin elasticity.

In the following years, Raffaele's clinical course remained remarkably stable. Both imaging studies and laboratory tests showed no evidence of disease. His overall health, although compromised by several chronic conditions, remained relatively stable for nearly a decade before deteriorating irreversibly due to severe cardiac complications.

A few clarifications can further enrich this account, offering tools for more informed reflection:

1- Medical opinions and tumor staging clearly indicated a severe condition, with a poor prognosis. For this staging and cancer type, five-year survival is statistically below 10% (544);

2- Raffaele received exclusively oral vitamin C, never resorting to the more potent intravenous route;

3- Over time, the overall pharmacological burden decreased, contrary to the initial and rather grim expectations of an increase;

4- Renal function, carefully monitored every three months, consistently remained within normal limits, despite the severely impaired right kidney, which had already been largely non-functional before the initiation of the polytherapy based on vitamin C and other substances. This finding strongly challenges the belief that high-dose vitamin C can be nephrotoxic, an issue that will be examined in more detail in the following sections.

5- Liver, pancreatic, and thyroid function; coagulation indices; electrolytes; glucose and iron levels; complete blood count; tumor markers; inflammatory indices; and other routine parameters have remained within normal ranges for many years.

Raffaele's case therefore represents a clinically extraordinary story that also sheds light on a scientific perspective at odds with prevailing theories about the antitumor mechanisms of vitamin C. Contrary to the dominant belief that only high-dose intravenous vitamin C can exert significant anticancer effects, my father's case suggests a potentially broader and more inclusive reality, empirically supported by the dramatic clinical benefits achieved through oral administration alone.

This extraordinary case lends support to an emerging consensus shared by both contemporary specialists, such as Lo-Coco and colleagues, who asserted just a few years ago that "vitamin C may exhibit antitumor properties even when administered orally, provided the doses are sufficiently high" (529), and earlier proponents of orthomolecular medicine: high-dose oral supplementation warrants its own pharmacological identity and, consequently, greater clinical and scientific attention.

Raffaele's story invites a reassessment of the pharmacology of vitamin C: it cannot be ruled out that properly implemented oral administration may also possess antineoplastic properties, an insight that should encourage researchers to reconsider their research frameworks. Supporting this hypothesis is a growing body of evidence showing that certain key mechanisms, such as the modulation of HIF-1 alpha levels (404) and epigenetic properties (539), can also be activated through a well-structured oral supplementation regimen.

An emblematic case

"We believe that a new treatment agent that shows robust laboratory and animal evidence, coupled with minimal patient toxicity, deserves rigorous clinical investigation without concern that clinical trials might not be supported by industry or have potential to generate profits. Indeed, patients deserve no less" (430). These are the closing remarks by Drisko, Serrano, Spruce, Chen and Levine in an instructive case report published in 2018 in the journal "Anti-Cancer Drugs" (430), detailing the extraordinary clinical course of a patient diagnosed with terminal pancreatic cancer, specifically, stage IV poorly differentiated pancreatic ductal adenocarcinoma.

Defying a prognosis of mere months, this patient experienced an unexpectedly long survival, nearly four years from diagnosis in March 2007. According to the authors, this outcome was attributed solely to monotherapy with vitamin C, since the patient had consciously refused chemotherapy. The pharmacological regimen based on vitamin C, administered intravenously at doses ranging from 75 to 125 g approximately 2.5 times per week throughout the course of the illness (nearly four years), for a total of about 500 infusions, achieved what conventional treatments, according to statistical consensus, would not have been expected to: markedly prolonged survival, accompanied by a satisfactory quality of life. Moreover, laboratory markers, including renal function, which is often a focus of safety concerns, remained stable throughout the entire course of treatment.

In summary, this case concerned a disease that, although initially highly aggressive and marked by extensive liver metastases, entered a state of continuous regression. By January 2011, thanks to vitamin C therapy, the numerous liver metastases had disappeared and the primary lesion had undergone substantial regression.

However, a questionable clinical decision, namely, the placement of a biliary stent in response to a suspected recurrence later ruled out by imaging, interrupted this remarkable regression and set in motion a fatal sequence of events, culminating in septic shock. In hindsight, the intestinal perforation that precipitated the patient's clinical decline was ultimately linked to this procedure. A retrospective analysis suggested that the rise in liver enzymes, which prompted the stent placement, might instead have been caused by self-administered megadoses of vitamin D.

Regardless of technical considerations, this case inspires thought-provoking insights. One in particular stands out: if the biliary stent had not been placed, it is plausible that the patient, four years after a devastating diagnosis, could have continued to live even longer, supported by ascorbic acid therapy. Only God could know for how long.

What we, mere mortals confined by our fleeting existence in a small corner of the cosmos, do know is that research into ascorbic acid for cancer has reached a critical point, one that now appears to demand the highest priority.

I would like to make one final remark: although no specific data are available, it is reasonable to assume that during his terminal decline, from the stent-related intestinal perforation to death by septic shock, the patient may no longer have received the megadoses of vitamin C to which he had become accustomed. This could explain why sepsis, one of the potential targets of vitamin C therapy, unfortunately prevailed.

Chapter 9
Vitamin C In The Treatment Of Other Conditions

Diabetes

Let us now turn to diabetes, a disease that affects approximately 10% of the global adult population and continues to show an increasing incidence (554). An increasing body of evidence supports the link between vitamin C and diabetes, already partially illustrated in previously discussed studies (76). A fundamental starting point is the well-established fact that hyperglycemia induces oxidative stress. A second critical aspect lies in the widespread vitamin C deficiency observed in individuals with diabetes, suggesting the potential benefit of supplementation. Furthermore, it is known that the maximum absorption of vitamin C, particularly in its oxidized form DHA, occurs during states of glucose deficiency, reflecting the competitive interaction between these two structurally similar molecules within GLUT transporters.

Several studies have examined diabetes through the lens of vitamin C, yielding interesting hypotheses and promising findings. A notable example is a 2017 observational study (353) that investigated fasting blood glucose, body mass index and smoking status, showing that all three considerably influence ascorbate levels. In addition to oxidative stress, the study identified chronic inflammation, a hallmark of diabetes, as another destabilizing factor affecting ascorbate levels. This low-grade systemic inflammation is driven by the chronic activation of the innate immune system commonly observed in both diabetes and obesity. It is worth noting that the study provided further confirmation of the inverse correlation between fasting glucose and plasma ascorbate levels, a relationship well-established in the literature (353). This strong inverse correlation can be interpreted in two ways. On one hand, numerous investigations have reinforced vitamin C's prophylactic properties. For instance, in the large-scale EPIC-Norfolk study (510), researchers concluded: “Dietary measures to increase plasma vitamin C may be an important public health strategy for reducing diabetes prevalence”.

On the other hand, the inverse correlation between glucose and ascorbate reflects its biological properties, since its levels in diabetic patients appear to be proportional to the severity of the disease (256). The result, ultimately, is a coherent and well-structured picture.

To enrich this discussion, we turn to a study published in the prestigious journal "The Lancet" in 2015 (254). A brief preamble and a definition are necessary. Firstly, since SVCTs are not expressed in erythrocytes, these cells must internalize DHA via GLUT transporters, requiring subsequent intracellular reduction into ascorbic acid. This recycling process, although essential, results in limited intracellular concentrations. Secondly, erythrocyte deformability refers to the ability of red blood cells to change shape in order to pass through narrow passages, such as tight capillaries.

In this context, the study (254) reported a very noteworthy finding: a direct correlation between erythrocytic ascorbate concentration and erythrocyte deformability. In practical terms, higher vitamin C levels are associated with greater red blood cell elasticity. This new relationship highlights notable microvascular implications of erythrocytic ascorbate, since its low levels may lead to an increase in red blood cell rigidity, impairing their ability to pass through capillaries. This, in turn, may result in local hypoxia, a condition that tends to cause considerable vascular damage.

The study also provided statistical evidence of an inverse correlation between plasma glucose concentrations, both in humans and in mice, and erythrocytic ascorbate levels (254), reflecting the competition between glucose and DHA within GLUTs, a potential determinant factor of erythrocyte function.

Therefore, repeated episodes of hyperglycemia, characteristic of poorly controlled diabetes, can completely deplete erythrocyte ascorbate, consequently reducing red blood cell deformability to the point of causing marked rigidity. This, in turn, contributes to diabetic microangiopathy, a complication characterized by substantial capillary alterations that primarily affect the kidneys (diabetic nephropathy) and the retina (diabetic retinopathy).

In summary, competition between DHA and glucose for erythrocyte GLUTs may initiate a cascade: hyperglycemia → impaired ascorbate transport → red blood cell rigidity → diabetic microangiopathy. This proposed mechanism offers a potential etiological explanation for a complication whose origins remain unclear. If the role of erythrocyte ascorbate in microangiopathy is confirmed, it could emerge as a potential biomarker for the management of diabetes and its complications.

Yet, as the authors of the 2015 Lancet study lament (254): "Surprisingly, modern hematology textbooks contain no description of vitamin C in red blood cells". This omission is striking and, given the journal's scientific authority, points to an urgent need to reassess or update current understanding of vitamin C. Its complex physiology, distinctive pharmacokinetics, and emerging pharmacological roles deserve greater emphasis in medical education. The involvement of ascorbate, both erythrocytic and systemic, in the pathophysiology of diabetes exemplifies a long-overdue paradigm shift. This shift could illuminate the therapeutic potential of vitamin C and emphasize the clinical relevance of both plasma and intracellular measurements, which are frequently overlooked.

Overall, the study "Low Red Blood Cell Vitamin C Concentrations Induce Red Blood Cell Fragility: A Link to Diabetes Via Glucose, Glucose Transporters, and Dehydroascorbic Acid" (254) identifies novel dynamics in diabetes pathophysiology, indicating that maintaining adequate ascorbate levels may contribute to the prevention of common diabetic complications.

Vitamin C is not solely a preventive agent; it also exerts specific pharmacological effects beyond correcting deficiencies or preventing complications. For instance, a double-blind, placebo-controlled study (255) evaluated the effect of combining vitamin C (500 mg orally, twice daily) with metformin, the standard first-line treatment for type 2 diabetes, over a 12-week period. The combination therapy outperformed metformin alone in lowering fasting and postprandial glucose, and glycated hemoglobin. The authors concluded: "Both drugs can be used in combination to maintain good glycemic control in type 2 diabetes" (255). Notably, the modest dosage used (500 mg twice daily) still produced hypoglycemic effects, prompting speculation that higher doses might enhance therapeutic outcomes, especially given the profound ascorbate deficiency commonly observed in diabetic individuals (477), (256), (374). Indeed, final vitamin C levels in the study remained low (25.5 micromoles post-treatment vs. 14.8 micromoles pre-treatment), suggesting that the dose was largely insufficient for complete repletion (255).

Other investigations (256), (374) have reported deficiencies in diabetic patients. A 2021 comparative study (256) found that plasma vitamin C levels in individuals with diabetes were half those of the control group (12.5 micromoles vs. 26.7 micromoles), reinforcing the alarming conclusion of the previously discussed study (255): diabetes may induce subclinical scurvy.

The hypoglycemic effects of vitamin C have been confirmed by several studies, including a recent meta-analysis of 20 randomized, controlled clinical trials (478), (353). A key finding from these studies is that the duration of treatment plays a crucial role in determining outcomes. Short-term interventions, in fact, may underestimate the true potential of vitamin C, a concept also supported by research on sepsis, where longer intravenous treatments (at least 5 days) have been shown to be more effective than shorter ones (394).

A 2017 multicenter randomized study (446) compared three groups over 12 months: metformin + placebo, metformin + vitamin C (500 mg/day orally), and metformin + aspirin. Despite the conservative dose, the vitamin C group had double the probability of reducing glycated hemoglobin compared to metformin alone, and a tenfold greater likelihood (compared to the aspirin group) of lowering diabetes-related risk factors. The study suggests that even modest doses of vitamin C can yield substantial benefits.

A recent review and meta-analysis, published in the influential journal "Diabetes Care" in 2021 (504), confirmed vitamin C's efficacy and also offered a critical view of current scientific research: "While short-term studies suggest that vitamin C supplementation may improve glycemic control and blood pressure in people with type 2 diabetes, it cannot yet be recommended as a therapy until larger, longer-term, high-quality studies confirm these findings" (504). Given that the average publication year of the 28 studies analyzed is 2011, critical questions arise: why delay further research?

What factors continue to hinder the validation of a compound that is safe, affordable, biologically versatile, frequently deficient in individuals with diabetes, and potentially effective in glycemic control?

The ongoing stagnation in vitamin C research appears ethically concerning and scientifically discouraging.

From a theoretical standpoint, the molecular mechanisms by which vitamin C influences glucose metabolism remain poorly understood. The prevailing hypothesis suggests a modulatory effect on insulin secretion or sensitivity. Vitamin C's antioxidant effect on pancreatic beta cells supports this idea (255). Recent studies (257) indicate that vitamin C supplementation may stimulate production of a quartet of protective molecules: prostaglandin E1, prostacyclins (anti-platelet prostaglandins), nitric oxide, and lipoxin A4 (a vasodilatory-antioxidant lipid mediator). These mediators may safeguard pancreatic beta cells and endothelial tissue against endogenous and exogenous toxins (257). Therefore, vitamin C is believed to contribute to the management of diabetes and hypertension by supporting this anti-inflammatory and vasodilatory molecular network. This hypothesis is shared by the eminent Indian immunologist and endocrinologist Undurti Narasimha Das, who advocates for further scientific evaluation (257).

Vitamin C may also offer benefits during acute hypoglycemia. A reputable study found that its intravenous administration during insulin-induced hypoglycemia in type 1 diabetes can reduce oxidative stress, inflammation and endothelial dysfunction (509).

This section concludes with a look at gestational diabetes, for which the literature is limited but fairly consistent. Some studies, such as one published in "Reproductive Medicine" (258), suggest an inverse correlation between vitamin C levels and gestational diabetes risk, while others highlight a dose-dependent response (259). For example, in one study, women with plasma vitamin C levels < 42.6 micromoles/L had a twelvefold higher risk of gestational diabetes than those > 63.3 micromoles/L (258). Similarly, a 2004 study (487) found that women with levels < 55.9 micromoles/L had triple the risk compared to those with levels > 74.6 micromoles/L. Therefore, even in this context, maintaining plasma levels above 80 micromoles/L could be genuinely protective.

An additional favorable element, which moreover has greater scientific reliability, is contained in a recent meta-analysis, in which the authors state in their conclusions that: "Low vitamin C exposure during pregnancy may increase the risk of gestational diabetes mellitus. Given these findings, it could be beneficial for pregnant women to increase their intake of vitamin C-rich foods and to ensure adequate blood vitamin C levels as a preventive measure against gestational diabetes mellitus" (594).

Let us return to plasma levels. During pregnancy, the biosynthesis of vitamin C increases significantly in animals capable of producing it, suggesting that pregnant women have a particular need to compensate for GULO inactivity. It is no coincidence that several studies have indeed shown a substantial decline in vitamin C levels throughout pregnancy. A Nigerian study involving 400 women (368) reported plasma concentrations of 11.3 micromoles/L in the first trimester, 28.4 micromoles/L in the second, and 19.9 micromoles/L in the third. This pattern has been confirmed by studies from Brazil (556) and Uganda (555).

Vitamin C also appears to protect against premature rupture of membranes (PPROM), a condition in which the amniotic sac breaks before the onset of labor, potentially leading to preterm birth and increasing the risk of infection for both mother and baby. Multiple studies (488), (489), (490), (521) confirm an inverse correlation between ascorbate levels and PPROM risk. One study (490) was particularly conclusive: "Ascorbic acid concentration was low in women with PPROM. Therefore, vitamin C supplementation should be mandatory alongside iron and calcium during pregnancy".

One of the most remarkable features of vitamin C is its effectiveness even at low doses. In a study involving 170 Iranian women, for example, even the microscopic dose of 100 mg per day proved effective in reducing the incidence of PPROM (521).

To conclude, several general points merit clarification. Vitamin C's hypoglycemic, antihypertensive, and hypocholesterolemic effects must not be seen as substitutes for a healthy lifestyle. These properties should instead support and encourage healthy habits.

Moreover, compared to conventional pharmacotherapies, which can cause excessive reductions in blood glucose, blood pressure, or cholesterol, vitamin C acts more gently, modulating elevated levels without triggering dangerous counter-effects such as hypoglycemia or hypotension. While this characteristic is advantageous in terms of safety, it may also limit its standalone therapeutic efficacy, thereby highlighting its role as a valuable adjunct.

Vitamin C may also help reduce the need for certain treatments, and limit their side effects. This benefit is increasingly supported by scientific data. Its promising synergies with amiodarone, metformin, statins, beta-blockers, fluoxetine, propofol, levodopa, antineoplastics, and hydrocortisone have been documented in several preliminary studies, suggesting potential clinical relevance that unquestionably warrants further investigation.

Finally, the correlations between vitamin C and several risk factors, such as hypertension, impaired fasting glucose, hypercholesterolemia, obesity, and endothelial dysfunction, suggest a central role in metabolic syndrome, a cluster of conditions that represents a significant cardiovascular threat. Recent meta-analyses (377), (522) have confirmed the inverse correlation between plasma ascorbate levels and the risk of metabolic syndrome.

Eye diseases

The quotient of 50, obtained by dividing the average ascorbic acid content in the aqueous humor by its plasma concentration, is sufficient to highlight the crucial role of vitamin C for ocular health. This role becomes even more evident when we turn our attention to the animal kingdom, where a clear preference for local accumulation has been observed in species more inclined to diurnal life (260). This phenomenon points to the strong protective power that ascorbic acid can provide against sunlight: the cornea, the lens (a structure that appears unsaturable through dietary intake (410)), and all other ocular tissues benefit from a formidable defense capable of shielding against the oxidative dangers of UV light. One of the many available examples?

A recent study (506) conducted on 138 healthy individuals, divided into two groups based on their plasma levels (< 34 micromoles/L, > 34 micromoles/L), yielded results supporting the importance of ascorbic acid in retinal diseases, showing that higher plasma levels enhance the eye's protective mechanisms in multiple ways.

From a broader perspective, various elements support the view that vitamin C is essential for protecting ocular tissues from photo-oxidative damage. It should therefore come as no surprise that the literature highlights its importance in the prevention and treatment of numerous ocular diseases. Let us begin with the most widely known condition: cataracts, a disorder characterized by the loss of lens transparency, which significantly impairs visual capacity. While many epidemiological studies support a correlation between vitamin C intake and a reduced risk of cataracts (261), others have found no such link. For example, the comprehensive study titled "A randomized, placebo-controlled, clinical trial of high-dose supplementation with vitamins C and E and beta carotene for age-related cataract and vision loss: AREDS report no. 9" (262) produced disappointing results. Nearly 5000 participants aged 55-80 were randomly assigned to receive a daily tablet containing various antioxidants (vitamin C 500 mg, vitamin E 400 IU, beta-carotene 15 mg) or no antioxidants. Data collected over an extended observation period revealed no positive effect: "The use of a high-dose formulation of vitamin C, vitamin E, and beta-carotene in a cohort of relatively well-nourished older adults had no apparent effect on the 7-year risk of development or progression of age-related lens opacity" (262). What could be the explanation for these negative results?

It is not unreasonable to attribute the lack of efficacy to both the weak therapeutic approach adopted and the age group included in the study, which is typically characterized by low ascorbic acid levels (SVCTs are believed to lose efficiency with age (63)). However, the issue becomes rather absurd when we consider the wording in the study's title, "high dose", which is quite misleading. Referring to an oral dose of 500 mg as "high" seems truly inappropriate. Surely, the pioneers of vitamin C would have had much to say about that!

So how, then, should we describe the doses used in oncology studies?

The misuse of the term "high dose", and this deserves a brief digression, is unfortunately common in the literature. A paradigmatic example is the study titled "High-dose oral vitamin C partially replenishes vitamin C levels in patients with Type 2 diabetes and low vitamin C levels but does not improve endothelial dysfunction or insulin resistance" (477), focusing on diabetic patients. In it, 800 mg/day was administered orally for four weeks. This is the so-called "high dose" of vitamin C, an amount that proved insufficient to adequately restore plasma levels in the diabetic participants. The evidence is unequivocal: at the end of four weeks of "high-dose" supplementation, the average plasma concentration, though increased, still failed to surpass the sufficiency threshold of 50 micromoles/L.

Therefore, based on findings from (477), and especially from a previously discussed paradigmatic trial (255), it would be misleading to conclude that high oral doses of vitamin C are ineffective in managing diabetes. Instead, what logic suggests is a general principle already outlined: although often labeled as "high" or "robust", standard oral supplementation (500-1000 mg/day) is, in many cases, insufficient to ensure adequate plasma levels in patients with pre-existing conditions, and therefore inadequate to induce any meaningful clinical response.

Consequently, especially in light of the prevailing ideological confusion, it becomes increasingly necessary to formally define the concept of a "high dose of vitamin C". Therefore, I would like to take the liberty of proposing a working definition of high-dose vitamin C. Specifically:

– High-dose oral vitamin C: application of the dynamic flow model or bowel tolerance method;

– High-dose intravenous vitamin C: dosage no less than 300 mg/kg.

This is a symbolic statement, intended to highlight the need for objective criteria to make clinical evaluations more analytical and to avoid unfair judgments that further diminish vitamin C, a compound already often misunderstood. "I took high doses of vitamin C, 800 mg per day, and noticed no benefit". What could be more inconsistent than a statement like that?

Returning to epidemiological studies on cataracts, it is surely no coincidence that a meta-analysis (263) published in the journal "Acta Ophthalmologica" in 2016 concluded: "Higher vitamin C intake and plasma ascorbate may be inversely associated with cataract risk. Vitamin C intake should be encouraged for primary cataract prevention".

Other studies have confirmed this: in a large Italo-American investigation (411), the results not only reaffirmed the protective efficacy of high plasma levels ("In agreement with some previous studies, we found that high plasma vitamin C levels are associated with reduced cataract prevalence", the authors state), but they also highlighted an asymmetry that further increases the value of vitamin C. Indeed, findings in (411) reveal a troubling tendency for vitamin E to increase cataract risk, an "unexpected" discovery, as scientists describe it, which consists of a direct correlation between high vitamin E intake and an increased risk of cataract. To conclude, one might ask: could this unexpected correlation help explain the negative results of the study "A randomized, placebo-controlled, clinical trial of high-dose supplementation with vitamins C and E and beta carotene for age-related cataract and vision loss: AREDS report no. 9" (262)?

Before moving forward, it is worth revisiting the asymmetries noted in (411) concerning the vitamin C-vitamin E relationship. This is not the only instance in which vitamin C has shown protective effects, while vitamin E has displayed negative trends. Another example?

A large prospective study (500), involving 3919 individuals monitored over 11 years, revealed a similar scenario, this time within a more challenging clinical context. The data identified an inverse correlation between ascorbic acid and heart failure, while also suggesting that a high intake of vitamin E may increase the risk of heart failure.

As for a therapeutic approach in ophthalmology, the few available studies have reported intriguing results, often proportional to circulating levels. A case in point is the study titled "Efficacy of Systemic Vitamin C Supplementation in Reducing Corneal Opacity Resulting from Infectious Keratitis" (354), which highlights how inadequate the so-called "high doses" of 500-800 mg actually are. To evaluate the effectiveness of vitamin C in reducing corneal opacity caused by infectious keratitis, the researchers employed two strategies: oral supplementation at 3 grams and intravenous infusions at 20 grams. As expected, intravenous administration proved more effective, although oral treatment still performed better than placebo. A provocative question remains: what kind of results would we have seen with only 500-800 mg?

Overall, a clear pattern seems to emerge: while studies using low doses generally yield modest or null results, those using vitamin C more vigorously tend to produce positive results. Therefore, I propose the following mathematical proportion: pharmacological intake : nutritional intake = fist : caress. In short: what makes the difference is not just the weapon used, but the cleverness with which it is employed!

In 2011, researchers examined SVCT polymorphisms from an ophthalmological perspective. Among the various polymorphisms screened, a study published in "Molecular Vision" (264) identified one that may significantly increase the risk of glaucoma: RS1279683, a polymorphism in the SLC23A2 gene, which markedly reduces intracellular vitamin C concentrations.

It is noteworthy that glaucoma, a group of eye diseases characterized by chronic, progressive damage to the optic nerve, was the focus of scientific attention in the 1960s, when studies suggested that high doses of vitamin C could reduce its main risk factor/indicator: intraocular pressure (523). This fact, inexplicably overlooked for decades, has recently resurfaced with new insights, particularly through the identification of a specific vitamin C metabolite known as methylascorbate. This compound has been recognized as a potentially crucial factor in the metabolic regulation of intraocular pressure (265), and it is therefore believed that its use may help reduce intraocular pressure. "Our study shows that vitamin C metabolism is involved in the regulation of intraocular pressure", the researchers stated at the end of a 2019 study published in "Redox Biology" (265). This valuable insight also generates regret for the marginalization of the early intuitions seen decades ago by pioneers in the field.

An interesting study (369) documented widespread ascorbic acid deficiencies in patients with glaucoma, clearly in line with existing literature and intriguingly linked by the authors to the well-known inverse association between ascorbate levels and uric acid levels. In fact, the study outlined an AA-uric acid-glaucoma triangle, characterized by interdependent relationships, suggesting that AA supplementation may reduce both uric acid levels and glaucoma risk. Ultimately, the authors attributed clinically promising potential to vitamin C: "A possible alternative treatment for normal-tension glaucoma".

In addition to this hypothesis, the study (369) reaffirmed the high sensitivity of vitamin C to pathological states: the unchanged levels of vitamins A and E observed in patients with glaucoma further underscore the uniqueness of vitamin C, reinforcing the idea that its use may be beneficial, if not essential, whenever a disease condition is present.

Vitamin C in Dermatology

As previously emphasized in the section on immune functions, the essential role of vitamin C in maintaining skin health is well-established. Its function as a cofactor in collagen synthesis (a fundamental component of dermal fibers), its ability to stimulate collagen gene expression in fibroblasts (99), its potent antioxidant properties, and its role in skin barrier formation processes place this molecule at the forefront among nutrients crucial for dermatological health. This topic is particularly interesting as it introduces an alternative mode of administration. What exactly does it involve?

The well-known limitations of oral vitamin C bioavailability can be bypassed in dermatological practice through direct topical application, thereby enabling highly effective treatments and high-quality anti-aging interventions. In fact, ascorbic acid has long been incorporated into cosmetic products, particularly facial serums designed to protect the skin from sun damage and oxidative stress.

It is important to note that topical use adheres to the general principles of vitamin C, although in this context the dose-response relationship shows a certain degree of variability. Specifically, the optimal range is considered to be 10-20%. Several studies have documented a sigmoid-like pattern, similar to that of oral pharmacokinetics, wherein concentrations above 20% generally do not yield additional clinical benefits in facial serums (266). This has led to a practical guideline: for optimal efficacy, a facial serum should contain an AA concentration within this specified range.

Let us now shift the focus to the prevention and treatment of skin diseases, beginning with porphyria cutanea tarda (PCT). This condition is a disorder of heme production that mainly affects the skin, making it particularly sensitive to sunlight and prone to damage. As a potent antioxidant, vitamin C is hypothesized to inhibit the oxidation of a specific enzyme involved in heme synthesis, thus emerging as a potential therapeutic option for PCT (269).

A small-scale study conducted in the mid-1990s reported significant findings in this regard: 62% of patients were found to be deficient (plasma levels < 11 micromoles/L) during the acute phase of the disease. These results suggest that ascorbic acid deficiency may represent a key pathogenic factor in PCT (267). Furthermore, the same study monitored eight patients during remission and revealed a concerning scenario: half of the individuals remained vitamin C deficient even after the acute phase, an outcome that places PCT among the disorders that most severely deplete vitamin C (267). Therefore, PCT may serve as a valuable scientific model for studying the pathophysiological mechanisms responsible for vitamin C depletion during disease.

Turning to atopic dermatitis, a chronic, relapsing inflammatory skin disorder, it is essential to highlight vitamin C's relevant role in ceramide biosynthesis, stimulating their production via three distinct biochemical pathways (269). But what are ceramides?

These lipid molecules act as cell signaling agents and, more importantly, serve as a key structural component of the epidermal barrier. This latter function provides tangible evidence that vitamin C can substantially improve epidermal barrier integrity, an aspect commonly impaired in several dermatological conditions, including various forms of dermatitis (268).

Further evidence of vitamin C's important role comes from a 2016 study (268), which reported a strong inverse correlation between the severity of atopic dermatitis and both plasma AA levels and ceramide concentrations. In this study, 80% of patients with atopic dermatitis exhibited hypovitaminosis C, while those with severe forms of the disease showed a clear deficiency. As in the case of PCT, these findings suggest a pathophysiological role for vitamin C deficiency in various forms of dermatitis.

Let us now turn our attention to melanocytes, epidermal cells responsible for producing melanin, the pigment that determines skin color. Vitamin C has long been hypothesized to modulate melanin production, or melanogenesis, opening therapeutic avenues in melanoma management. This hypothesis stems from in vitro studies demonstrating that AA reduces melanogenesis in specific melanoma models, and it has been further supported by animal research showing that ascorbic therapy effectively reduces disease progression (269).

The relationship between vitamin C and melanoma appears to be particularly strong. It has been proposed that vitamin C may hinder melanoma progression through at least two mechanisms: the strengthening of the extracellular matrix and the inhibition of HIF-1 alpha. Several studies have identified HIF-1 alpha as a key factor in melanoma carcinogenesis, thereby indirectly supporting the potential role of vitamin C (270). Epigenetic mechanisms also warrant attention: some research has shown that vitamin C may hinder melanoma progression by promoting DNA demethylation (271).

Overall, the wide range of pharmacological effects attributed to vitamin C has led some authors to openly propose it as a highly promising drug for the treatment of melanoma (271). Surprisingly, this potential therapeutic role does not necessarily require supraphysiological concentrations, as even levels achievable through oral supplementation may be effective, thereby supporting those researchers who advocate for a potential oncological role of orally administered vitamin C. "This result suggests that vitamin C at physiological levels (0.1 millimoles) attenuated the malignant transformation of melanoma cells. Taken together, our results demonstrate that vitamin C at physiological concentrations may significantly reduce the malignant phenotype of A2058 cells in vitro, by inhibiting migration and transformation, although not suppressing proliferation. Therefore, vitamin C at physiological concentrations may be considered a safe and clinically valuable therapeutic option", affirm the authors of the notable article "Epigenetic reprogramming of melanoma cells by vitamin C treatment", published in the esteemed journal "Clinical Epigenetics" in 2015 (271).

Specifically, the numerical value of 0.1 millimoles/L corresponds to 100 micromoles/L. This brings us to a critical point: although 100 micromoles/L represents a physiological concentration and theoretically falls within the nutritional range, achieving such levels in cancer patients through oral intake likely requires intensive and repeated dosing, exclusively supported by a dynamic flow model. Put more explicitly: even the "simple" rebalancing of plasma levels may necessitate specialized supplementation protocols in oncology patients. The dynamic flow model may offer an optimal solution. In fact, although robust data are lacking, there is strong suspicion that conventional supplementation (500-1000 mg/day) is inadequate to maintain plasma concentrations of 100 micromoles/L in patients with melanoma. Limited supporting evidence includes findings showing that even 800-1000 mg/day of oral vitamin C failed to raise plasma levels above 30-40 micromoles/L in diabetic patients (255), (477).

In summary, while maintaining optimal physiological levels of vitamin C may prove beneficial in melanoma, this goal does not appear to be achievable through diet or standard vitamin C supplements alone.

Looking ahead, the dermatological benefits of vitamin C extend beyond oncology. An intriguing finding concerns the potential link between psoriasis, a recurrent, clinically intense inflammatory skin condition, and the HAT therapy protocol developed by Marik for the treatment of sepsis. A complex clinical case handled in his intensive care unit (272), a 45-year-old woman with a history of psoriasis, hospitalized for widespread skin rash and severe respiratory failure, was initially diagnosed with acute respiratory distress syndrome via imaging. A subsequent dermatologic consultation confirmed a severe psoriatic flare-up, leading to a combined treatment plan involving cyclosporine and HAT therapy. The response was rapid and dramatic: the patient was weaned off respiratory support within 24 hours of treatment initiation and discharged shortly thereafter (272). Marik later described this as a "dramatic response to the combination of low-dose systemic corticosteroids, intravenous vitamin C and thiamine".

Remaining within the context of psoriasis, a recent study identified a novel vitamin C-related compound: DDH-1, a highly permeable derivative that demonstrated significant anti-inflammatory effects and disease resolution in certain animal models (273).

However, the future of dermatological innovation increasingly lies in the hands of epigenetics. A 2020 study published in the "Journal of Investigative Dermatology" (274) reported reduced expression of TET enzymes in skin stem cells from patients with psoriasis. Could a reparative strategy, aimed at counteracting downstream damage when the primary cause is incurable, be relevant in this case?

According to the authors of the study, the answer is yes. The improvements observed following the restoration of TET enzyme expression suggest that DNA demethylation, a process known to be promoted by vitamin C, may represent a key mechanism for the safe and effective treatment of psoriasis. The authors describe it as "a therapeutically relevant approach that has so far been underappreciated" (274).

From sun protection to chronic inflammatory skin diseases and even melanoma, vitamin C proves to be much more than a simple nutrient: it is emerging as a versatile ally in modern dermatology, with exciting potential still waiting to be fully explored.

Vitamin C as an antihistamine

During the acute phases of allergic inflammation, the production of reactive oxygen species considerably contributes to the persistence of pro-inflammatory conditions. It is therefore evident that oxidative stress plays a crucial role in the pathogenesis of allergic diseases and, at the same time, represents a potential therapeutic target.

However, this objective has gradually taken a backseat due to a growing number of studies that have revealed an additional physiological role of ascorbate, deeply involved in the modulation of allergic reactions. A prospective multicenter observational study (275) described the clinical effects of moderate intravenous doses of vitamin C in the treatment of 71 patients during the acute phase of an allergic reaction, providing results that update existing knowledge on the subject. It is worth noting that Cathcart (45) was the first to highlight the antihistamine properties of vitamin C. This multicenter study confirmed its antihistamine and antiallergic potential, indicating that intravenous administration at moderate doses (7.5 g) is capable of relieving both respiratory and skin symptoms associated with allergic reactions (275). This effect is plausibly due to vitamin C's ability to positively influence histamine levels, a concept consistent with both the intuitions of the pioneers and some contemporary studies. One such study, published in 2013 (276), demonstrated that intravenous administration of 7.5 g can significantly reduce histamine concentrations. The measurements conducted on the 89 enrolled patients were so compelling that the authors concluded: "Intravenous infusion of ascorbic acid clearly reduced serum histamine concentrations and may represent a therapeutic option for patients with symptoms and conditions associated with pathologically elevated histamine levels" (276).

It is important to emphasize a key point: vitamin C's modulation of histamine levels appears to be a biologically grounded, physiological mechanism rather than a pharmacological one, despite the fact that AA was used pharmacologically in the referenced studies. This assertion is strongly supported by animal studies, which consistently show that any increase in histamine levels is associated with a rapid and significant rise in endogenous ascorbate biosynthesis (444), (445), (378), (277). Essentially, the antihistamine and antiallergic properties of vitamin C could be attributed to the correction of hypoascorbemia, rather than to a direct pharmacological effect. This influential hypothesis was first proposed by Stone, several decades ago.

The inverse correlation between AA and histamine has been further confirmed by numerous studies consistently showing a strong negative relationship between vitamin C levels and histamine concentrations (276), (278),

(359). Moreover, some research has focused on the mathematical characterization of this interaction (275), (278), specifically analyzing the rate of incremental change in histamine levels as a function of plasma ascorbate. Put simply, histamine levels tend to increase exponentially, that is, sharply, when plasma ascorbate falls below 57 micromoles/L (275), (278). This model has potential clinical implications. It suggests that maintaining plasma vitamin C levels above 57 micromoles/L could be particularly beneficial for patients with a predisposition to allergic conditions. But if an individual is not predisposed to allergies, would this recommendation still be plausible?

To answer this question it is useful to consider a serious clinical condition: anaphylaxis, a severe and potentially life-threatening allergic reaction. A 1988 study (279) investigated the effect of intravenous vitamin C on anaphylaxis in guinea pigs and found a greatly reduced incidence of anaphylactic shock in pretreated animals, along with milder symptoms in the few that did develop a reaction: “Animals treated with 281 mg/day of sodium ascorbate rarely developed anaphylactic shock, or when they did, it was of lesser severity” (279).

These findings suggest that prophylactic administration of vitamin C could serve as an effective preventive measure against anaphylaxis, and may therefore be potentially useful in high-risk clinical scenarios, such as the administration of a previously untested drug.

Although very few studies have investigated this promising direction, the available data and various biological plausibilities reinforce the logic of maintaining consistently elevated plasma vitamin C levels (as proposed by the dynamic flow model), a regimen that may offer valuable protection against unpredictable real-life risks, including exposure to potentially fatal allergens.

The allergy field also highlights the considerable gaps that remain in our understanding of vitamin C. While its antihistamine properties have been acknowledged for decades, the underlying mechanisms remain largely unexplained, pushing research into new exploratory directions. Personally, I believe that future advances in elucidating the dynamics of vitamin C within the immune system will be the most fruitful avenues for clarification. For instance, could the pronounced antihistaminic effect be mediated via distinct epigenetic pathways, such as the functional modulation of TREGs?

Recent findings (280), however, have shifted attention toward specific derivatives of ascorbic acid with notable antiallergic potential. As stated in an article published in the journal "Molecules" (280): "These results suggest that 2-Me-6-N-Palm-AA could be a promising therapeutic candidate for allergic diseases".

As is evident, research on ascorbic acid continues to progress, albeit slowly, along multiple lines of investigation, ranging from the pharmacological properties of its metabolites and derivatives to its increasingly intriguing epigenetic implications.

Gastrointestinal diseases

In this section, we'll explore the role of vitamin C in the prevention and treatment of various gastrointestinal diseases, beginning with those affecting the stomach. This role has been recognized for several decades, thanks to two early pioneers, Crescenzo and Cayer, who used the depletion-repletion method to design a series of studies in the mid-1940s (484). Their work led to the discovery that ascorbic acid deficiency is very common among patients with peptic ulcers, lesions affecting the lining of the stomach or duodenum due to exposure to stomach acid.

This finding prompted further research into the role of vitamin C in the prevention and progression of such conditions, extending the focus to other gastric disorders marked by significant vitamin C depletion, including atrophic gastritis, a distinct chronic form of stomach inflammation. One of the main causes of ascorbic acid depletion in atrophic gastritis is its rapid degradation within the gastric mucosa, a process triggered by abnormally high pH levels, which are in turn linked to the typical hydrochloric acid deficiency. In addition, excessive bacterial growth has also been identified as a major contributing factor.

Other researchers, such as Kendall and Chinn, accumulated additional evidence suggesting that bacterial overgrowth associated with achlorhydria or hypochlorhydria (absence or deficiency of hydrochloric acid in gastric juice, respectively) plays a crucial role in the destruction of ascorbic acid. This hypothesis aligns with the symptoms of gastric ulceration, which include hemorrhages similar to those observed in acute scurvy (281).

A groundbreaking discovery that strengthened the association between gastritis/ulcers and low levels of ascorbic acid was the identification of the bacterium Helicobacter pylori in 1982. This infection has proven to be a major factor in gastric pathology, not only because it is now recognized as the primary cause of associated gastritis and peptic ulcers, but also as a major risk factor for gastric cancer.

From an epistemological standpoint, the H. pylori paradigm highlights the institutional challenges involved in accepting new and disruptive scientific paradigms. The association between H. pylori and gastritis/ulcer was initially rejected, even ridiculed, by many within the medical establishment. This skepticism stemmed from the long-held belief that bacteria could not survive the acidic environment of the stomach. It was only through the perseverance of Warren and Marshall, who were later awarded the Nobel Prize in Medicine in 2005 for their discovery, that the theory gained full acceptance, ultimately overturning the prevailing doctrine that stress and spicy foods were the primary causes of ulcer development.

Leaving the digression aside, it is important to highlight that it is now well documented that individuals infected with H. pylori have low levels of ascorbic acid, as demonstrated by numerous studies, including the large-scale U.S. National Health and Nutrition Examination Survey (282). The depletion of ascorbic acid appears to be primarily caused by H. pylori-induced gastritis, which triggers a chain reaction that converts a substantial portion of ascorbic acid first into dehydroascorbic acid, which is then rapidly further oxidized into irreversible metabolites such as diketogulonic acid (281).

In summary, gastritis and hypochlorhydria are the two main factors inducing the conversion of AA into irreversible compounds, while also hindering ascorbate recycling. More precisely, the pH of the stomach is directly correlated with the rate of irreversible AA conversion (281). This dynamic was confirmed by researchers who studied hundreds of patients with H. pylori infection, showing that elevated gastric pH and epithelial damage resulting from the infection are the main drivers of AA concentration decline in the stomach (281). In addition to changes in gastric pH, both bacterial overgrowth and local inflammation, which represents an intense source of reactive oxygen species, are considered primary factors contributing to the depletion of ascorbic acid.

Overall, there is no doubt that various gastric disorders, particularly H. pylori infection, impair the bioavailability of vitamin C. But to what extent?

A study involving 1106 individuals in the UK and published in the "European Journal of Gastroenterology & Hepatology" (480) reported that H. pylori-positive individuals had plasma vitamin C concentrations 35% lower than H. pylori-negative individuals.

Even more striking are the results from a five-year study involving 452 Korean children (417): "In Korean children, data show that vitamin C levels in whole blood, plasma, and gastric juice, as well as gastric juice pH, are closely related to the severity of H. pylori infection and histological changes in the stomach. These data suggest that vitamin C may play a role in determining infection and progression, and that its supplementation could be an important axis in the management of H. pylori infection in children", the authors concluded. This is both alarming and "encouraging", highlighting the potential therapeutic benefits of ascorbic acid.

The direct correlation between gastric pH and the irreversible conversion rate of ascorbic acid becomes clinically relevant in the pharmacological context of proton pump inhibitors (PPIs), a widely used class of gastroprotective agents that reduce the production of gastric hydrochloric acid. This raises a logical question: could PPI-induced hypochlorhydria reduce the gastric concentration of ascorbic acid?

Unfortunately, yes. Several authors have reported that suppression of gastric acid secretion through PPI therapy is associated with the irreversible conversion of ascorbic acid, leading to a scenario in which reduced gastric, plasma and tissue levels of AA become virtually inevitable (281), (283). This observation warrants closer examination. It is therefore reasonable to hypothesize that long-term PPI use may progressively deplete AA concentrations, potentially leading to its deficiency. Given the widespread and prolonged use of PPIs worldwide, this possibility calls for careful scientific evaluation. What has been described represents a rare yet significant case of negative interaction between vitamin C and pharmacological agents, capable of markedly reducing both gastric and systemic levels of ascorbic acid. As a result, its antioxidant and anti-inflammatory functions, essential for maintaining the integrity of the gastric mucosa and overall physiological balance, may be compromised during prolonged therapy with PPIs.

We now turn to AA's protective value against H. pylori infection. Some studies have reported increased infection risk following severe dietary restrictions. One such study showed that limiting daily AA intake to only 40 mg increased the risk of infection twelvefold compared to an intake of 120 mg (281).

As for its therapeutic potential, several in vitro studies have shown promising results, indicating that AA can inhibit various H. pylori strains (281). This finding is consistent with the well-documented antibacterial properties of vitamin C. Preliminary clinical studies support this evidence: one trial involving patients with H. pylori infection reported remarkable findings because the experimental group, treated with 5 g of oral AA daily for four weeks as monotherapy, achieved a 30% eradication rate, compared to 0% in the control group (447). Although conducted in 1998, this study remains significant as it demonstrated the anti-H. pylori effects of high-dose oral ascorbate, a therapeutic approach that has been rarely explored in clinical settings.

A 2005 clinical trial (482) attempted to replicate the findings of (447), but was unsuccessful, perhaps due to some methodological inconsistencies. The authors themselves acknowledged potential inaccuracies due to concurrent PPI use. Moreover, unlike (447), this study did not assess gastric and plasma AA levels before and after treatment. In contrast, (447) included AA measurements at three distinct time points, baseline, end of treatment and four weeks post-treatment, offering greater reliability. Interestingly, the authors of (482) noted that some patients who chose to extend AA therapy beyond four weeks eventually achieved full eradication.

Unfortunately, scientific research has since shifted its focus elsewhere, choosing not to further explore the potential of high oral doses. As a result, the anti-H. pylori potential of ascorbic acid has been relegated to an adjunctive role, with the dosage drastically reduced. Regarding combination therapies, the use of ascorbic acid has shown positive results despite very low dosages. For example, a randomized study involving 312 patients found that adding 500 mg of oral ascorbic acid to the standard treatment regimen improved eradication rates from 48.8% to 78% within four weeks (284).

We will now explore vitamin C's prophylactic role in gastric cancer prevention. A large study (285) involving patients with precancerous gastric lesions tested various therapeutic combinations, including H. pylori eradication agents, oral AA (1 g twice daily) and beta-carotene. The results, while varied, demonstrated the effectiveness of AA over a period of 72 months.

In the field of chemoprevention, namely, the use of natural compounds or drugs to prevent carcinogenesis, AA may also act independently, particularly at the gastric level. Indeed, some studies have shown that even modest AA supplementation may potentially suppress precancerous conditions such as intestinal metaplasia (485). Notably, AA's chemopreventive action is not solely attributable to its antioxidant properties. A substantial part of its protective effect stems from its ability to inhibit the formation of nitrosamines, carcinogenic compounds formed by the reaction of nitrites and amines. AA achieves this by converting nitrites into nitric oxide (NO), a mechanism first reported in the early 1970s in "Science" (483). Thus, NO reappears in this context, raising the question: can AA-mediated conversion of nitrites into NO constitute an independent, BH4-unrelated pathway for enhancing NO synthesis?

According to a recent clinical study (434), the answer is yes. Oral administration at a daily dose of 1 g for four weeks increased NO concentrations while simultaneously reducing nitrite and lipid levels in hypercholesterolemic subjects.

The ability of ascorbic acid to neutralize nitrites depends on a three-dimensional configuration involving gastric/plasma AA levels, nitrite concentration, and gastric pH. Notably, increased nitrosamine formation is associated with a reduced ratio of gastric AA to nitrites; in this context, elevated gastric pH leads to the rapid conversion of AA into irreversible metabolites and the concurrent accumulation of nitrosamines. This is consistent with studies showing that PPI therapy (once again!) in H. pylori-infected individuals can exacerbate gastric inflammation, increase nitrite levels, and reduce AA concentrations (481), (281), (287).

This raises the following question: could correcting the ascorbic acid depletion induced by PPIs provide anti-inflammatory and anti-nitrosamine benefits?

One study (481) suggests exactly this: oral supplementation with AA (1200 mg/day) prevented the exacerbation of H. pylori-associated gastritis induced by PPIs. Remarkable, isn't it?

Vitamin C could therefore counteract the damage caused by PPIs themselves, drugs that, paradoxically, impair its gastric accumulation.

The inhibition of nitrosamine formation further expands the range of physiological functions attributed to AA, highlighting its significant role in cancer prevention. Nitrites, commonly used as preservatives in processed meats, canned foods, and dairy products, pose an increased health risk when exposed to unhealthy cooking practices such as frying or high-temperature processing, which enhance their conversion into carcinogenic nitrosamines.

In summary, the fundamental role of vitamin C in the prevention of gastric cancer is well established and supported by a substantial body of scientific evidence, including epidemiological studies. Several investigations have demonstrated a statistically significant inverse correlation between plasma vitamin C levels and the risk of developing gastric cancer (486), (418).

These findings support a consideration that deserves a brief but essential summary: substantial evidence highlights a dual gastroprotective role of vitamin C, both as a nitrosamine inhibitor and as an anti-H. pylori agent. Paradoxically, this role is antagonized by the very class of widely prescribed drugs known as proton pump inhibitors (PPIs), commonly referred to as "gastroprotectants". However, this antagonism is unidirectional: while PPIs deplete ascorbic acid, appropriate supplementation can mitigate some of the side effects associated with their use.

However, the above should not be misinterpreted or misused; rather, it must be carefully contextualized. In cases where PPI therapy is truly necessary, evidence suggests that ascorbate supplementation should be considered a rational and potentially highly effective strategy. Moreover, when we consider the negative impact of PPIs on vitamin B12 absorption, also linked to altered gastric acidity, the idea of a broader supplementation strategy becomes all the more reasonable.

From a broader perspective, the impairment of ascorbate absorption caused by gastric disorders highlights an important concept: ascorbic acid supplementation may not only help address the underlying gastrointestinal condition, but more importantly, support the systemic functions associated with it. The stomach serves as a symbolic and critical gateway: any compromise in gastric absorption can hinder the plasma accumulation and tissue distribution of ascorbate.

This principle can be extended to all conditions in which vitamin C levels are at risk, regardless of whether the underlying pathology can be directly addressed. In such cases, supplementation becomes essential, particularly in the presence of depleting factors such as chronic stress, illness, or gastrointestinal malabsorption, to prevent the wide range of complications associated with vitamin C deficiency, especially when these factors are persistent.

This section on the stomach concludes with a clinical study (420) highlighting a different role of vitamin C: as a bioavailability enhancer for drugs. This synergistic effect, reminiscent of the well-known interaction between vitamin C and levodopa, was also observed with levothyroxine, a synthetic hormone analogous to T4 used in the treatment of hypothyroidism. When gastrointestinal disorders are present, the absorption of levothyroxine can be significantly impaired.

Even a daily dose of 500 mg can improve serum T3, T4 and TSH levels by enhancing levothyroxine bioavailability. As noted by Jubiz and Ramirez, authors of the study published in "The Journal of Clinical Endocrinology & Metabolism" (420): "In patients with hypothyroidism and gastrointestinal disease, vitamin C improves abnormalities in serum free T4, T3, and TSH concentrations. This approach is therefore useful in managing these patients".

Following this detailed examination of gastric processes, we now turn our attention to the pancreas. We begin with acute pancreatitis, a potentially life-threatening inflammatory condition, which is marked by a highly predictable finding: low plasma AA levels that characterize its progression. These levels were found to be strikingly low in a 1993 study published in the "British Journal of Surgery" (288), which documented a "disproportionate reduction in plasma vitamin C concentrations".

Ten years later, researchers explored a therapeutic approach (289), clearly distinguishing between physiological repletion and supraphysiological dosing. The prestigious "World Journal of Gastroenterology" published the study, which involved 84 patients with acute pancreatitis, who were divided into two treatment groups: one receiving 10 g of intravenous AA daily for 5 days, and the other receiving 1 g of intravenous AA daily for the same duration. As expected, the high-dose group (10 g) showed better symptom control and shorter hospital stays (289).

Once again, we are left with the usual methodological questions: what results might have emerged if a placebo group had been compared to a group treated with just 1 g/day of AA?

The answer appears evident, and it highlights a long history of uncertain interpretations and methodological errors that have often obscured the potential of vitamin C: "High-dose vitamin C is therapeutically effective against acute pancreatitis. Potential mechanisms include enhancing antioxidant capacity, blocking plasma lipid peroxidation, and improving cellular immune function", the authors stated (289), reaffirming the dual antioxidant and anti-inflammatory role of vitamin C, which seems to depend on supraphysiological concentrations for full efficacy.

The anti-inflammatory potential of vitamin C has recently gained further scientific validation. An animal model (290) provided additional evidence supporting the hypothesis that high-dose ascorbate mitigates pancreatic damage in acute inflammation by enhancing the so-called NRF2 pathway. NRF2 is a transcription factor involved in the regulation of genes encoding cytoprotective antioxidant enzymes. It serves as a central hub in cellular defense systems, capable of counteracting even the most challenging environmental stressors. By binding to antioxidant response elements (AREs), NRF2 triggers a cascade of protective effects such as the stimulation of HO-1 and the inhibition of the NLRP3 inflammasome, which has also been implicated in Parkinson's disease therapy (469). A growing body of evidence supports the significance of the AA-NRF2 axis, generating considerable scientific interest. For instance, in a rat model of sepsis (393), high-dose vitamin C significantly enhanced NRF2 expression, thereby reducing inflammation and cognitive decline.

This section concludes with a recent meta-analysis that reviewed the literature on pancreatitis (474). Although only two of the included clinical studies used intravenous administration, the one previously mentioned (289) and another that administered an average daily dose of 1.28 g for seven days, combined with high-dose selenium and NAC (475), the overall assessment was positive, particularly in terms of reduced hospital stay duration (474).

The next focus is the liver. A 2019 study (291) described an experiment in which mice were pharmacologically induced to develop liver toxicity in order to evaluate the protective efficacy of vitamin C. The results indicated that its administration protected liver tissue by modulating hepatocellular inflammatory responses.

A well-established body of literature supports the hepatoprotective potential of vitamin C. Evidence ranges from protection against cholestatic liver injury (292) to the modulation of complex cytoprotective pathways, such as the attenuation of NF-kB signaling (293), including defense against hazardous toxins like arsenic (294). This last result is particularly relevant, as it highlights the detoxifying ability of vitamin C.

Focusing now on hepatic steatosis, a randomized clinical trial (295) demonstrated substantial benefits in managing the most common liver disease worldwide: non-alcoholic fatty liver disease (NAFLD), a condition characterized by lipid accumulation in hepatocytes followed by inflammatory damage not related to alcohol consumption. In this study, a 12-week course of oral AA supplementation at 1 g per day significantly improved liver function among participants (295). This effect was attributed to improved glucose metabolism, modulation of the gut microbiota (to be discussed later), and upregulation of adiponectin, a protein synthesized by adipose tissue with important biological functions and an inverse association with blood pressure and LDL cholesterol levels.

These findings transversally support an interesting correlation between vitamin C and adiponectin, a connection further reinforced by recent studies. One of these, published in 2022 in "Molecular and Cellular Endocrinology" (425), is particularly impactful because it reported that AA administration can increase adiponectin secretion in a clinically meaningful way.

Epidemiological data also favor vitamin C. An analysis involving 4494 subjects, published in 2021 in "Frontiers in Nutrition", exemplifies the potential of vitamin C for liver health, while also validating its complex physiological role (505). The study found a strong inverse correlation between plasma vitamin C levels and NAFLD risk. Importantly, protection increased even at levels far above the deficiency threshold of 11 micromoles/L. Specifically, the 50.5-67 micromoles/L plasma range was significantly more protective than the 30.9-50.5

micromoles/L range. This same range, 50.5-67 micromoles/L, was also found to be associated with a 71% reduction in the statistical risk of developing hepatic cirrhosis, a severe degenerative pathology marked by irreversible disruption of hepatic architecture (505).

Despite numerous promising clinical and preclinical findings, as well as established mechanistic foundations, some uncertainty remains regarding the pathways underlying the hepatoprotective effects of vitamin C. In this context, its antioxidant and anti-inflammatory functions are thought to exert a highly beneficial immunomodulatory impact on the structure and function of liver tissue (296).

We close the hepatic section with a potentially forward-looking study on cancer (297). This study puts forth a novel hypothesis: in assessing the efficacy of vitamin C against cholangiocarcinoma, a highly aggressive bile duct cancer, the expression level of SVCT2 may serve as a predictor of therapeutic response. The study revealed an inverse correlation between SVCT2 expression and tumor resistance to the cytotoxic effects of ascorbic acid, as reduced SVCT2 expression led to greater resistance. This suggests that increasing the local concentration of AA may enhance cytotoxicity against malignant cells.

In general, I believe that future research should strongly focus on strategies to upregulate SVCT transporters, as this could be the most effective way to achieve the best clinical outcomes.

We now turn our attention to intestinal disorders, where we encounter yet another major contributor to ascorbate depletion. Patients with inflammatory bowel diseases (IBDs) are at elevated risk of nutritional deficiencies, including vitamin C deficiency. At least three factors contribute to this phenomenon: increased metabolic demands, the damaging influence of reactive oxygen species and, most significantly, malabsorption due to local inflammation (298). This latter mechanism has been the focus of numerous studies, which have linked it to reduced expression of the SVCT1 transporter, a reduction attributed to the high levels of TNF alpha released during the inflammatory response.

In essence, intestinal malabsorption presents several challenges, including a particularly relevant vicious cycle: intestinal inflammation → reduced levels of ascorbic acid → exacerbation of inflammation. Low AA levels can therefore significantly aggravate the inflammatory state. This is the central thesis put forth by several researchers (298): "Given the essential role of vitamin C in preventing and mitigating oxidative stress and inflammation, TNF alpha–mediated suppression of AA absorption (and thus tissue levels) may initiate a vicious cycle, whereby inflammation induces vitamin C deficiency, which in turn worsens the inflammation".

Therefore, in addition to chronic stress, pregnancy, chronic diseases, genetic defects in SVCT transporters, and gastric disorders, intestinal malabsorption must be recognized as another significant factor contributing to ascorbic acid depletion. This condition should not be underestimated, as it can severely impair the absorption of a broad range of essential nutrients, with consequences that extend well beyond vitamin C metabolism alone.

As in other contexts, in intestinal diseases vitamin C supplementation should not be considered merely as an indirect or supportive measure. It is well known that vitamin C can modulate the intestinal microbiota, the vast and complex population of bacteria that physiologically colonize the gut. This influence raises several important considerations, chief among them the biological relevance of the gut-brain axis, an intriguing field, primarily mediated by the immune system, which will be briefly discussed later (575).

Equally important is the interplay between the gut microbiota and the body's redox balance, which plays a critical role in maintaining cellular homeostasis and regulating inflammatory responses (576). In this context, an animal study (299) demonstrated that an antioxidant blend containing vitamin C helped restore microbial balance, suggesting that redox homeostasis is essential for intestinal health. Further supporting evidence came from a 2021 clinical study (371), which found that even a short-term intervention with ascorbic acid (1 g/day for two weeks) modulated the gut microbiota by promoting the growth of beneficial bacterial genera, particularly lactobacillus and bifidobacterium species.

The therapeutic potential of vitamin C is remarkably broad. Its ability to inhibit NF-kB, a key mediator in the IL-15/NF-kB axis implicated in the pathogenesis of celiac disease, has led to the hypothesis that vitamin C supplementation may exert beneficial anti-inflammatory effects in managing the condition. This idea was supported by a 2012 in vitro study, in which the authors proposed high-dose vitamin C as an adjunctive therapy for various inflammatory bowel diseases (391).

When it comes to therapeutic efficacy in intestinal disorders, the available literature remains unfortunately limited. One of the few studies (300) examined the use of high-dose intraperitoneal vitamin C (4 g/kg) in an animal model of ulcerative colitis, demonstrating a marked anti-inflammatory effect. On the one hand, the reduction in inflammatory biomarkers was so substantial that the authors called for further investigation. On the other hand, the experimental setting offers an important translational insight: the suppression of pro-inflammatory cytokines at a dose typically used in oncology models (4 g/kg, suggestive of pro-oxidant activity) reinforces the favorable safety profile of vitamin C, even at very high concentrations.

Taken together, these findings highlight the need for deeper clinical exploration: high-dose vitamin C may offer underutilized therapeutic potential in inflammatory bowel disease, warranting rigorous, targeted human studies.

Heavy metal detoxification

Numerous studies have investigated a distinctive property of vitamin C, first recognized by Klenner over seventy years ago: its ability to alleviate metal-induced toxicity. High levels of metals can generate large amounts of free radicals, causing damage to DNA bases and lipid peroxidation. However, these effects can be suppressed through the appropriate use of molecules such as vitamin C and other antioxidants like glutathione and its precursor N-acetylcysteine (NAC). These molecules are extremely beneficial in this context: they form a powerful antioxidant barrier and also promote chelation, a key chemical process through which metal ions are bound and neutralized by chelating agents. These agents can sequester heavy metals such as mercury and lead, facilitating their excretion through urine.

The dual ability of vitamin C to neutralize oxidative stress and promote chelation has attracted increasing scientific attention since the early work of Jungeblut and Klenner, forming a body of preliminary evidence supporting the potential detoxifying role of ascorbic acid. This body of evidence has been reinforced by several contemporary studies that have explored a variety of toxic exposures.

One of these studies evaluated the toxic effects of cadmium chloride, mercury chloride, and their combined administration, showing that ascorbic acid therapy can protect the kidneys, which are particularly sensitive to chemical intoxication (301). Other studies have focused on lead, a metal historically known for its antagonistic interaction with vitamin C. Due to its chemical and physical properties, lead is notoriously difficult to eliminate from the body, resulting in prolonged renal excretion times. A 2013 animal study (302) highlighted this antagonism, showing that high doses of vitamin C increased lead excretion in a dose-dependent manner: an oral dose of 2 g/kg facilitated lead elimination much more effectively than 500 mg/kg, in the context of acute intoxication.

The relationship between vitamin C and lead extends beyond acute exposure. Epidemiological studies (432), (303) have increasingly revealed a statistically significant inverse correlation between vitamin C concentrations and blood lead levels. This is a finding of considerable importance, as lead poisoning can cause long-term health complications and represents a serious public health issue, particularly for children. Several scientific reports, including a major UNICEF study, have highlighted the widespread prevalence of abnormal lead levels among children (511), (512), suggesting that the public health impact could increase alarmingly over time. These results bring attention to the value of vitamin C's biological versatility, highlighting its potential effectiveness even in chronic lead exposure.

This concept is supported by a relevant study (304) in which vitamin C was tested against a dual toxic challenge: lead exposure combined with radiation. In this model, two groups of mice were exposed to lead and then subjected to high-dose radiation; one group was pretreated with intravenous AA at a dose of 400 mg/kg. The pretreatment proved particularly effective in the liver, where cellular damage was markedly reduced thanks to the preservation of glutathione, mediated by high-dose vitamin C therapy. This highlights its important sparing role during oxidative storms (first-line ROS sink), a property that in this case helped maintain glutathione, an essential molecule for liver integrity. In addition to confirming its hepatoprotective activity, the study also hinted at the radioprotective potential of vitamin C, which will be discussed shortly.

Animal studies are numerous and generally positive. But what about humans?

Some clinical evidence does exist, although the small sample sizes and administered doses reflect the usual “quantitative limitations”, further constrained by their historical context (432). In fact, the first two studies date back to the pioneering era of Jungeblut, in 1939 and 1941 respectively (432). These studies yielded promising results and inspired later investigations, including a 1978 study by the team of Papaioannou, in which battery industry workers exposed to high levels of lead experienced a significant reduction in blood lead levels following combined treatment with ascorbic acid and zinc (432).

Overall, these preliminary results appear promising, though largely overlooked, placing science in a rather cryptic position. Ahmad and Liu have recently attempted to shed light on this enigma through an insightful review (432), whose conclusions convey the bitterness of lost time. “Our understanding of AA-Pb interactions remains limited, and we are far from fully appreciating this vitamin’s utility as an effective therapeutic agent. Further studies are necessary to confirm AA's prophylactic effects in both animal models and human subjects exposed to Pb, as well as to elucidate the protective mechanisms involved. With this review, we hope to reignite scientific interest in this essential, water-soluble, and virtually non-toxic vitamin as a neuroprotective agent, not only in Pb-induced neurotoxicity but also in other neuropathologies”, the authors state (432).

“Reignite” is the key word: something, indeed, seems to have been extinguished.

In recent years, ascorbate has been proposed as a potentially useful pharmacological agent for the management of paraquat poisoning, a common herbicide whose ingestion can lead to serious complications such as liver dysfunction and kidney failure. Such intoxication is notoriously difficult to treat due to the lack of specific therapies. However, a retrospective study indicated that high-dose vitamin C therapy might improve survival rates and reduce the risk of acute kidney injury (365).

This brings us back to the pioneering insights of McCormick and Klenner, whose innovative ideas and various clinical observations often led to the resolution of extremely complex cases, highlighting those clinical potentials of vitamin C that, even today, unfortunately still struggle to be considered even remotely plausible by a large part of the scientific community.

Radioprotection

One of the increasingly interesting aspects of vitamin C concerns its potential anticancer properties, as well as its ability to mitigate the adverse effects of cancer treatments. A notable example is a phase 1 study (305) published at the end of 2018 in the prestigious journal "Cancer Research", which evaluated the effectiveness of intravenous vitamin C during radiotherapy for pancreatic cancer. The goal was to assess its radioprotective properties and potential synergistic effects with radiotherapy. In line with previous findings, the results confirmed that pharmacological ascorbate can protect surrounding healthy tissues from radiation-induced damage, which in turn reduces the overall toxicity of radiotherapy. Furthermore, a significant survival benefit was documented, indicating that high-dose ascorbic acid enhances the cytotoxic effects of radiation against cancer cells. As the 16 authors state: "Our study demonstrates that pharmacological ascorbate selectively radioprotects normal cells and radiosensitizes tumor cells". "These findings suggest that pharmacological ascorbate enhances radiation-induced cytotoxicity in pancreatic cancer cells while potentially protecting surrounding healthy tissue. This makes pharmacological ascorbate an optimal adjunct for treating locally advanced pancreatic adenocarcinoma" (305).

Radioprotection and radiosensitization, an expression of refined pharmacologic intelligence.

These results reinforce the versatility, oncological relevance, and radioprotective properties of the molecule, consolidating previous studies that link the radioprotective effects of AA to its remarkable ability to reduce the massive oxidative stress triggered by radiation exposure.

One such study (306) explored vitamin C's effects on radiation-induced gastrointestinal syndrome in mice, a condition characterized by severe nausea, vomiting, diarrhea, dehydration, and electrolyte imbalance. The results provided valuable insights into the pathogenic mechanisms and allowed for longitudinal comparisons with other areas of research. The key interpretation lies in a notable asymmetry: while oral therapy administered after radiation exposure proved ineffective, high-dose oral pretreatment significantly alleviated gastrointestinal symptoms and improved survival. Two plausible explanations can be considered for the failure of post-exposure therapy. First, radiation-induced intestinal damage may have impaired AA absorption to the extent that plasma levels remained extremely low. Second, even in the absence of structural damage, it is known that the intestine inherently limits the achievement of plasma concentrations necessary to address acute pathology. This leads to an increasingly unequivocal conclusion: acute conditions require higher plasma concentrations than those needed for prophylactic pretreatment. Indeed, when high-dose post-radiation therapy was administered intraperitoneally, even 24 hours after exposure, the results improved considerably. In addition to preventing bone marrow dysfunction, this intensive treatment also enhanced survival (306).

The protective effect of various antioxidants was evaluated in another insightful animal model (373), which once again highlighted the unmatched efficacy of vitamin C, proving to be more radioprotective than antioxidant vitamins E and A. Furthermore, vitamin C also demonstrated protective effects when administered 24 hours after exposure to high doses of ionizing radiation, thus revealing broad therapeutic potential: "This study showed that vitamin C can be administered up to 24 hours after exposure to high levels of ionizing radiation, offering protection in life-threatening scenarios", the authors state (373).

Therefore, vitamin C once again emerges not only as a preventive, but also as a true therapeutic agent, a concept still unfamiliar to parts of the scientific community. It is worth reiterating: vitamin C can act as a powerful pharmacological agent, uniquely combining multifunctionality, efficacy, affordability and safety. However, these characteristics have not been sufficient to attract clinical research, as evidenced by the scarcity of clinical studies on vitamin C-mediated radioprotection. Within this investigative gap lies a compelling clinical study (307), published in "Nuclear Medicine and Biomedical Imaging", involving patients undergoing standard radioactive treatment for thyroid disease (hyperthyroidism). A single daily oral dose of 1 g, administered for one week, was sufficient to reduce oxidative stress caused by therapeutic radiation. The authors concluded: "According to our study results, vitamin C reduces radiation-induced oxidative stress, suggesting that supplementation may benefit patients undergoing therapeutic radiation procedures" (307).

In addition to promoting vitamin C as a radioprotective agent, these findings suggest a broader clinical application. For instance, prophylactic use of vitamin C could be explored in diagnostic settings involving ionizing radiation, such as computed tomography (CT). Prophylactic supplementation may offer two significant advantages: attenuating the harmful effects of radiation and protecting the kidneys during contrast-enhanced imaging, preventing contrast-induced acute nephropathy, a condition characterized by acute kidney injury following radiologic contrast administration. Two benefits for the price of one, at a very modest cost. A systematic review published in the reputable "American Journal of Cardiovascular Drugs" reached similar conclusions, highlighting vitamin C's potential in reducing the risk of contrast-induced acute kidney injury during radiologic procedures (356).

Chapter 10
Practically C

Natural or synthetic vitamin C?

At first glance, the question of the optimal source of vitamin C may seem complex. Over time, however, it has proven to be far more straightforward than its intricate premises suggest. We will examine this alongside another widespread belief: the stereotype that vitamin C in its natural form confers superior benefits.

Considering Stone's perspective based on the correction of hypoascorbemia, the issue appears straightforward, since it is practically impossible to reach the amounts needed to replicate the fortunate condition of animals solely through diet, the true natural source of vitamin C. For example, to obtain one gram of vitamin C from food, one would need to consume about 700 grams of fresh peppers, an amount that the human digestive system would struggle to handle.

An alternative to plant-based foods can be found in the category of "natural" supplements. This definition, however, is rather vague, since natural supplements are generally produced by combining synthetic products derived from plant sources with biologically active compounds found in nature, such as flavonoids, a class of polyphenolic compounds widely found in plants, which act as pigments and exhibit well-documented antioxidant and anti-inflammatory properties. The goal is clearly to improve the problematic intestinal absorption of vitamin C in a "natural" way.

But there's a catch.

Studies have offered interesting insights, although they must be analyzed with a crucial distinction in mind: animal studies vs. human studies. In animal models, several experiments have shown improved vitamin C absorption in the presence of flavonoids (308), (309). In one specific animal model, kiwi extract, known for its rich flavonoid content, proved superior to synthetic vitamin C, resulting in higher concentrations in plasma, leukocytes, heart, liver, and kidneys (310). Overall, a range of animal studies supports the idea that certain bioactive compounds (including, but not limited to, flavonoids) can increase vitamin C levels in plasma and tissues (310). In this context, nature seemed to prevail, as in most of these animal studies plant-derived vitamin C showed greater bioavailability (310). All quite clear and, to some extent, predictable.

Now comes the surprise: in stark contrast to animal studies, human studies have shown no significant differences in bioavailability between synthetic vitamin C and that derived from fruit or plant-based preparations (310). But bioavailability is not the only area where discrepancies between human and animal studies emerge. In comparative clinical trials, synthetic formulations and natural sources such as kiwi and other fruits have demonstrated very similar pharmacokinetic profiles (311).

While this may seem paradoxical, given the widespread belief that the natural is superior to the synthetic, there are rational explanations. One of the most plausible explanations is the typical presence of glucose in plant-based foods, which can compete with vitamin C, particularly its oxidized form DHA, for transport into cells. Vitamin C is generally better absorbed in the absence of glucose. This, in turn, indirectly influences strategies for synthetic intake: consuming glucose and vitamin C at the same time may reduce intracellular uptake.

The most important conclusion is the disparity between animals and humans: only in humans do chemistry and nature appear equivalent in terms of absorption, bioavailability and biological value. However, this evidence should neither be abused nor misunderstood, but rather placed in its proper context. It is evident that consuming vitamin C as part of whole foods is preferable, due to the additional presence of other beneficial compounds, such as flavonoids. At the same time, it is equally clear that correcting hypoascorbemia solely through diet is impossible. No one disputes that a healthy diet, based primarily on an abundant and varied intake of plant-based foods, is essential for health. But this does not mean it can fully meet all our needs. The numerous biological and pharmacological properties of vitamin C strongly support this view, suggesting that its presence in nature is insufficient to fully express its potential.

The liposomal formulation

A new method of vitamin C administration has recently emerged as a significant development in the scientific landscape: the liposomal route, made possible by advances in modern biomedical technologies. Liposomes are spherical vesicles composed of one or more phospholipid bilayers enclosing an aqueous core. This architecture enables the encapsulation of both hydrophilic (within the core) and lipophilic (within the bilayer) molecules, protecting them from degradation and enhancing their bioavailability and intracellular uptake.

The pharmacokinetic properties of liposomal delivery make this approach particularly useful in contexts where molecules have difficulty accumulating and persisting in the body, allowing for a slower and more efficient release. Therefore, liposomes represent a valuable tool for the delivery of drugs or bioactive substances that require sustained release over time. Among these, of course, is vitamin C, whose oral administration presents clear challenges in terms of both intestinal absorption and systemic retention.

In recent years, liposomal vitamin C has been investigated in a series of comparative studies that measured its plasma concentrations against traditional oral or intravenous administration. Results have been largely consistent. A 2016 study (312), published in "Nutrition and Metabolic Insights", compared four administration methods: placebo, 4 g via standard oral route, 4 g liposomal, and 4 g intravenous. The study found that the liposomal route outperformed standard oral supplementation, although intravenous administration produced plasma concentrations so high that the advantage of the liposomal form appeared minimal by comparison (see figure).

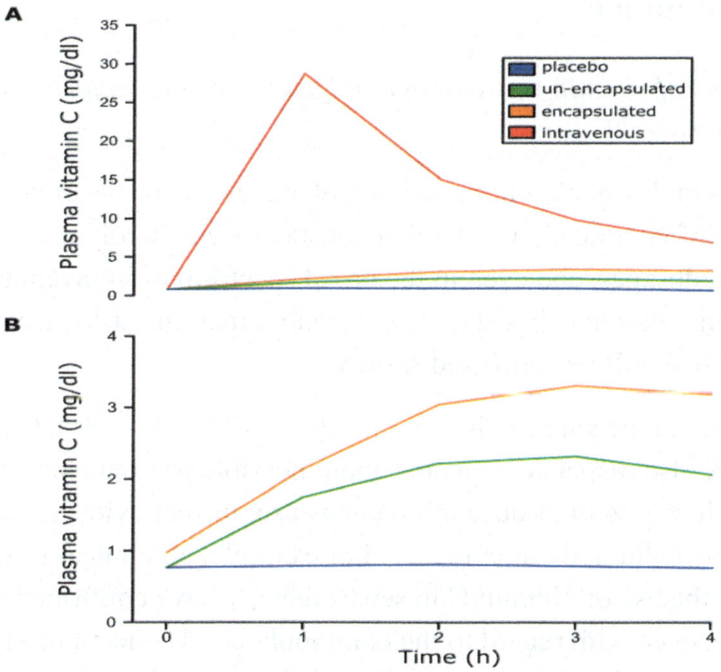

graph adapted from (312)

However, this seemingly small difference could still be meaningful when compared to standard oral delivery, at least according to other recent evaluations. A 2021 analysis (313) reported a 1.77-fold higher bioavailability for liposomal vitamin C compared to the standard oral form, while another study published in the "Journal of Microencapsulation" (314) found a 1.7-fold higher antioxidant capacity for the liposomal formulation.

Overall, the evidence appears to confirm the superiority of liposomal delivery compared to traditional oral supplementation, making it preferable in specific contexts. Two scenarios do not appear to be included among these: the management of acute illnesses, in which the intravenous approach generally remains irreplaceable, and low-income populations, for whom liposomal supplements are less accessible due to their generally higher cost compared to standard formulations.

Safety of vitamin C

'The safety of vitamin C is a double-edged sword: it comforts patients but complicates research'

Throughout this book, one reassuring element has consistently emerged: the safety profile of vitamin C, which other substances can hardly match. Across all ranges of oral dosages, and even in the broad spectrum of intravenous administration, vitamin C has shown wide safety margins, aside from some "exceptions" that will be addressed shortly.

In addition to the studies already introduced (72), (73), (86), (87), (88), many of which have also dispelled concerns about possible pro-oxidant effects theoretically linked to high-dose intravenous use, further evidence can be added, forming a truly solid body of evidence. For example, all clinical studies investigating the use of vitamin C in sepsis therapy have confirmed its strong safety profile, even with regard to the commonly cited concern of kidney stone formation. Kashiouris, L'Heureux, Cable, Fisher, Leichtle and Fowler were quite clear (177): "A hypothetical side effect of intravenous vitamin C is an increased risk of oxalate kidney stones, but to date, this has not been demonstrated in any clinical study".

Even when infused at doses far exceeding those used in sepsis treatment, vitamin C appears to remain safe, including from a renal perspective. Notably, even the very high doses of 100 g showed no clinically negative effects on key blood parameters, vital signs, coagulation profiles, or cardiac electrical activity (424), (367), (243). The same applies to concerns regarding blood glucose: the severe hyperglycemia observed after high-dose intravenous vitamin C administration was traced back to laboratory artifacts, since glucose meters tend to misinterpret structurally similar molecules such as vitamin C and glucose (424), (367).

Overall, there is solid justification to stamp all ascorbate-based therapies with an authoritative "safety certificate" (424), (367), (243).

The safety topic also spans both time and space across the scientific literature, with roots dating back decades. In 1995, Bendich and Langseth published a comprehensive review (413), establishing two pivotal conclusions regarding oral supplementation: "A thorough review of the literature indicates that populations with long-term intake of vitamin C levels above the RDA (> 60 mg/day) from food and/or supplements have reduced risk of cancer at various sites, cardiovascular disease, and cataracts. The safety of vitamin C intake above the RDA is confirmed in eight placebo-controlled double-blind studies and six non-placebo clinical trials where up to 10000 mg of vitamin C per day was consumed for up to 3 years" (413).

A decade later, a comprehensive evaluation (315) examined the effects of vitamin C and its mineral derivatives: sodium ascorbate (ascorbic acid/sodium ratio 8:1), calcium ascorbate (9:1), and magnesium ascorbate (12:1). In these compounds, ascorbic acid is bound to different minerals, producing stable salts that maintain the same biochemical activity as ascorbic acid. The study further strengthened the safety profile of vitamin C, extending it to these mineral ascorbates.

What about kidney stones?

One of the commonly mentioned precautions with vitamin C supplementation is the potential risk of kidney stones. However, this risk appears to be overestimated, as the scientific literature is far from consistent. A large 2019 meta-analysis (316) found that low-dose ascorbic acid supplementation (< 1500 mg/day) was associated with an increased incidence of kidney stones in men, but not in women. In contrast, "high-dose" supplementation (> 1500 mg/day) showed no increase in risk in either sex. Surprisingly, this finding revealed an increased risk only in men, and only at lower intake levels. This meta-analysis confirmed a pattern first observed in the large 1997 Harvard prospective follow-up study (317): vitamin C intakes above 1500 mg/day were associated with a lower risk compared to lower doses.

In 2013, a study conducted exclusively in men reported that a daily intake of 1 g could double the risk of kidney stones (318). Thus, based on the most robust studies, the risk appears relatively selective and moderate, predominantly affecting the male subgroup at daily intakes below 1500 mg. This raises an important question: could these findings provide further arguments to support the use of dynamic flow?

Moreover, the fact that higher doses (> 1500 mg) do not appear to increase the risk of kidney stones provides a rational basis for designing more "ambitious" clinical trials. In fact, using doses higher than the commonly employed 500-1000 mg could offer two clear benefits: allowing vitamin C to exert its effects more effectively, while at the same time steering participants away from the potential risk of kidney stones.

The debate over vitamin C and kidney stones was addressed in a significant one-year prospective study (319) published in the prestigious journal "Antioxidants". This investigation, involving 157 patients receiving high-dose ascorbic acid infusions, aimed to clarify the relationship between massive vitamin C intake and the risk of kidney stones over a relatively long observation period. The results were surprisingly conclusive, contradicting alarmist opinions: no patient (yes, not a single one) developed kidney stones during the observation period, despite 8% having a prior history. Another noteworthy finding also emerged: the majority of patients showed no deterioration in renal function. "We also observed no substantial changes in mean serum creatinine or eGFR among those who underwent follow-up renal function testing" (319).

Overall, the evidence seems to clear vitamin C of the accusation of promoting kidney stone formation, and moreover does not at all support the alarming claims that its high-dose use could impair kidney function, a conclusion that is, after all, consistent with my father's clinical experience (424), (243).

With regard to the primary marker of renal function, creatinine, it is worth highlighting the findings reported in a large U.S. evaluation (409): "We examined the relationship between serum antioxidant vitamin levels and serum creatinine levels, as well as hypercreatininemia risk, in a representative sample of 6629 non-Hispanic whites, 4411 non-Hispanic blacks, and 4480 Mexican Americans aged 18 and older who participated in the Third National Health and Nutrition Examination Survey. Serum vitamin A levels were positively and significantly associated with serum creatinine, while serum vitamin C levels were inversely and significantly associated". This statement, published in the prestigious "American Journal of Kidney Diseases", needs no further comment. It clearly illustrates the asymmetry between vitamin C and vitamin A with respect to creatinine, adding to the other asymmetries favourable to vitamin C discussed above. Indeed, the data suggest that maintaining adequate levels of vitamin C supports kidney health. Statistically, plasma levels above 25 micromoles/L have been associated with a 30% reduction in the risk of hypercreatininemia, reaffirming that vitamin C, at least at physiological levels, cannot impair kidney function. Surprisingly, the study also indicated that high levels of vitamin A may be harmful (409).

Even more noteworthy, and more recent, is a 2024 study (588) which identified elevated plasma vitamin C levels as a potential nephroprotective factor, demonstrating strong inverse correlations with creatinine and other renal-specific parameters. This association was particularly pronounced in the elderly population, the group most vulnerable to kidney disease: "An appropriate increase in serum vitamin C levels may hold promise for protecting renal function, particularly among older individuals" (588).

Let's return to kidney stones: a general overview suggests a slight increase in risk associated with low-dose oral supplementation. However, the logic can be disorienting: should we advise against a generous intake of fruits and vegetables, given the possibility that high consumption of plant-based foods could lead to dietary doses theoretically compatible with kidney stone formation?

On this point, it appears that no such recommendations exist, unlike the frequent concerns raised with supplementation.

Alongside the "emergency" of kidney stones, another debatable approach persists: the tendency to attribute harmful renal effects to supra-dietary intakes, especially in the presence of preexisting kidney disease. Yes, a debatable approach. And we will examine it in depth, as the accusation is serious and deserves to be analyzed through a complete body of evidence in which causal relationships and scientific data can be fully expressed.

Let's start from an undeniable fact: like most diseases, kidney failure, also known as chronic kidney disease, is associated with low plasma vitamin C concentrations, marked oxidative stress, inflammation and endothelial dysfunction (320), (321). Furthermore, it has been observed that patients with advanced kidney disease, those who therefore require hemodialysis, suffer from an even more severe vitamin C depletion, a fact that further supports the theoretical principles of its biology. In fact, several studies have even found a deficiency status in many patients undergoing hemodialysis (321), (323). Low vitamin C levels, greater susceptibility to cardiovascular events, persistent oxidative stress, and chronic inflammation (with some studies showing strong inverse correlations between AA levels and key inflammatory biomarkers in dialysis patients) together provide strong biological plausibility for restoring plasma levels, far outweighing the potential risks of nephrolithiasis (321).

In this context, another potential benefit emerges, particularly useful for a significant proportion of patients with kidney failure: the improvement of anemia, a complication that often accompanies this disease. This benefit has been observed in some clinical evaluations in which plasma ascorbate was positively associated with hemoglobin levels (323). Vitamin C may therefore play a supportive role in managing renal anemia, a common complication largely driven by reduced erythropoietin production.

But there's more: its supplementation seems to meet all the criteria to be considered highly advantageous for patients with kidney disease. It has demonstrated the ability to improve the erythropoietic response (remember that AA reduces ferric iron to ferrous iron and functionally modulates the iron-transferrin absorption pathway) and increase oxygen saturation (323). Impressive, isn't it?

However, this is still not enough to convince the scientific community, as there are currently no recommendations for AA supplementation in patients with chronic kidney disease (321).

Perplexity rises when thinking back to October 2021, when a very interesting study (397) revealed extremely concerning data. In addition to once again confirming the main theorem of vitamin C (hemodialysis patients had lower plasma concentrations than non-dialysis patients), the study reported an alarming figure: a single hemodialysis session led to a drop of about 40% in plasma vitamin C levels, further depleting the already scarce reserves in these patients. These data strongly support the hypothesis that vitamin C may be completely depleted in hemodialysis patients. Doshida and colleagues share this view, making very explicit statements: "Total plasma ascorbate levels in patients with chronic kidney disease not on dialysis and those undergoing dialysis were 27.1 ± 13.9 and 12.0 ± 6.2 micromoles, respectively. Since the risk of developing scurvy increases at ascorbate concentrations below 11 micromoles, it is likely that many dialysis patients develop scurvy. In fact, globally, many dialysis patients have been found to have scurvy" (397).

Thus, a serious threat from a dark past seems to reemerge among patients undergoing hemodialysis: frank scurvy, not merely one of its subclinical forms. It is the same affliction that once devastated the lives of countless sailors, taking advantage of the limited scientific understanding of the time. A long time has passed since Lind's pioneering work, and yet we must point out that the danger still looms over today's "modern sailors" (such as patients with advanced kidney disease), an underestimated risk that, fortunately, is easily preventable, making a certain degree of skepticism only natural.

But there is also a constructive side, which proposes an operational criterion: according to some experts, ascorbic therapy in dialysis is considered advisable when plasma ascorbate levels fall below 30 micromoles/L, probably because below this threshold the risk-benefit ratio remains clearly positive (321).

We now turn to a study (322) published in the "Clinical Kidney Journal", which offers what could be seen as a near-Copernican shift in perspective. In their work, Karahan, Afsar and Kanbay examined the issue from the opposite angle, highlighting the potential risks posed by low AA levels in patients with kidney failure. Specifically, the authors highlighted a direct association between asymmetric dimethylarginine (ADMA), an endogenous inhibitor of nitric oxide synthase (the enzyme that synthesizes NO via BH4), and a worse prognosis in chronic kidney disease. This association, well characterized biochemically (ADMA tends to reduce endothelial NO production, consequently impairing vascular homeostasis), has been confirmed by several studies linking elevated ADMA levels to increased cardiovascular disease and mortality (322), (578). In light of this, reducing ADMA levels could represent a promising therapeutic strategy for patients with chronic kidney disease, especially considering the persistent combination of oxidative stress and inflammation that afflicts them.

Surprisingly, some studies have suggested that adequate vitamin C supplementation may reduce ADMA levels, thereby providing additional support for these patients (579). As the researchers write, "Ascorbic acid may be a promising agent in chronic kidney disease through the reduction of oxidative stress and ADMA levels" (322).

Overall, these findings lead to an important conclusion: vitamin C supplementation is not only generally safe for the kidneys, but may also offer tangible benefits for people with chronic kidney disease. In this regard, we must not forget its potential nephroprotective effects, which have emerged in several critical scenarios such as sepsis, reperfusion injury, radiation damage and hemorrhagic shock, conditions in which high doses of vitamin C have built a powerful and multifaceted antioxidant and anti-inflammatory shield.

Moreover, recent studies have reported new benefits, further enriching the list of synergistic effects that this molecule has with various drugs. A case in point is the powerful antibiotic vancomycin, whose administration can cause acute kidney injury. Pharmacological vitamin C has been shown to be effective in reducing its pronounced nephrotoxicity, especially in critically ill patients. "High-dose intravenous vitamin C can significantly reduce vancomycin-induced nephrotoxicity and shorten hospital stays. When vancomycin is used in critically ill patients, AA may be co-administered to prevent or reduce drug-induced kidney damage, improve the therapeutic effect, and reduce toxicity", explained the authors of a retrospective study on 245 patients (414). Thus, not only effective kidney protection, but also solid antibacterial support, consistent with the crucial role of vitamin C in neutrophil function.

The second-to-last study we will highlight, although not offering new insights, has symbolic significance because it takes us back to the classic dilemma in ascorbic acid research. The authors of an article in the "World Journal of Clinical Urology" (323) agree that patients with chronic kidney disease may benefit from vitamin C supplementation, expressing the hope for further clinical research to "confirm its potential benefits, optimal dosage, and possible side effects".

In summary, the typical scarcity of ascorbic acid in patients with chronic kidney disease, combined with the severe oxidative stress and chronic inflammation characteristic of the condition, highlights the need to ensure adequate ascorbemia, an imperative that seems to clearly outweigh the fear of kidney stones.

We now close the renal section with information from one of the most authoritative journals in the world, "Nature". In 2015, it published a meta-analysis (380) whose results once again challenge the alarmist rhetoric surrounding vitamin C. Drawing on data from a dozen epidemiological studies, the analysis reached a conclusion of significant epidemiological relevance: vitamin C intake is associated with a reduced risk of kidney cancer.

From the kidneys, we move on to the gut. It was Robert Cathcart who first observed that mild diarrhea is the main sign of intestinal saturation, and therefore not really a side effect. This indicator can help determine the optimal oral intake and serves as a useful guide for the well-known bowel tolerance (40).

In fact, a discomfort associated with oral ascorbic acid can occur, and it may affect a considerable part of the population. Thc culprit is its slight acidity, which can exacerbate underlying gastric issues, problems that are increasingly common worldwide. In such cases, considering buffered salt forms such as sodium ascorbate and calcium ascorbate could be a smart strategy. An important study on calcium ascorbate (324) strongly supports this hypothesis. This mineral ascorbate has demonstrated the ability to reduce the mild gastric acidity caused by ascorbic acid, in rats. Interestingly, the study (324) also found that calcium ascorbate had greater bioavailability than ascorbic acid, both in the short term and beyond 24 hours (see figure).

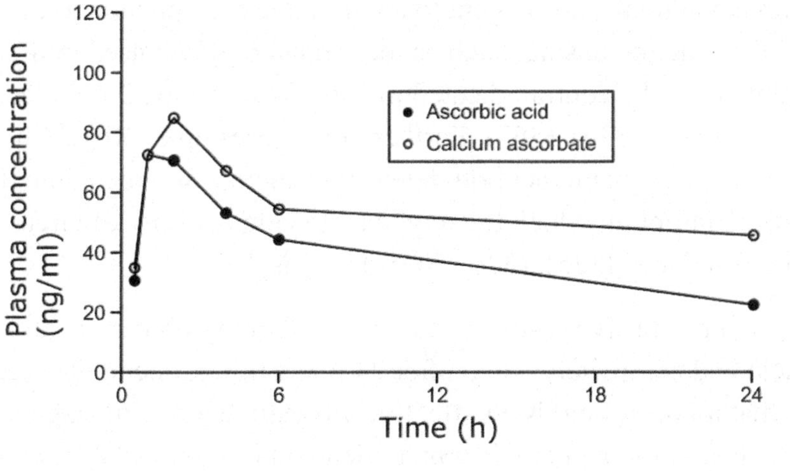

graph adapted from (324)

This suggests a vitamin C "enhancer", a molecule potentially capable of increasing its bioavailability. But one swallow does not make a summer, and the fact that the study is based on animal models only reinforces this conclusion. This implies that, although the data suggest a solution to the problematic intestinal absorption of supra-dietary doses, further investigation is necessary. It should also be noted that any enthusiasm may be tempered by the well-known limitations of calcium itself, whose excess can be quite toxic.

Continuing the analysis of potential toxicities, it is necessary to revisit the long-debated issue of favism, which may be responsible for hemolytic anemia in individuals with G6PD deficiency exposed to high-dose infusions (230). The epistemological preamble offered earlier provides an ideal basis to grasp all the nuances of the issue. Let us start with an objective fact: hemolytic anemia associated with vitamin C has been reported in very few cases, and almost exclusively in clinical situations where the administered dose exceeded 50 g intravenously (230), (325). As previously mentioned, the destruction of red blood cells (hemolysis) seems to be closely dependent on extremely high concentrations. A recent study by Marik attempted to clarify the matter, providing essential distinctions. According to his analysis, intravenous vitamin C at moderate doses is not harmful in terms of hemolysis, and may even be beneficial. In fact, it could serve as a treatment of choice for drug-induced hemolytic anemia in patients with G6PD deficiency (325).

In a striking reversal, the perception of vitamin C in G6PD deficiency has shifted from a potential causal agent to an effective therapeutic tool. Evidence indicates that moderate dosing, such as the typical 6 g/24 h used in the HAT protocol, should not be contraindicated in patients with G6PD deficiency, as it is likely to be harmless (325), (367). Furthermore, doses up to 30 g/24 h have been shown to effectively counteract both hemolytic anemia and methemoglobinemia, a dangerous condition in which the oxygen-carrying capacity of circulating hemoglobin is reduced (325), (326). Surprising, isn't it?

"Here we present five cases of acquired methemoglobinemia, all treated with ascorbic acid and completely cured after 24 hours of treatment. Our series highlights that ascorbic acid is an effective alternative in the management of acquired methemoglobinemia when methylene blue is unavailable, and suggests that ascorbic acid infusion may be indicated in patients with glucose-6-phosphate dehydrogenase deficiency", states an article published in the "American Journal of Therapeutics" (326).

A careful overall analysis seems to reveal a single factor potentially responsible for adverse effects: very high intravenous dosages, theoretically associated with pro-oxidant effects. However, apart from cancer treatment, a condition that may indeed require pro-oxidant mechanisms for AA to act effectively, there are currently no other known diseases that require such extreme dosages.

Once again, the urban legends surrounding vitamin C have been debunked through a rational approach that quantifies the actual extent of the phenomenon. As mentioned, it is unfortunately not uncommon to encounter a media-scientific drama over the connection between G6PD and vitamin C ("red blood cell rupture"), without the matter receiving a proper scientific framework. Why spread a fear that seems unjustified?

Further support for this thesis comes from seminal research by Winterbourn, published in 1979 in the authoritative "British Journal of Haematology" (381). His work anticipated Marik's evidence by forty years, providing therapeutic data for vitamin C at slightly supraphysiological concentrations. In addition to confirming the safety of physiological levels, Winterbourn emphasized the effectiveness of moderately elevated levels, noting that AA could protect red blood cells by replacing depleted glutathione due to G6PD deficiency (381). The question then arises naturally: would it not be more constructive to promote the effectiveness of moderate intravenous doses as a potentially valuable resource to counteract "red blood cell rupture", rather than raising concerns about potential risks that, in any case, seem to be linked to astronomical doses?

Let us now shift our focus to the potential problems related to iron excess. Regarding the risks associated with iron overload and potential oxidative effects, it is worth returning to a previous point, namely, the demonstrated safety of vitamin C even in individuals with elevated iron levels (131).

It is useful to recall the two hypothetical concerns about AA's ability to increase iron absorption: the excessive accumulation of this mineral, which could potentially damage organs, and a pro-oxidant state that might result from the simultaneous presence of high levels of iron and ascorbate (observed in vitro).

Some studies (131), (360) have documented AA's regulatory role in the pathway that enhances iron absorption, with the increase in iron appearing to be regulated by strict protective mechanisms. To further confirm its non-toxicity, it is worth citing the results of a 2000 in vivo study (375). This study evaluated guinea pigs fed high or low doses of ascorbate, with or without prior iron loading, to assess potential oxidative effects related to the reduction of transition metals. The results showed that:

1- AA acts as an antioxidant for lipids even in the presence of iron overload;

2- Iron overload, while not causing oxidative damage to lipids, can delay growth and damage certain tissues;

3- Iron overload combined with low ascorbemia can lead to further pathophysiological alterations, particularly elevated plasma triglycerides and lipid peroxidation markers.

As is evident, the arguments against ascorbate supplementation remain shrouded in a cloud that seems more magical than scientific. Speaking of magic, one should not overlook the hepatoprotective properties of vitamin C, which has been shown to protect the liver from uncontrolled iron accumulation (360).

So, in animals, the verdict seems clear. But what about humans?

Nine healthy volunteers participated in a study (384) in which they were assigned to three different treatment combinations: 2 g of AA orally, 150 mg of iron, and finally 2 g of AA orally + 150 mg of iron. The study, published in "Annals of Nutrition and Metabolism", offered little comfort to alarmists, confirming previous animal data: not even a trace of oxidative damage was detected, even days later.

Ultimately, it is conceivable that a pro-oxidant scenario arising from the simultaneous presence of high levels of iron and vitamin C could only materialize in the presence of extremely high ascorbemia, something achievable only through intravenous administration. The discrepancies between in vivo studies and the small subset of in vitro studies showing pro-oxidant effects should therefore not be alarming. One must also consider the efficiency with which endogenous antioxidant systems can neutralize many oxidants. But how likely is it that a high plasma concentration could overwhelm these systems and trigger oxidative effects on healthy cells?

A reliable answer can be found in phase 1 clinical trials, which are specifically designed to assess safety and tolerability. Judging from phase 1 studies focused on cancer treatment, where massive intravenous infusions of vitamin C were consistently found to be non-toxic (424), (367), (243), the likelihood appears low. It is further reduced when we look at other experimental settings, such as studies on burn victims, in which "slow-release" megadoses (110 g via continuous intravenous infusion over 24 hours) yielded distinctly antioxidant responses (181).

Carr and Frei further bolstered the concept with a review that compiled additional reassuring evidence regarding the "iron problem", as well as broader considerations (496). "We found convincing evidence that vitamin C provides antioxidant protection to lipids in animal and human biological fluids, both with and without iron supplementation. Although data on protein oxidation in humans are limited and inconclusive, the available animal data consistently show an antioxidant role for vitamin C. Data on in vivo DNA oxidation are inconsistent and conflicting, but some discrepancies may be due to flawed experimental design and methodology", the authors report (496). A telling statement, suggesting that many of the pro-oxidative scenarios reported in the literature may in fact be virtual, or simply the result of flawed experimental designs.

We have now reached the moment of the overall conclusions, once again favorable to vitamin C. A comprehensive evaluation paints a scientific picture in which its side effects, apparently rare and generally insignificant, represent mere microscopic traces compared to the full extent of its potential. As has been emphasized several times, one of these traces, perhaps the most remarkable, is its ability to act very aggressively, although probably only in the context of tumor cells (pro-oxidant effect), thereby transforming a potentially harmful action into a selective therapeutic weapon aimed directly at cancer (424), (86), (110), (181), (367), (243).

A general analysis, therefore, leaves little justification for the apprehensive, if not outright alarmist, tone adopted by some sources when discussing high-dose vitamin C. It reveals a media narrative increasingly distorted by a conceptual reversal of scientific truths. And so, the ghosts of the past resurface: from the fierce battle that unjustly silenced Pauling and Cameron, to the potential polio breakthrough dismissed by an experiment Klenner described as "unscientific".

Not to mention the collective inattention that marred Lind's extraordinary discovery, delaying by over 40 years the adoption of simple measures that could have eradicated scurvy. After all, Lind was considered a second-tier scientist, certainly not on the level of Pauling. And yet, even the double Nobel laureate was not spared from criticism, often lacking any solid logical basis.

The parallel with aspirin

Is there anyone who has never taken aspirin?

Acetylsalicylic acid, the active ingredient of the famous aspirin, is a molecule with a rich history. Its most notable pharmacological property is its non-steroidal anti-inflammatory action, distinct from that of adrenal hormones known as corticosteroids. The stories of aspirin and vitamin C are fascinating because they intertwine in ways that offer particularly intriguing epistemological insights. Synthesized in the laboratory in 1897, aspirin was immediately hailed as a sort of enfant prodige. It was rapidly adopted in clinical practice despite the incomplete understanding of its mechanisms of action, which would only be clarified many years later. Its effectiveness in alleviating inflammation was so evident that everything else was momentarily set aside. At the beginning of the 20th century, when medicine had few tools to address rheumatic and inflammatory diseases (powerful steroidal anti-inflammatories, for example, would be discovered much later), aspirin truly seemed like a godsend for many patients. In this context, it appeared rational to consider its clinical use, as indeed occurred, even though several key conceptual questions remained unanswered.

Now, let us project this line of thought into the present day and replace aspirin with vitamin C. What picture emerges?

Mathematicians might call this a change of coordinates, a transformation that reveals striking parallels with the history of aspirin, generating a series of considerations that could be relevant for clinical practice. Research on vitamin C has shed light on a wide range of physiological and pharmacological processes, from antitumor mechanisms to immunomodulatory effects, from its potent antioxidant action to its role in synthesizing essential compounds such as collagen, catecholamines and carnitine. Thousands of studies have been enthusiastically conducted by researchers around the world, often producing encouraging, though at times disappointing, results. Despite this, many issues remain shrouded in mystery. Consider, for example, the mechanisms regulating AA-mediated neuromodulation and the size of its therapeutic window, both areas where our understanding remains limited.

If the future remains uncertain, the past of vitamin C is, paradoxically, still chained to many enigmatic biases. Here we must recall the bold genius of Dr. Klenner, a man of extraordinary intuition and vision as deep as the ocean, qualities supported by numerous robust arguments. Among these, one of his most valuable suggestions deserves to be emphasized once again: his advice to emergency physicians to promptly administer vitamin C in critical situations, even before beginning diagnostic procedures. In this light, we cannot overlook another pioneer: Irwin Stone, the first to connect vitamin C deficiency to increased susceptibility to a wide range of diseases. Therefore, it seems entirely reasonable to ask a question that is fully justified by logic: is it not time to seriously reconsider vitamin C with the goal of achieving formal clinical recognition?

Let us be clear: this is, of course, only my opinion, albeit one supported by a substantial body of literature and by an increasingly plausible evidentiary framework. And it is also an opinion that sees no downside, even when stretched to the limits of imagination. This is because vitamin C not only lacks significant toxicity, but is also desperately needed by patients' bodies, whose illnesses are often so severe that they voraciously consume virtually all the vitamin C present in the blood and tissues. Does that sound like an exaggeration?

This finding has been observed in many hospitals, starting with a study conducted at a Canadian university clinic, where 60% of patients were in a state of hypovitaminosis and 19% were deficient (327). In another hospital study (407), the authors reported striking figures and evident gaps, not only regarding vitamin C: "In conclusion, this research confirms several previous studies documenting a very high prevalence of hypovitaminosis C and D in hospitalized patients with acute illnesses. Since this information appears almost exclusively in nutrition journals, it remains unknown to most physicians". Given the numerous fundamental biological roles played by these vitamins, such statements are indeed alarming.

It is important to emphasize that these data have been widely confirmed by other studies. An observational study (328) conducted in a general medicine ward of an Australian hospital, for example, revealed that 76.5% of 149 patients had plasma levels < 28 micromoles/L, also showing an inverse correlation between ascorbic acid levels and major inflammatory biomarkers.

In elderly patients, the situation appears even more severe: 88% of patients had very low levels (mean level: 18 micromoles/L), and a striking 44% had levels almost incompatible with life (< 6 micromoles/L). These are the figures from a study conducted in a geriatric ward during the period 1999-2000 (465), which also found that patients coming from nursing homes were admitted to hospital with a mean concentration of 6.8 micromoles/L. These are unequivocal, almost unbelievable, numbers that force us to confront a harsh reality: scurvy is far from eliminated. Perhaps it has changed its appearance to confuse rigid minds, or perhaps it has undergone a radical transformation to mislead even the sharpest thinkers. Or perhaps it is right before our eyes, unchanged and as clear as day. While these are all speculations still awaiting confirmation, statistics from intensive care units, dialysis wards, and nursing homes leave little room for doubt and suggest the chilling hypothesis that scurvy is still with us.

Very recently, a notable and methodologically rigorous scoping review of studies conducted in high-income countries provided strong evidence supporting the association between hospitalization and critically low ascorbemia. The review analyzed 2494 serum samples, revealing that 27.7% had vitamin C concentrations in the scurvy range (< 11.4 micromoles/L) (596).

Let us turn to the duration of hospital stays. While it may seem obvious to associate ascorbate deficiency with prolonged hospitalization, a point highlighted in some of the previously mentioned studies (497), (165), (328), I believe it is useful to present the data explicitly. This is part of a broader dynamic in which taking obvious facts for granted can become a significant issue. As George Orwell aptly observed, "Sometimes the first duty of intelligent people is the restatement of the obvious".

Everything discovered over the years by scientific research, particularly regarding the influence of vitamin C on the length of hospital stays, converges with certain of its characteristics (ready availability, low cost and minimal toxicity), all of which seem to justify its clinical use in the hospital setting. This scenario closely recalls the bold early adoption of aspirin in clinical practice, despite the limited scientific knowledge of the time. With vitamin C, however, although high-quality clinical trials are still lacking in many experimental areas, we are far more advanced scientifically than we were with aspirin in the early 1900s. It is not a magic potion, but a substance with numerous physiological properties and broad multidirectional pharmacological potential. It is therefore reasonable to assert that its use could provide meaningful support in a wide range of clinical scenarios, from the simplest to the most severe, particularly in the hospital setting, where cases characterized by the simultaneous presence of multiple pathologies are common, a feature typically seen among the elderly, the demographic who are moreover particularly vulnerable to vitamin C deficiency.

What reasons prevent the systematic measurement of plasma ascorbate levels in hospitals?

Systematic monitoring, as is done for other substances such as sodium, potassium, and folic acid, would reveal the widespread state of hypovitaminosis among patients, paving the way for restorative therapies that could lead to clinical improvements and shorter hospital stays, thereby also reducing management costs. Why, then, does vitamin C stubbornly remain locked in its "nutritional prison"?

Here we return to the classic dichotomy: the conflict between nutritional and pharmacological use, which has created enormous conceptual confusion. This confusion persists today, obscuring the multidirectional pharmacological potential of vitamin C, a remarkable property that some technically describe as pleiotropic, meaning it influences multiple physiological processes.

Let us continue by illustrating the pharmacological interactions between aspirin and vitamin C. Since the 1980s, it has been known that the two molecules interfere with each other at the level of gastrointestinal absorption (329). More than interference, it is more accurately a kind of friction that, like proton pump inhibitors, is unilateral: while aspirin impairs vitamin C absorption, in the opposite direction there is a positive interaction, as it has been observed that vitamin C can reduce the toxicity and the dosage required for aspirin therapy. One of many supporting studies was published in the authoritative "Journal of Neuroimmunology" (330): "These experiments suggest that combining aspirin with ascorbic acid offers a novel approach to enhance COX-2 sensitivity to aspirin, enabling anti-inflammatory treatment at lower doses, thereby avoiding the typical side effects of high-dose aspirin therapy" (330).

It is worth noting that this unilateral interaction has been confirmed by multiple lines of evidence. In a compelling clinical trial (331), for example, vitamin C demonstrated the ability to protect the primary site of aspirin-induced toxicity, the gastric mucosa. The authors concluded: "Vitamin C combined with acetylsalicylic acid, unlike acetylsalicylic acid alone, protects the human gastric mucosa, probably through attenuation of oxidative stress and pro-inflammatory cytokines" (331).

All this, incidentally, highlights a little-appreciated aspect of vitamin C: cytoprotection, the ability of a substance to shield a mucosal surface from the harmful effects of environmental or pharmacological agents. This is supported by consistent evidence, at least with regard to the cytoprotective effect that vitamin C can have on the gastric mucosa (462), (463), (464).

To conclude this section on interactions, we turn to HIF-1 alpha. A 2016 study (332) examined the protective effects of the aspirin-vitamin C combination against heart damage caused by chronic intake of corn syrup. The authors found that this combination may reduce cardiac damage through various mechanisms, particularly by increasing SIRT-1 expression and, most importantly, by significantly lowering HIF-1 alpha levels.

And so we reach the end of this section, which has highlighted the "kindness" of vitamin C. Its attitude toward aspirin appears genuinely kind, unaffected by the friction that makes aspirin a threat to vitamin C bioavailability. The enhancement of aspirin's effects and the mitigation of its toxicity fully justify this kindness.

After all, if we give weight to the words of Muhammad, "Kindness is a sign of faith", then we should place immense faith in vitamin C, even though the scientific evidence supporting this extraordinary molecule hardly needs metaphysical reinforcement. But perhaps this is precisely the point: it might be investigative faith that harmonizes the scientific landscape of ascorbate. Indeed, even if we do not know how much faith and courage have in common, history teaches us that courage has often been essential in alleviating pain and suffering in times when hope was scarce. This reference clearly applies to the wager known as aspirin, a wager that has paid off handsomely despite the scientific mystery that long surrounded it. With vitamin C, however, we may not even need a wager. It seems more like one of those sure bets, that is, situations of financial arbitrage that generate profits without excessive risk. I repeat: profits without excessive risk.

Is there an optimal dosage of vitamin C?

As you may have guessed, we are approaching the final sections of the book, and for that reason, I believe the time is ripe to clearly address the delicate issue of the optimal daily dosage.

Before we begin, let's lay out some fundamental premises: we'll start with a few functional preliminaries, presented within a specific communicative philosophy. This is an inductive approach, built on objective elements, logical reasoning, and plausible interconnections. We've already emphasized that intravenous administration is not viable as a standard supplementation method. It should be considered only under medical supervision and primarily for acute cases. Based on this, we'll focus our attention on the only practical option under ordinary conditions: oral intake. We will also distinguish between a healthy, unstressed individual and someone who is either ill or subjected to ongoing stress of any kind.

Let's start with the statistics: several studies have extended the numerous inverse associations discussed throughout this book, analyzing them in terms of mortality. A prospective Chinese study (333) tracked the risk of death from all causes, heart disease, and cancer over a 16-year period. The results were highly revealing: higher plasma concentrations of vitamin C were associated with lower mortality, particularly from cancer and cardiovascular events.

This study supports the findings of another investigation (334) published in the prestigious journal "The Lancet", which reported: "Plasma ascorbic acid concentration was inversely related to mortality from all causes and from cardiovascular disease and ischemic heart disease in both men and women". This finding expands on an earlier study on heart failure (501), whose significance lies not only in the fact that a 20 micromoles/L increase in plasma concentration was linked to a 20% reduction in all-cause mortality risk, but also because the correlation appeared independent of various factors such as age, blood pressure, blood cholesterol, smoking habits, and diabetes (334). The journal's credibility and the large sample size (nearly 20000 participants) lend strong weight to these findings, though they do not rule out the influence of a broader underlying mechanism. This is suggested by the phrase: "The relationship with mortality was continuous across the whole distribution of ascorbic acid concentrations" (334), which makes it conceivable that even a moderate supraphysiological level (such as 150-250 micromoles/L, achievable through dynamic flow intake) might be inversely related to mortality. Simply put: a plasma level of 250 micromoles/L might reduce the risk of death more effectively than any other level achievable through oral intake.

When it comes to global vitamin C deficiency, available assessments are not encouraging. For instance, the National Health and Nutrition Examination Survey (NHANES, USA) reported hypovitaminosis in nearly 20% of individuals aged 6-19 during the 2003-2004 period (335). Concerns deepen when we learn that nearly one-third of Mexican children aged 0-2 were deficient (335). From Mexico, where 40% of women of childbearing age were found to have low levels (350), we move to Nigeria, a country where, according to a hospital analysis, almost 80% of pregnant women suffer from marked hypovitaminosis (368).

Even in the West, the numbers are concerning, particularly among low-income populations. In the United Kingdom, hypovitaminosis has been observed in 40%, and deficiency in 20%, of the low-income population (336).

Among the most vulnerable demographic, elderly individuals (62), (63), the situation worsens. A large study (350) focusing on elderly Indians found alarming figures: 73.9% in the northern region and 45.7% in the southern region were deficient.

In general, it seems clear that vitamin C deficiency incidence depends on various factors, including economic status, smoking, education level, access to fresh produce, geographic pollutants, and stress exposure, each highly variable and significant.

As mentioned earlier, we can identify six distinct levels of vitamin C intake. To make things clear, we will initially consider conditions of full health, absence of chronic stress, and no underlying ascorbate deficiency. Here is the classification:

1- Daily intake of 10-15 mg, the minimum amount required to prevent scurvy;

2- Daily intake of 70-100 mg, consistent with the RDA. This level offers solid protection against scurvy;

3- Daily intake of 200-300 mg, sufficient to saturate plasma under optimal health and no stress, maintaining plasma levels of 70-80 micromoles/L over time (22), (65);

4- Daily intake of 70-100 mg with periodic 500-1000 mg supplements, a common practice that prevents scurvy and produces plasma peaks of 3-4 hours;

5- Daily intake of 200-300 mg with periodic 500-1000 mg supplements. This maintains 70 micromoles/L in plasma, with transient peaks;

6- Daily intake of 3 g every 4 hours, which achieves high and sustained plasma concentration (220-250 micromoles/L). This is probably the maximum achievable through oral intake and can be defined as "dynamic flow under full health conditions and without underlying stress or deficiencies" (22), (337).

As stated earlier, this analysis initially considers a condition of full health and absence of stress. So, let us begin with a few questions:

How many people truly meet this condition?

How many regularly monitor their ascorbate levels?

How many successfully avoid stress, whether physical trauma, intense exercise, psychological strain, poor diet, environmental pollution, electromagnetic radiation, smoking, medications, or infections? And how many undergo regular medical checkups to rule out chronic disease and ensure an optimal state of health?

It is easy to see that very few people actually meet all these criteria, especially when considering unavoidable sources of stress such as pollution. Under these ideal circumstances, it is reasonable to say that a modest intake (levels 2-3) would be sufficient. However, advocates of microdoses should not celebrate just yet, for two main reasons.

First, it is difficult to rule out the presence of SVCT polymorphisms, which could significantly impair ascorbate transport across various tissues, potentially rendering intake levels 2 and 3 inadequate. Second, even in an ideal life scenario, characterized by a healthy diet, no smoking or alcohol, stress management practices such as yoga and meditation, living in the countryside, regular checkups, light daily exercise, a positive mindset, a fulfilling job, and a supportive partner, what would happen if one experienced physical trauma or an accident?

Let us recall Stone's personal experience: he credited saturated tissue ascorbate levels with protecting him from life-threatening complications after his car accident.

What happens if one contracts a dangerous pathogen, considering that suboptimal ascorbate levels impair immune responses to viral or bacterial invasions?

What happens if one is bitten by a venomous insect? (think of the inverse correlation between histamine and vitamin C).

How would your body cope with the physical and mental stress of certain jobs?

What about cold, humidity, or prolonged sun exposure?

Even environmental and atmospheric pollutants, often unavoidable, must be taken into account. Consider carbon monoxide, lead (recall the inverse correlation with AA), particulate matter, and even cosmic rays, high-energy particles from space. "Cosmic rays? Really?" someone might ask. But scientific evidence is clear: vitamin C may act as a powerful radioprotective agent in space. Several studies (421) have identified it as mitigating radiation-induced damage, with efficacy observed even when administered hours after exposure, making it potentially valuable for space missions, where astronauts are exposed to ionizing radiation, cosmic rays, and solar wind.

We have thus listed a series of highly stressful factors that can lower vitamin C concentrations, our primary defense against oxidative stress (427), (528). This stands in contrast to animals, in which the modulation of endogenous synthesis constantly ensures vitamin C homeostasis.

Therefore, even under perfect conditions, it is reasonable to assume that the ideal steady state of 70 micromoles/L (achievable through level 3, with a diet rich in vegetables) could be compromised by daily life. Sudden, unpredictable stress can cause ascorbate losses even in the healthiest organism, a phenomenon that could potentially lead to deficiency.

Here is another illustrative example: suppose one is at level 3 intake and encounters a dangerous pathogen. This could cause severe depletion of ascorbate in both plasma and leukocytes. Logic suggests that a plasma concentration of 220-250 micromoles/L would offer greater protection than 70 micromoles/L, not only because post-infection levels would remain higher, but because a higher baseline might directly confront the threat, slowing its progression through multiple biological mechanisms. It is plausible that such levels could better meet the increased demands of leukocytes, particularly neutrophils, which can increase vitamin C transporter expression by up to tenfold during acute infection (378). So, is it reasonable to constantly maximize plasma levels up to the oral threshold of 220-250 micromoles/L?

A definitive answer is difficult to give, but such a strategy could provide the best defense. In the event of pathogenic invasion, these plasma levels would decline more gradually, reducing the risk of deficiency.

Consider Partipilo's antiviral conjecture: viruses cause rapid vitamin C depletion and exploit long incubation times. The conclusion? The only useful preventive strategy might be the dynamic-flow approach.

In short: vitamin C as both a preventive and proactive model, a spontaneous paradigm in the animal kingdom. Once again, vitamin C: the ultimate anti-stress agent.

Strengthening our ascorbate levels could indeed be beneficial, and the strong prophylactic effect demonstrated in potentially lethal acute scenarios provides further support. We have repeatedly observed this phenomenon in conditions such as ischemia, viral infections, anaphylaxis, severe trauma (Stone's car accident, hemorrhagic shock models), and complications such as postoperative atrial fibrillation, with encouraging results in both incidence and severity (124), (145), (160), (165), (184), (279).

Overall, the positive results of the preventive model support the importance of maintaining high plasma concentrations, a strategy that could help buffer the sharp decline that follows acute conditions.

So here's a curious question: if a time traveler warned you of an imminent medical crisis, say, a stroke or severe trauma, would it change the way you think about vitamin C?

Would it be reasonable to face such events with a high plasma level, ideally the highest achievable by oral means?

With 250 micromoles/L in the blood, tissues would be more fortified and better equipped to withstand sudden adverse events. The logic is clear: the unpredictable nature of diseases and traumas justifies the continuous intake of AA (dynamic flow), just as epileptics must take anticonvulsants on an ongoing basis, in a purely conceptual sense, because the onset of seizures cannot be predicted. Independently of this analogy, it is noteworthy that, in epilepsy itself, some evidence suggests substantial benefits of vitamin C, likely due to its multifaceted neuroprotective effects (422).

Returning to the numerous inverse associations between plasma ascorbate and the risk of various diseases, these associations strengthen the arguments in favor of higher levels. Considering daily stress, it is plausible to state that the cumulative effect of small, constant stressors could eventually lead to a subtle ascorbate deficiency, an increasingly common scenario in modern life, and that level 6 could effectively counteract this.

Another aspect: under ideal conditions, level 3 appears to saturate plasma and favourite tissues. But what about other organs?

Clinical data reveal asymmetries between white blood cells and muscles, the lens and aqueous humor, suggesting different pharmacokinetic behaviors in areas not favored by vitamin C (401), (410), (431), (537). This seems consistent with animal models (69), (363), which indicate that organs such as the heart, lungs, liver, and kidneys may require much higher doses for saturation compared to plasma, brain, and leukocytes. It is therefore reasonable to imagine that these vital organs could absorb ascorbate almost indefinitely, possessing a broader "receptive substrate". This could provide prophylactic benefits if level 6 were implemented: if one of these organs were to become diseased, likely producing strong local oxidative stress and alterations in SVCT, its tissue concentrations could decrease more slowly in the presence of level 6, making the antioxidant and anti-inflammatory defenses less weakened and likely leading to less severe clinical outcomes. Therefore, could a cardiac concentration of 0.6 millimoles be more protective than the typical 0.3 millimoles during an acute cardiovascular event?

Probably yes. It is indeed plausible that a higher ascorbate concentration could better neutralize ROS, more effectively reduce cardiovascular inflammation, and validly support the synthesis of essential substances such as vasopressors, epigenetic modulation, and vascular integrity (note that full BH4 defense appears to require endothelial saturation (438), (149), (527)). Overall, this could further weaken the idea that plasma or leukocyte saturation alone can determine the optimal dosage.

In other words, based on current evidence, we do not have sufficient proof to claim that plasma (or leukocyte) levels are a reliable indicator of ascorbate homeostasis. In fact, available data suggest we must look well beyond plasma and white blood cells.

Some researchers (67) even hypothesize that supraphysiological local concentrations may have unknown functions. Others (363) propose a model in which certain vital organs require full saturation to function optimally, likely due to epigenetic mechanisms: "The recent identification of the key role of ascorbate in the alpha-hydroxylation of HIF-1 alpha and in histone demethylase regulation highlights the need for adequate ascorbate levels in all tissues to properly control metabolism and gene expression".

In addition to all this, it should be remembered that vitamin C is first and foremost an antioxidant, the primary one, which supports the following theory that will be explored later: the maximum local antioxidant efficacy could be linked to local saturation.

Let us return to the preventive model. Even a lifestyle that is slightly less than ideal, a bit of stress, an imperfect diet, intense exercise, and indirect exposure to pollutants would continue to push us toward the dynamic flow. In these cases, levels 2-3-4-5 might not provide adequate protection against everyday disturbances, whereas level 6 could. In essence, level 6 helps correct our genetic defect, hypoascorbemia, protecting us from excessive vulnerability to the many stressors of life. This brings us closer to the animal world, where nature relies heavily on vitamin C to preserve health.

Let us revisit the idea of vitamin C as a stress hormone, taking inspiration from animals under stress which, unlike humans, use cortisol in a probably more efficient and balanced way (25), (175). Could levels 1-2-3-4-5 mimic this dynamic?

Probably not. Only consistently high concentrations could modulate cortisol optimally, avoiding its excesses, as some scientists argue. Therefore, high AA levels could produce a stress response that is dynamic yet balanced, keeping cortisol within physiological limits and preventing the many harmful metabolic consequences associated with chronic cortisol excess. What numerical data support these fascinating assumptions?

One study found that fish producing vitamin C have a 1.6-fold increase in cortisol during stress, while species that do not produce it showed a 20.2-fold increase during the same type of stress (175). Other studies confirm that animals deficient in vitamin C present higher baseline cortisol levels regardless of stress conditions, a fact that supports vitamin-C-mediated cortisol modulation. This dynamic also appears to apply to humans. A randomized controlled trial (26) demonstrated that oral supplementation of 3 g/day effectively reduced cortisol and blood pressure under stress, supporting the idea of increasing vitamin C intake during any type of stress.

Let us consider the WHO definition of stress: "The health epidemic of the 21st century". A rapidly spreading and increasingly global problem, which, however, could find a valuable ally in vitamin C, thanks to its remarkable, though unfortunately underestimated, anti-stress properties. Could our inability to synthesize large amounts of ascorbate under stress be the reason why we are constantly "stressed"?

Could this explain why so many diseases are linked to stress?

Persistently low vitamin C levels during chronic stress could indeed be harmful, as they could increase cortisol levels, causing oxidative stress, immunosuppression and hyperglycemia (effects that are therefore the opposite of those offered by adequate vitamin C levels), providing a stress response opposite to that of animals. Could this be the reason why stray animals, despite having no pharmacological support, seem to handle crises better than we do?

Overall, we have highlighted hypotheses, insights and numerous compelling data, which considerably enhance the biological value of vitamin C when considered beyond its nutritional role.

Another factor to consider is the hidden risk of SVCT polymorphisms, a subtle threat that can significantly reduce AA accumulation in blood and tissues without obvious initial signs. Could this be another reason to consider the maximum sustainable oral intake of vitamin C?

As for levels 4 and 5, the situation is not much different from lower levels. Unlike dynamic flow, these levels fail to ensure stable plasma and tissue concentrations, mainly because supplementation with a single dose raises levels for only a few hours. Based on these premises, it is reasonable to consider single daily doses to be of limited effectiveness, even though they are widely used both in the general population and in scientific research.

The issue becomes even more complicated (or simpler, depending on the point of view) in the case of a diagnosed illness: the need for vitamin C would probably increase in proportion to its severity. The authors of the fundamental report "Dynamic Flow: A New Model for Ascorbate" (337), Hickey, Roberts, and Cathcart, write: "Diseased tissues can generate a large number of free radicals, thereby leading to a significant increase in the maximum rate of intestinal absorption. Under such conditions, dynamic flow cannot be achieved with normal intakes. The intake necessary to sustain plasma levels during illness can increase to as much as 200 grams or more. In severe illness, achieving dynamic flow corresponds to achieving the bowel tolerance already described by Cathcart. In cases of severe illness, the intravenous route may be necessary to maintain a reducing state in damaged tissue" (337).

In other words, the three scientists emphasized the major difference between health and illness. While there are models to achieve stable and high levels under healthy conditions (through dynamic flow), there is no such clear theoretical framework for disease. In fact, disease can alter pharmacokinetics in profound but not yet well-defined ways. However, this uncertainty does not represent a major obstacle: the logic and scientific material presented here support the idea that a sick person needs much more ascorbate than a healthy one. For this reason, Hickey, Roberts, and Cathcart propose the following:

1- In the absence of illness or stress, ordinary dynamic flow may be the optimal solution;

2- In the presence of illness, a reinforced dynamic flow, close to bowel tolerance, could be the most effective solution (mild diarrhea or slight gastrointestinal discomfort are the usual indicators of bowel tolerance, the authors note);

3- In severe illness, the intravenous route may become necessary to fully support vitamin C physiology.

These are the convictions of Hickey, Roberts and Cathcart. Although there is no scientific certainty, there are at least two points in favor of their theory: their ideas are biologically plausible (despite possible debate over the exact numbers) and consistent with their extensive clinical experience.

Cathcart proposed an effective analogy, comparing dynamic flow to the introduction of a vital electron fluid that passes through the body and, depending on the physiological needs related to stress and disease, is retained solely to meet the redox demand of the moment. Any excess, on the other hand, would be naturally excreted in the urine because vitamin C is markedly water-soluble.

In simple terms: without the ability to continuously measure plasma and tissue levels and in the absence of a solid theoretical model to define optimal ascorbic acid therapy, it is reasonable to argue that patients may benefit from the use of dynamic flow. This is a systematic approach based on a simple idea: "Give as much as possible and let the body absorb what it needs, confident that there will be no significant risks".

Before concluding this section, two clarifications are in order.

First, level 2 (intake corresponding to the recommended daily allowance) has not been examined in detail here, as it is clearly weaker than levels 3-4-5.

Second, from an epistemological standpoint, any evaluation of the therapeutic efficacy of vitamin C can only be deemed fully valid if accompanied by precise details of the therapeutic protocol employed. Although vitamin C exhibits substantial pharmacological potential, it differs from conventional pharmaceuticals not only in terms of its therapeutic window. A robust assessment must consider both dosage and timing (for instance, 8 g administered as a single dose may be less effective than 2 g given every six hours). Accordingly, broad statements such as "Vitamin C is ineffective against influenza" lack logical and scientific validity unless they specify the route of administration, timing, and dosage. A rigorous evaluation of ascorbic acid therapy should, therefore, encompass five essential parameters:

(1) route of administration;
(2) dosage;
(3) frequency over 24 hours;
(4) duration of treatment;
(5) timing of intervention.

Each of these parameters has a significant impact on the pharmacokinetics and potentially on the efficacy of vitamin C. The omission of even one of these factors weakens the scientific validity of any study or claim. For this reason, in my view, many studies on oral supplementation ought to be reconsidered, as they omit one or more of these essential elements.

In light of these reconsiderations, I believe that the often-repeated claim "a diet rich in fruits and vegetables provides all the vitamin C one needs" is influenced by several misconceptions that are not supported by science. Multiple lines of evidence challenge this notion, starting with the possible presence of SVCT polymorphisms, almost always overlooked, and extending to the widespread failure to monitor plasma levels and, more importantly, intracellular concentrations. As Michels, Hagen, and Frei pointed out (60): "Measurement of dietary intake of vitamin C is an imprecise measure of body status. Future studies should rely exclusively on direct measurement of circulating or cellular vitamin C levels to accurately determine total vitamin C status".

It is increasingly evident that plasma and tissue concentrations should guide both experimental and clinical decision-making, following the same logic by which physicians prescribe hypoglycemic agents based on elevated blood glucose levels. What, after all, is unusual about this?

One might consume large quantities of vitamin C assuming saturation, or eat copious amounts of vegetables presuming to have achieved optimal plasma levels, but without actual measurements, these remain mere assumptions. How can science rest solely on opinion?

What is needed are data and certainties, not conjectures. This leads us to strongly question a broader common belief: "A rich, varied, and balanced diet provides all the nutrients we need". It would be naïve to think that vitamin C transporters are the only ones subject to genetic polymorphisms. Thiamine and vitamin D, to cite just two relevant examples, appear to face the same issues (520), (577).

As for determining the optimal daily dosage, this calls for personal consideration that incorporates all the points addressed in this section. Factors such as stress levels, the presence of disease, body weight, genetic polymorphisms, lifestyle, and diet define the specific needs of each individual. Estimating the optimal dosage thus requires careful personalization, a goal difficult to achieve without sophisticated testing and measurements. Alternatively, one may turn to Cathcart's concept of bowel tolerance, an empirical approach that currently represents one of the few practical methods available to guide vitamin C intake according to individual needs.

The antioxidant effect is truly dose-dependent

The prophylactic model, which considers dynamic flow to be the only effective means of restoring a reactive attitude towards any threat, is by no means the only rational basis for the high concentration theory. Throughout the book, several reasons have been identified in its support, some as mere hypotheses, others tending towards certainty. For example, favouring a plasma concentration of 220-250 micromoles/L obtainable through dynamic flow, rather than the 70 obtainable with a plant-rich diet, is likely to result in higher-than-normal levels of ascorbic acid in some vital organs (heart, liver and kidneys), thereby triggering stronger epigenetic and coenzymatic ascorbic activity, as suggested by some researchers (363). Above all, it could enhance the quality of antioxidant protection.

Is there concrete evidence for the dose-dependent principle of antioxidant function?

It would appear so. The numerous studies in which higher doses produced stronger pharmacological effects, thus supporting the plausibility of a dose-dependent doctrine, constitute a solid body of empirical evidence. Similarly, numerous inverse correlations between plasma levels and disease risk and/or mortality support the idea that maximising concentrations may offer additional benefits.

There is even direct evidence showing that supraphysiological concentrations (such as the widely cited 250 micromoles/L in plasma) may elicit a more effective response than simple physiological saturation. Findings from laboratory, animal, and clinical studies have progressively consolidated a crucial hypothesis of some scientists (438), (439), (440), (441), (442), (443): "Normal extracellular concentrations of ascorbic acid (30 to 150 micromoles/L) are unlikely to prevent the interaction of NO with superoxide under physiological conditions" (438). This suggests that complete ascorbate-mediated neutralisation of a powerful oxidant such as superoxide requires supraphysiological levels. Jackson, Xu, Vita and Keaney Jr., authors of an interesting article published in the authoritative journal "Circulation Research" entitled "Ascorbate prevents superoxide-nitric oxide interaction only at very high physiological concentrations" (438), have gathered several pieces of evidence supporting this theory, framing the antioxidant capacity of AA as dose-dependent.

For example, it has been hypothesized that in order to fully counteract certain toxic effects of superoxide, particularly the NO-superoxide interaction that leads to peroxynitrite formation, ascorbemia levels around 10 millimoles/L may be necessary (438). Of course, reaching 10 millimoles/L is only possible through intravenous administration. But that's not the point. When looking for the optimal dose, which is what really matters, intravenous administration is impractical in everyday life. This makes the dynamic flow approach even more important. In other words, 250 micromoles/L might eliminate more ROS than plasma saturation alone. This view is consistent with the role of a fundamental pillar of many metabolic processes: tetrahydrobiopterin (BH4), known to be a cofactor in the synthesis of catecholamines, serotonin, and nitric oxide, a biologically crucial vascular mediator. As shown, various studies suggest that the maximum antioxidant protection of BH4 is achieved at ascorbic acid concentrations that produce endothelial saturation (527).

It is important to note that the dose-dependent antioxidant principle has also been observed clinically. For example, a "supplementation" of 180 mg in 33 volunteers increased antioxidant activity in the skin by 15% compared to a dose of 100 mg (439). Of course, one might think that 180 mg is a rather modest amount and that, as plasma saturation is approached, the antioxidant effect may stabilise in a sigmoidal curve. But the evidence seems to suggest otherwise. In one study (442), three levels of ascorbic acid supplementation (0, 500 mg, 1 g) in elderly diabetic patients revealed a vertically dose-dependent (non-sigmoidal) trend: 500 mg doubled intracellular glutathione levels compared to placebo, while 1 g tripled them and also significantly increased the vitamin E content in LDL.

In short, there is considerable evidence supporting dose-dependence, some of which extends to broader contexts. Take, for example, an interesting 2002 analysis published in "Toxicology Letters" (441) clearly showed a direct correlation between vitamin C and total antioxidant status (TAS), considered the best overall indicator of the body's antioxidant system, in individuals exposed to toxic substances.

Even among healthy participants, the pattern remained consistent: dose-dependent antioxidant responses were repeatedly observed. In a study published in "The American Journal of Clinical Nutrition", antioxidant capacity increased progressively in response to supplementation with 250, 500, 1000, and 2000 mg of vitamin C (508). This observation carries an important implication: because the anti-inflammatory effect is largely subordinate to the antioxidant effect, it is likely to follow a similar dose-dependent pattern. Supporting this view, some experts note that "the effects of ascorbate on inflammatory cytokines are concentration-dependent" (110).

Therefore, everything seems to fit, from the logic underlying the correction of hypoascorbemia to the hypothesis that certain vital organs, such as the heart, liver, and kidneys, are capable of absorbing large amounts of ascorbic acid. This ability would allow the dynamic flow to produce significant antioxidant and anti-inflammatory benefits. Consider, for example, the aqueous humour and the lens, two areas where clinical data have shown that dietary intake alone is unable to achieve saturation. A more effective oral dose (such as the 2 g needed to saturate the aqueous humour) could increase antioxidant protection in these areas prone to high oxidation, producing improvements consistent with epidemiological findings on cataract incidence.

Further support comes from pharmacological data, in which administrations reaching supraphysiological levels (not necessarily intravenously) have often produced results so interesting as to suggest even greater efficacy with higher doses. We might even have, indirectly, a concrete answer to the question about physiological, slightly supraphysiological, and millimolar levels in protocols for critically ill patients. Based on the available data, merely restoring physiological levels seems to be the weakest strategy, and probably insufficient, especially considering how easily critical conditions can trigger a storm of ROS.

Overall, the arguments in favor of the dynamic flow approach appear at least plausible, while the evidence regarding the dose-dependence of the antioxidant effect appears solid.

Possible research developments

An analytical overview of the scientific landscape surrounding ascorbic acid shows the enormous effort made by researchers worldwide to refine our understanding of its physiology, pharmacokinetics, and pharmacology. It also highlights potential future directions in scientific research, which is currently at a critical juncture, partly hindered by specific factors, including its extremely low economic cost.

Over the decades, studies have been characterized by a deeply ingrained pattern: the use of low doses (often less than one gram), combined with the additional drawback of single daily administration. These two elements, not fully aligned with the pharmacokinetic principles of oral administration, may have obscured some of the clinical effects of ascorbic acid, making it difficult to pursue a more refined investigative approach.

It is logically undeniable that the use of higher and more evenly distributed doses, as required by the pharmacokinetics of high-dose administration, would have created the optimal conditions for analytically verifying the efficacy of AA in various clinical contexts, at least with regard to oral administration. Hickey and Roberts' statements largely support this thesis: “60 years of vitamin C research have been largely wasted due to confusion between nutritional and pharmacological intake and a misunderstanding of pharmacokinetics. High-dose studies must take into account the biphasic pharmacokinetics of ascorbate. The dosage regimen should focus on achieving sustained plasma levels” (23).

The hope, therefore, is that future studies will move in this direction, possibly focusing on the use of dynamic flow, the most effective form of oral administration. However, even a more moderate regimen, for example 1 g every 8 hours, could be of scientific interest and potentially more feasible for clinical research.

Another feature of most clinical studies is the lack of plasma level measurements. This omission may have contributed to an underestimation or misinterpretation of the potential pharmacological effects of vitamin C. Therefore, considering a range of variables such as SVCT dysfunctions (with a clearly multifactorial aetiology, including genetic, inflammatory, metabolic and age-related components), stress, gastrointestinal malabsorption, drug use and other factors, I believe that the gold standard of clinical research on vitamin C should be based on plasma level measurements rather than, as is unfortunately still the case, on the administered dose.

In line with this, future studies should aim to clarify various aspects of pharmacokinetics, such as the variation in intracellular distribution based on the amount taken and plasma concentration. In this regard, it would not be surprising if the initial indications provided by some valuable animal studies (69), (363) were confirmed, namely that some vital organs may require higher doses than the plasma saturation point.

As mentioned earlier, an interesting line of research could focus on SVCT transporter polymorphisms and dysfunctions, with particular attention to the physiological and pathophysiological mechanisms regulating their activity. An insightful article published in "Aging and Disease" (338) reviewed the existing literature on altered SVCT expression, highlighting that aging, oxidative stress, and inflammatory factors are strongly associated with SVCT alterations. The authors even hypothesised an interesting link to a highly relevant issue: COVID-19. Specifically, Patterson, Isales and Fulzele hypothesised that transporter dysregulation and genetic polymorphism are two key factors in the development of severe cases of COVID-19 (338). "Future clinical studies should be designed and conducted taking into account all these factors, particularly the expression and polymorphism of vitamin C transporters"; "Furthermore, it is urgent to investigate the direct relationship between serum/plasma vitamin C levels and the severity of COVID-19 infection" (338). This 2021 article also reported the launch of several clinical trials to test the efficacy of pharmacological vitamin C in treating COVID-19 infections. Growing evidence, including recent scientific developments (395), (433), supports this efficacy, particularly in the treatment of severe forms of COVID-19.

To conclude this discussion on COVID-19, it is worth noting that pharmacological vitamin C appears to possess several biological tools to counter the notorious "cytokine storm", which is considered the main factor responsible for the typical worsening of COVID-19 infections that often require mechanical ventilation (339). In this regard, an important study published in the journal "Internal and Emergency Medicine" (395) highlighted the effectiveness of high-dose intravenous vitamin C in significantly lowering the rates of mechanical ventilation and cardiac arrest. Specifically, patients with severe COVID-19 treated with vitamin C showed reduced percentages of mechanical ventilation and cardiac arrest compared to controls (52.9% vs. 73.1%, and 2.5% vs. 9.1%, respectively), following intravenous administration of 3 g every 6 hours for 7 consecutive days.

Overall, the role of pharmacological vitamin C in COVID-19 appears promising, having demonstrated efficacy and remarkable adaptability in the management of severe cases of infection. This is confirmed by a review published at the end of 2021 (433), which notes: "To date, 12 studies on vitamin C and COVID-19 have been published, including five randomized controlled trials and seven retrospective cohort studies. The current level of evidence from RCTs suggests that intravenous vitamin C intervention may improve oxygenation, reduce inflammatory markers, shorten hospital stay, and decrease mortality, particularly in severely ill patients. High-dose oral vitamin C may improve recovery rates in milder cases. No adverse events have been reported in clinical trials involving COVID-19 patients treated with vitamin C. Larger-scale RCTs will provide further evidence on vitamin supplementation in COVID-19 patients".

Further positive trends come from two recent meta-analyses. The first, from 2024 (592), concluded: "High-dose vitamin C supplementation can alleviate inflammatory response and hinder the aggravation of COVID-19", highlighting mainly its strong anti-inflammatory properties. The second, from 2023 (593), highlighted potential survival benefits: "Overall, evidence from RCTs suggests a survival benefit for vitamin C in patients with severe COVID-19. However, we should await data from large-scale randomized trials to affirm its mortality benefits".

The versatility of vitamin C clearly extends well beyond respiratory infections and related complications. For instance, a review focused on the potential use of DHA for stroke management presents multiple positive preclinical findings and strong biological plausibility, highlighting a promising area of clinical research that could offer innovative therapeutic solutions in a context where treatment options remain limited (216).

Moving on to genetics, recent discoveries in epigenetics are opening exciting prospects, given the emerging role of vitamin C as a mediator between the genome and the environment. Its activation of DNA demethylation via TET enzymes could help shape cellular reprogramming, with potentially notable clinical implications, including the development of personalized epigenetic treatments for cancer patients.

Remaining in the oncological field, identifying tumors that may be more vulnerable to vitamin C, particularly those with KRAS or BRAF mutations, or with very low catalase activity, could represent a highly interesting area of research. A 2022 phase 3 study is of notable clinical value as it demonstrated that the addition of high-dose intravenous vitamin C significantly improved the effectiveness of standard chemotherapy in the treatment of colorectal cancer with KRAS mutations (586).

Regarding the nervous system, although the importance of vitamin C in neurophysiology is universally recognized, its clinical applications remain poorly defined. We know that it supports the differentiation, maturation, and survival of neurons, and that it is a neuromodulator of the glutamatergic, cholinergic, dopaminergic, and GABAergic systems (GABA is the main inhibitory neurotransmitter that regulates neuronal excitability). However, despite these biological plausibilities, there is currently a lack of solid scientific evidence supporting vitamin C-based therapies for the treatment of major neurological disorders (340).

Research should also explore new technologies to overcome one of the main problems of oral vitamin C: its low bioavailability. Liposomal technology represents a promising step in this direction, although not yet a decisive one. It is worth noting that various attempts to improve absorption through auxiliary molecules, particularly flavonoids, have failed, helping to debunk the myth of "natural vitamin C". In an animal study (324), combining vitamin C with calcium slightly improved bioavailability. However, the toxicity of high calcium doses limits the use of calcium ascorbate to just a few grams per day, bringing the issue back into focus.

Continuing along this line, I believe an interesting path lies in the in-depth study of the interactions that vitamin C can produce when combined with other biologically active substances. In one study, the combination of vitamin C, resveratrol, and beta-glucans (natural polysaccharides with notable immunomodulatory properties) effectively suppressed tumor growth in various models (341). Interestingly, this trio also showed strong detoxifying properties, counteracting the oxidative and immunosuppressive effects of certain toxic agents (376). The triad also highlighted the value of resveratrol. A 2020 study (342) revealed a surprising finding: the addition of resveratrol improved intracellular accumulation of vitamin C. The authors attributed this result to enhanced DHA transport and improved intracellular recycling (342).

Overall, it is by no means far-fetched to imagine that synergistic interactions with bioactive substances could represent a vast and fertile field of scientific research. The goal could be twofold: to identify compounds that enhance the effectiveness of vitamin C and those whose biological effects are enhanced by it. For example, some studies have shown greater bioavailability of certain polyphenols following AA intake, particularly the fascinating green tea catechins (343). Other research, dependent on future technologies, focuses on chitosan microspheres. These are sophisticated biodegradable polymer-based carriers that could improve the entire pharmacokinetic profile. In a noteworthy study, incorporating AA into chitosan microspheres increased the bioavailability of certain bioactive compounds added afterward. This included the well-known curcumin, a molecule with exceptional biological potential but characterized by very poor intestinal absorption (344).

In conclusion, the research path on vitamin C remains rich in promise, provided that future investigations can overcome the methodological and conceptual barriers that still persist. Such progress would not only represent a milestone for science, but also open new opportunities to integrate this molecule into broader strategies aimed at supporting a long, healthy, and high-quality life.

A quality life

I must confess to a certain sense of disorientation: the completion of this book, my first literary work, is now clearly on the horizon, stirring a whirlwind of conflicting emotions. I can't help but think of the reader, a wonderful presence that created a virtual connection, from which my desire for clarity in writing emerged, a challenging goal considering the depth of the content. Here, a seemingly trivial yet tremendously helpful factor stepped in, allowing me to reach a state closely resembling mental serenity. I have discovered that the early hours of the morning are the most productive, as they offer an atmosphere of utmost tranquility, almost mystical, woven with silence and wonderful aromas, including the scent of coffee lovingly prepared by my dear wife. This extraordinary atmosphere cannot be replicated during the rest of the day and is incredibly conducive to writing.

Indeed, this "magic" of the early morning gifted me with rare moments of serenity and presence of mind. Yes, mental serenity and presence of mind, two essential elements for a quality life. Elements that inevitably invoke a vital factor involved in physical, mental, genetic, and even gut microbiota interactions: nutrition. Particularly fascinating is the mutual interaction between diet and microbiota: while diet can modify the microbiota's composition and function, the microbiota, in turn, selects from the diet the components most aligned with its needs, from vitamins to key precursors of neurotransmitters. Two of these neurotransmitters, serotonin and GABA, modulate neural signaling in the enteric nervous system, the so-called second brain, influencing both brain function and behavior (576). Fascinating, isn't it?

After all, it's estimated that nearly 90% of serotonin is produced in the gut! (524).

These data, which strengthen the link between microbiota composition and neuropsychiatric disorders, underscore the importance of a healthy diet and offer hope that many issues may be addressed through an appropriate dietary approach. It is therefore not surprising that modulation of the microbiota, a process that primarily requires a diet rich in vitamins, minerals and fiber, may help counter some of the major threats to quality of life, such as stress and anxiety.

The widely shared recommendations emphasizing the fundamental role of a healthy diet are therefore becoming increasingly compelling, not only for achieving and maintaining physical fitness but also for adequately supporting mental well-being.

Returning to the disturbances that can threaten life's quality and serenity, it's worth repeating that proper use of vitamin C can mitigate the negative effects of our genetic deficiency, helping maintain psychophysical balance under stress. We have shown how an adequate presence of vitamin C can buffer the consequences of both physical and psychological stress, a capacity attributed to its remarkable adaptogenic properties (26). This ability, akin to the "hormonal response" observed in fortunate mammals (175), has been enigmatically sidelined, when in fact it likely deserves to be central in discussions on human health, increasingly under siege from the monster known as chronic stress.

In addition to alleviating stress, vitamin C's close involvement in neurophysiology suggests it may also have a positive effect on anxiety. In one of the few available studies (345), a randomized, double-blind, placebo-controlled trial demonstrated efficacy in reducing anxiety, even with a modest dose of 500 mg. "This suggests that a diet rich in vitamin C could be an effective addition to medical and psychological treatments for anxiety and could improve academic performance", the authors noted (345).

More broadly, it is plausible that stress and anxiety can be substantially alleviated through a targeted therapeutic strategy primarily involving diet and vitamin C supplementation. This strategy also incorporates an additional element that both stress and anxiety seem to greatly fear: meditation, an ancient practice used to train the mind to focus on a single thought. An increasing number of studies have demonstrated its effectiveness in reducing key markers of stress, including cortisol, particularly in individuals chronically exposed to high levels of stress (346), (595).

Meditation, which is deeply intertwined with the well-known concept of the "here and now", is the perfect element with which to introduce the story of a personal experience I lived through in 2019-2020, a unique adventure, much like vitamin C itself, whose ultimate outcome brings together many of the themes explored in this book.

It all began in October 2019, when I put myself to the test with an experiment as bold as it was unpopular: spending the entire winter wearing only light summer T-shirts. These garments were to be worn continuously, 24 hours a day, regardless of location, temperature, humidity, or any other adverse environmental factors. The experiment, if it can be called that, was designed to assess the impact of my robust vitamin C supplementation on the consequences of continuous exposure to low temperatures, as well as to evaluate the quality of my mental resilience. Therefore, it was a fascinating challenge in which cold, wind, and humidity could easily have overwhelmed me from the very start. But that never happened, because the intense stress associated with these hostile elements was met with a powerful countermeasure: an increase in my already substantial vitamin C supplementation, which, by the end of the trial period, proved to be completely protective.

But is it truly plausible to credit this special countermeasure with having neutralized the potentially devastating effects of low temperatures?

It would seem so. In fact, multiple studies suggest that vitamin C supplementation is effective in significantly and multifacetedly limiting cold-induced stress. For example, an interesting study on volunteers (347) evaluated the effects of supplementation with vitamin C (500 mg/day) and vitamin E (400 mg/day) in response to cold exposure at high altitude (3700 m). It is worth recalling that high altitude tends to generate large amounts of reactive oxygen species due to lower atmospheric pressure and reduced oxygen concentration. Despite the low dosage, vitamin C, but not vitamin E, proved effective in supporting the so-called "cold-induced vasodilation", a still poorly understood bodily response that helps prevent cold-related damage (347). This finding confirms that vitamin C can counteract the negative effects of cold through several biological mechanisms: increased metabolism, antioxidant protection, improved microcirculation, and better peripheral blood flow.

The study also reinforced the uniqueness of vitamin C, which clearly outperformed vitamin E in terms of effectiveness even in this context (347). Similar results have been observed in other studies on volunteers, in which vitamin C, unlike vitamin E, also exerted neuroprotective effects by preserving normal ulnar nerve conduction under hypothermic conditions (nerve conduction is impaired by low temperatures) (423).

In conclusion, there appears to be a scientific basis for my victory over the cold, officially certified in the spring of 2020. Thanks to the power of vitamin C, my body endured the entire winter without showing the slightest sign of fatigue: no colds, infections, muscle cramps, cold-induced dermatitis, circulatory problems, or other ailments, an optimal state of health confirmed by regular biochemical and radiological examinations conducted afterwards. But meditation and mindfulness also played a part in this success, allowing me to mentally reinterpret the cold as a kind of friend with whom I could coexist peacefully, at times even finding myself missing it.

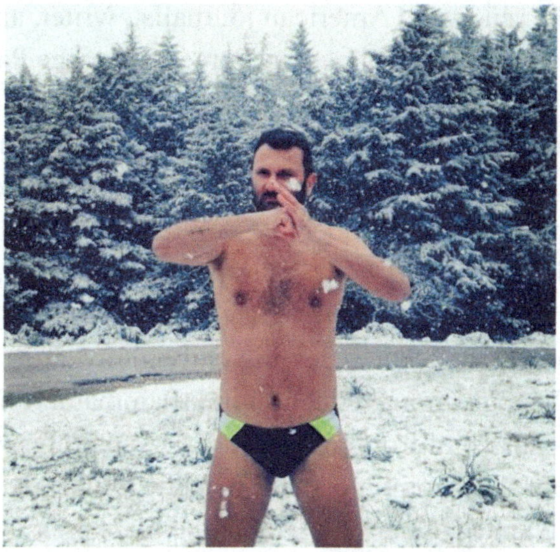

The author during a snowfall in the winter of 2021, in his beloved Mercadante Forest, Cassano delle Murge, Apulia, Italy

My experience represents a valuable application of the synergy that can arise from the targeted use of vitamin C combined with meditative practices, giving rise to a powerful tool capable of effectively counteracting a wide range of stressful situations. This tool, inherently dynamic, is open to further enrichment, for instance, the integration of holistic massage seems particularly effective, helping to complete a personal well-being framework I refer to as the MCM triad (Holistic Massage-Vitamin C-Meditation), through which alleviating stress could become surprisingly accessible.

Holistic thinking also teaches us that "All is One", and this "One" can begin with the material act of eating healthily and extend to the abstract, our thoughts, an abstraction that modern physics increasingly shows to have a material substance, capable of influencing the surrounding physical space. A healthy diet, high-quality sleep (incidentally, the journal "Nature" recently published a relevant study (587) showing an inverse correlation between vitamin C levels and sleep disturbances), personalized and targeted supplementation, a healthy lifestyle, a positive approach to everyday challenges, and a touch of good humor together form the foundations for enriching the experience of life.

Speaking of good humor and irony, I would like to conclude by recounting the key elements of another extraordinary adventure, this time, not my own. Norman Cousins, the renowned American journalist, writer, and peace activist, told in his book "Anatomy of an Illness as Perceived by the Patient", published around 1979, the story of his battle against ankylosing spondylitis, a severe form of arthritis that primarily affects the spine, causing stiffness and intense pain. Unfortunately, Cousins appeared to have one of the most aggressive forms of the disease, to the point of being bedridden. It should be noted that conventional drug therapies offered him little hope, both in terms of prognosis and symptom control. Eventually, encouraged by his dear friend Linus Pauling, Cousins turned to high-dose vitamin C therapy. He began receiving daily intravenous infusions of 25 grams, progressively achieving a reduction in inflammatory biomarkers and, most importantly, significant relief from his unbearable symptoms. Over time, this pharmacological approach, combined with what he himself called "Laughter Therapy", a practice aimed at constantly and openly expressing positive emotions, proved incredibly effective: Cousins regained full mobility and lived a dignified life for over 30 years after his diagnosis. In short, he astonishingly reversed the dire prognosis.

To this day, it remains unclear whether the healing factor, as Irwin Stone might have called it, was due exclusively to the massive doses of vitamin C or to its synergy with laughter therapy. We may never know. What is indisputable, however, is the extraordinary outcome, achieved against all odds. This is the kind of result worth sharing with those who, with a certain irritating sense of irony, or perhaps out of ignorance, tend to greatly underestimate the qualities of vitamin C. An irony often rooted in the archaic view of vitamin C as nothing more than a dietary supplement, an outdated perspective that, unfortunately, still echoes in some scientific circles. Raising awareness among what I like to call the "vitamin C superficialists" could prove a winning strategy, transforming their unfounded irony into thoughtful reflection and guiding them toward a new vision in which vitamin C and its theorems are no longer seen as unfounded postulates but rather as rigorously validated, or at least plausible, conclusions.

We cannot exclude the possibility that logic itself, defined by the brilliant philosopher Locke as "the anatomy of thought", which brings us back to Cousins' book, enabled him to overturn a desperate situation by adopting the following approach: what is there to lose in trying a therapy based on the "sure bet" of vitamin C?

Cousins' remarkable experience has also taught us the fundamental importance of laughter and positivity, through which we can fully enjoy moments of joy and face the darker ones with resilience, and with greater hope and confidence.

So, if you've made it this far in the reading, all that's left is to sincerely thank you for your generous dose of patience, and to wrap up with an observation that may seem playful: in the end, could it all be GULO's fault?

One final piece of advice: don't try to imitate my winter challenge, especially if you don't have complete faith in vitamin C. After all, vitamin C, in addition to being truly Nobel Prize-level science, is a story of trust, love, and perhaps even miracles. Yet let's hope it won't take a miracle to undo the damage caused by decades of unfounded prejudice, which have made some brilliant minds suspicious and formed an army of "truth enthusiasts". I consider myself one of them, and I hope I've provided the impetus needed to launch the long-awaited "Copernican revolution of vitamin C".

Specialists Hemilä and Chalker probably also agree, concluding their explanatory article published in the journal "Life" in 2022 as follows: "In this review, we demonstrated significant bias in many influential papers on vitamin C. We showed that many of these papers were cited uncritically in textbooks and reviews, assumed to be scientifically sound when in fact many had serious flaws. Prominent authors referred to them without any critical evaluation. We proposed conceptual explanations for the persistent and deep-rooted bias against vitamin C. This bias is regrettable because vitamin C is safe and inexpensive, and thus even its small effects are worth considering" (503).

A persistent and deep-rooted prejudice against a vital, safe and inexpensive substance. It is logically unacceptable, just like any position rooted in bias. Perhaps, in the end, what vitamin C needs most is not more data, but more open minds.

'If you help others, you will be helped, perhaps tomorrow, perhaps in one hundred years, but you will be helped. Nature must pay off the debt. It is a mathematical law and all life is mathematics'

Georges Ivanovič Gurdjieff

Bibliography

(1) Luong KV, Nguyễn LT. The beneficial role of thiamine in Parkinson disease. CNS Neurosci Ther. 2013 Jul;19(7):461-8. doi: 10.1111/cns.12078. Epub 2013 Mar 6. PMID: 23462281; PMCID: PMC6493530.

(2) DiNicolantonio JJ, Niazi AK, Lavie CJ, O'Keefe JH, Ventura HO. Thiamine supple-mentation for the treatment of heart failure: a review of the literature. Congest Heart Fail. 2013 Jul-Aug;19(4):214-22. doi: 10.1111/chf.12037. PMID: 23910704.

(3) Aranow C. Vitamin D and the immune system. J Investig Med. 2011 Aug;59(6):881-6. doi: 10.2310/JIM.0b013e31821b8755. PMID: 21527855; PMCID: PMC3166406.

(4) Time: "Medicine: Polio Clues", 18 Settembre 1939

(5) Jungeblut, C W. "VITAMIN C THERAPY AND PROPHYLAXIS IN EXPERIMENTAL POLIOMYELITIS." The Journal of experimental medicine vol. 65,1 (1937): 127-46. doi:10.1084/jem.65.1.127. PMID: 19870585; PMCID: PMC2133474.

(6) Jungeblut CW. INACTIVATION OF POLIOMYELITIS VIRUS IN VITRO BY CRYS-TALLINE VITAMIN C (ASCORBIC ACID). J Exp Med. 1935 Sep 30;62(4):517-21. doi: 10.1084/jem.62.4.517. PMID: 19870431; PMCID: PMC2133291.

(7) Wikipedia: "poliomielite"

(8) Wikipedia: "vaccino anti-poliomielite"

(9) Sabin, A B. "VITAMIN C IN RELATION TO EXPERIMENTAL POLIOMYELITIS: WITH INCIDENTAL OBSERVATIONS ON CERTAIN MANIFESTATIONS IN MACACUS RHESUS MONKEYS ON A SCORBUTIC DIET." The Journal of experimental medicine vol. 69,4 (1939): 507-16. doi:10.1084/jem.69.4.507

(10) Fred R. Klenner. "The Use of Vitamin C as an Antibiotic". The Journal of Applied Nu-trition, Volume 6, 1953, pp. 274-278.

(11) Fred R. Klenner. "The Treatment of Poliomyelitis and Other Virus Diseases with Vita-min C". Southern Medicine & Surgery, Volume 111, Number 7, July, 1949, pp. 209-214.

(12) KLENNER FR. Virus pneumonia and its treatment with vitamin C. South Med Surg. 1948 Feb;110(2):36-8. PMID: 18900646.

(13) Hemilä, Harri, and Pekka Louhiala. "Vitamin C may affect lung infections." Journal of the Royal Society of Medicine vol. 100,11 (2007): 495-8. doi:10.1177/014107680710001109

(14) KLENNER FR. Massive doses of vitamin C and the virus diseases. South Med Surg. 1951 Apr;113(4):101-7. PMID: 14855098.

(15) BERZIN' VK. Gipovitaminoz C kak faktor, snizhaiushchii priobretennyi immunitet k difterii ili prepiatstvuiushchii ego razvitiiu; eksperimental'nye issledovaniia [Vitamin C defi-ciency as a factor lowering acquired immunity to diphtheria and as a factor obstructing devel-opment of immunity; experimental investigations]. Zh Mikrobiol Epidemiol Immunobiol. 1955 Sep;(9):18-23. Russian. PMID: 13282443.

(16) BERZIN' VK, GLINSKAIA EV. Izuchenie vliianiia vitamina C na ustoichivost' im-muniteta k difterii u privitykh detel [Effect of vitamin C on resistance against diphtheria in vaccinated children]. Zh Mikrobiol Epidemiol Immunobiol. 1957 Dec;28(12):33-8. Russian. PMID: 13544563.

(17) BERZIN' VK. Izuchenie vozmozhnosti vosstanovleniia immuniteta k difterii u S-gipovitaminoznykh morskikh svinok vitaminizatsiei askorbinovoi kislotoi [Possibility of pro-duction of immunity against diphtheria by ascorbic acid in vitamin C deficient guinea pigs]. Zh Mikrobiol Epidemiol Immunobiol. 1957 Nov;28(11):103-7. Russian. PMID: 13544544.

(18) Claus W. Jungeblut. Inactivation of Tetanus Toxin by Crystalline Vitamin C (l-Ascorbic Acid). J Immunol September 1, 1937, 33 (3) 203-214.

(19) Dey PK. Efficacy of vitamin C in counteracting tetanus toxin toxicity. Naturwissen-schaften. 1966 Jun;53(12):310. doi: 10.1007/BF00712228. PMID: 5986216.

(20) Hemilä H, Koivula T. Vitamin C for preventing and treating tetanus. Cochrane Data-base Syst Rev. 2013 Nov 13;(11):CD006665. doi: 10.1002/14651858.CD006665.pub3. PMID: 24226506.

(21) Hemilä H. Vitamin C and Infections. Nutrients. 2017 Mar 29;9(4):339. doi: 10.3390/nu9040339. PMID: 28353648; PMCID: PMC5409678.

(22) Padayatty SJ, Sun H, Wang Y, Riordan HD, Hewitt SM, Katz A, Wesley RA, Levine M. Vitamin C pharmacokinetics: implications for oral and intravenous use. Ann Intern Med. 2004 Apr 6;140(7):533-7. doi: 10.7326/0003-4819-140-7-200404060-00010. PMID: 15068981.

(23) Hickey S, Roberts H. Misleading information on the properties of vitamin C. PLoS Med. 2005 Sep;2(9):e307; author reply e309. doi: 10.1371/journal.pmed.0020307. Epub 2005 Sep 27. PMID: 16173838; PMCID: PMC1236801.

(24) Gorton HC, Jarvis K. The effectiveness of vitamin C in preventing and relieving the symptoms of virus-induced respiratory infections. J Manipulative Physiol Ther. 1999 Oct;22(8):530-3. doi: 10.1016/s0161-4754(99)70005-9. PMID: 10543583.

(25) Marik, Paul E. "Vitamin C: an essential "stress hormone" during sepsis." Journal of thoracic disease vol. 12,Suppl 1 (2020): S84-S88. doi:10.21037/jtd.2019.12.64. PMID: 32148930; PMCID: PMC7024758.

(26) Brody S, Preut R, Schommer K, Schürmeyer TH. A randomized controlled trial of high dose ascorbic acid for reduction of blood pressure, cortisol, and subjective responses to psy-chological stress. Psychopharmacology (Berl). 2002 Jan;159(3):319-24. doi: 10.1007/s00213-001-0929-6. Epub 2001 Nov 20. PMID: 11862365.

(27) Odumosu A. Ascorbic acid and cortisol metabolism in hypovitaminosis C guineapigs. Int J Vitam Nutr Res. 1982;52(2):176-85. PMID: 7129799.

(28) Padayatty SJ, Doppman JL, Chang R, Wang Y, Gill J, Papanicolaou DA, Levine M. Human adrenal glands secrete vitamin C in response to adrenocorticotrophic hormone. Am J Clin Nutr. 2007 Jul;86(1):145-9. doi: 10.1093/ajcn/86.1.145. PMID: 17616774.

(29) Carr, Anitra C et al. "Ascorbate-dependent vasopressor synthesis: a rationale for vita-min C administration in severe sepsis and septic shock?." Critical care (London, England) vol. 19 418. 27 Nov. 2015, doi:10.1186/s13054-015-1131-2. PMID: 26612352; PMCID: PMC4661979.

(30) BURNS JJ, MOSBACH EH, SCHULENBERG S. Ascorbic acid synthesis in normal and drug-treated rats, studied with L-ascorbic-1-C14 acid. J Biol Chem. 1954 Apr;207(2):679-87. PMID: 13163053.

(31) CONNEY AH, BRAY GA, EVANS C, BURNS JJ. Metabolic interactions between L-ascorbic acid and drugs. Ann N Y Acad Sci. 1961 Apr 21;92:115-27. doi: 10.1111/j.1749-6632.1961.tb46111.x. PMID: 13695066.

(32) Mayland CR, Bennett MI, Allan K. Vitamin C deficiency in cancer patients. Palliat Med. 2005 Jan;19(1):17-20. doi: 10.1191/0269216305pm970oa. PMID: 15690864.

(33) White R, Nonis M, Pearson JF, Burgess E, Morrin HR, Pullar JM, Spencer E, Vissers MCM, Robinson BA, Dachs GU. Low Vitamin C Status in Patients with Cancer Is Associated with Patient and Tumor Characteristics. Nutrients. 2020 Aug 5;12(8):2338. doi: 10.3390/nu12082338. PMID: 32764253; PMCID: PMC7468872.

(34) Carr, Anitra C et al. "Hypovitaminosis C and vitamin C deficiency in critically ill pa-tients despite recommended enteral and parenteral intakes." Critical care (London, England) vol. 21,1 300. 11 Dec. 2017, doi:10.1186/s13054-017-1891-y. PMID: 29228951; PMCID: PMC5725835.

(35) Pauling, L. "The significance of the evidence about ascorbic acid and the common cold." Proceedings of the National Academy of Sciences of the United States of America vol. 68,11 (1971): 2678-81. doi:10.1073/pnas.68.11.2678. PMID: 4941984; PMCID: PMC389499.

(36) Bucher, Amanda, and Nicole White. "Vitamin C in the Prevention and Treatment of the Common Cold." American journal of lifestyle medicine vol. 10,3

181-183. 9 Feb. 2016, doi:10.1177/1559827616629092. PMID: 30202272; PMCID: PMC6124957.

(37) Rath M, Pauling L. Hypothesis: lipoprotein(a) is a surrogate for ascorbate. Proc Natl Acad Sci U S A. 1990 Aug;87(16):6204-7. doi: 10.1073/pnas.87.16.6204. Erratum in: Proc Natl Acad Sci U S A 1991 Dec 15;88(24):11588. PMID: 2143582; PMCID: PMC54501.

(38) Harakeh S, Jariwalla RJ, Pauling L. Suppression of human immunodeficiency virus replication by ascorbate in chronically and acutely infected cells. Proc Natl Acad Sci U S A. 1990 Sep;87(18):7245-9. doi: 10.1073/pnas.87.18.7245. PMID: 1698293; PMCID: PMC54720.

(39) Kodama M, Kodama T. Is Linus Pauling, a vitamin C advocate, just making much ado about nothing? (Review). In Vivo. 1994 May-Jun;8(3):391-400. PMID: 7803724.

(40) Cathcart RF. Vitamin C, titrating to bowel tolerance, anascorbemia, and acute induced scurvy. Med Hypotheses. 1981 Nov;7(11):1359-76. doi: 10.1016/0306-9877(81)90126-2. PMID: 7321921.

(41) Chen, Shuangdi et al. "Clinical Effect of Intravenous Vitamin C on Viral Myocarditis in Children: A Systematic Review and Meta-Analysis." Evidence-based complementary and alternative medicine : eCAM vol. 2019 3082437. 23 Apr. 2019, doi:10.1155/2019/3082437. PMID: 31178914; PMCID: PMC6507266.

(42) Cathcart RF 3rd. Vitamin C: the nontoxic, nonrate-limited, antioxidant free radical scavenger. Med Hypotheses. 1985 Sep;18(1):61-77. doi: 10.1016/0306-9877(85)90121-5. PMID: 4069036.

(43) Cathcart RF 3rd. Vitamin C in the treatment of acquired immune deficiency syndrome (AIDS). Med Hypotheses. 1984 Aug;14(4):423-33. doi: 10.1016/0306-9877(84)90149-x. PMID: 6238227.

(44) Cathcart RF. A unique function for ascorbate. Med Hypotheses. 1991 May;35(1):32-7. doi: 10.1016/0306-9877(91)90080-i. PMID: 1921774.

(45) Cathcart RF 3rd. The vitamin C treatment of allergy and the normally unprimed state of antibodies. Med Hypotheses. 1986 Nov;21(3):307-21. doi: 10.1016/0306-9877(86)90025-3. PMID: 2879212.

(46) Carter, Steven. "Origins of Orthomolecular Medicine." Integrative medicine (Encinitas, Calif.) vol. 18,3 (2019): 76-77.

(47) Foster HD, Hoffer A. Schizophrenia and cancer: the adrenochrome balanced morphism. Med Hypotheses. 2004;62(3):415-9. doi: 10.1016/S0306-9877(03)00319-0. PMID: 14975514.

(48) Hoffer A, Prousky J. Successful treatment of schizophrenia requires optimal daily doses of vitamin B3. Altern Med Rev. 2008 Dec;13(4):287-91. PMID: 19238764.

(49) Schizophrenia: A New Approach. II. Result of a Year's Research. Published online by Cambridge University Press: 08 February 2018. Abram Hoffer, Humphrey Osmond and John Smythies.

(50) HOFFER A. Nicotinic acid: an adjunct in the treatment of schizophrenia. Am J Psychi-atry. 1963 Aug;120:171-3. doi: 10.1176/ajp.120.2.171. PMID: 13963912.

(51) HUXLEY J, MAYR E, OSMOND H, HOFFER A. SCHIZOPHRENIA AS A GENETIC MORPHISM. Nature. 1964 Oct 17;204:220-1. doi: 10.1038/204220a0. PMID: 14212411.

(52) Hoffer A. Orthomolecular treatment for schizophrenia. I. J Pract Nurs. 1972 Aug;22(8):16-9. PMID: 4486647.

(53) OSMOND H, HOFFER A. Massive niacin treatment in schizophrenia. Review of a nine-year study. Lancet. 1962 Feb 10;1(7224):316-9. doi: 10.1016/s0140-6736(62)91259-x. PMID: 14482545.

(54) HOFFER A, OSMOND H, CALLBECK MJ, KAHAN I. Treatment of schizophrenia with nicotinic acid and nicotinamide. J Clin Exp Psychopathol. 1957 Apr-Jun;18(2):131-58. PMID: 13439009.

(55) Xu XJ, Jiang GS. Niacin-respondent subset of schizophrenia – a therapeutic review. Eur Rev Med Pharmacol Sci. 2015;19(6):988-97. PMID: 25855923.

(56) Lesperance ML, Olivotto IA, Forde N, Zhao Y, Speers C, Foster H, Tsao M, MacPher-son N, Hoffer A. Mega-dose vitamins and minerals in the treatment

of non-metastatic breast cancer: an historical cohort study. Breast Cancer Res Treat. 2002 Nov;76(2):137-43. doi: 10.1023/a:1020552501345. PMID: 12452451.

(57) Hoffer LJ, Levine M, Assouline S, Melnychuk D, Padayatty SJ, Rosadiuk K, Rousseau C, Robitaille L, Miller WH Jr. Phase I clinical trial of i.v. ascorbic acid in advanced malignan-cy. Ann Oncol. 2008 Nov;19(11):1969-74. doi: 10.1093/annonc/mdn377. Epub 2008 Jun 9. Erratum in: Ann Oncol. 2008 Dec;19(12):2095. PMID: 18544557.

(58) Padayatty SJ, Riordan HD, Hewitt SM, Katz A, Hoffer LJ, Levine M. Intravenously administered vitamin C as cancer therapy: three cases. CMAJ. 2006 Mar 28;174(7):937-42. doi: 10.1503/cmaj.050346. PMID: 16567755; PMCID: PMC1405876.

(59) Corpe CP, Tu H, Eck P, Wang J, Faulhaber-Walter R, Schnermann J, Margolis S, Pa-dayatty S, Sun H, Wang Y, Nussbaum RL, Espey MG, Levine M. Vitamin C transporter Slc23a1 links renal reabsorption, vitamin C tissue accumulation, and perinatal survival in mice. J Clin Invest. 2010 Apr;120(4):1069-83. doi: 10.1172/JCI39191. PMID: 20200446; PMCID: PMC2847422.

(60) Michels AJ, Hagen TM, Frei B. Human genetic variation influences vitamin C homeo-stasis by altering vitamin C transport and antioxidant enzyme function. Annu Rev Nutr. 2013;33:45-70. doi: 10.1146/annurev-nutr-071812-161246. Epub 2013 Apr 29. PMID: 23642198; PMCID: PMC4357493.

(61) Agus DB, Gambhir SS, Pardridge WM, Spielholz C, Baselga J, Vera JC, Golde DW. Vitamin C crosses the blood-brain barrier in the oxidized form through the glucose transport-ers. J Clin Invest. 1997 Dec 1;100(11):2842-8. doi: 10.1172/JCI119832. PMID: 9389750; PMCID: PMC508490.

(62) Lykkesfeldt J, Tveden-Nyborg P. The Pharmacokinetics of Vitamin C. Nutrients. 2019;11(10):2412. Published 2019 Oct 9. doi:10.3390/nu11102412. PMID: 31601028; PMCID: PMC6835439.

(63) Wilson JX. Regulation of vitamin C transport. Annu Rev Nutr. 2005;25:105-25. doi: 10.1146/annurev.nutr.25.050304.092647. PMID: 16011461.

(64) Kübler W, Gehler J. Zur Kinetik der enteralen Ascorbinsäure-Resorption zur Berech-nung nicht dosisproportionaler Resorptionsvorgänge [Kinetics of

intestinal absorption of ascorbic acid. Calculation of non-dosage-dependent absorption processes]. Int Z Vitamin-forsch. 1970;40(4):442-53. German. PMID: 5484426.

(65) Levine M, Padayatty SJ, Espey MG. Vitamin C: a concentration-function approach yields pharmacology and therapeutic discoveries. Adv Nutr. 2011;2(2):78-88. doi:10.3945/an.110.000109. Epub 2011 Mar 10. PMID: 22332036; PMCID: PMC3065766.

(66) Carr AC, Cook J. Intravenous Vitamin C for Cancer Therapy - Identifying the Current Gaps in Our Knowledge. Front Physiol. 2018;9:1182. Published 2018 Aug 23. doi:10.3389/fphys.2018.01182. PMID: 30190680; PMCID: PMC6115501.

(67) Padayatty SJ, Levine M. Vitamin C: the known and the unknown and Goldilocks. Oral Dis. 2016;22(6):463-493. doi:10.1111/odi.12446. Epub 2016 Apr 14. PMID: 26808119; PMCID: PMC4959991.

(68) Tveden-Nyborg P, Johansen LK, Raida Z, Villumsen CK, Larsen JO, Lykkesfeldt J. Vitamin C deficiency in early postnatal life impairs spatial memory and reduces the number of hippocampal neurons in guinea pigs. Am J Clin Nutr. 2009 Sep;90(3):540-6. doi: 10.3945/ajcn.2009.27954. Epub 2009 Jul 29. PMID: 19640959.

(69) Tsao CS, Leung PY, Young M. Effect of dietary ascorbic acid intake on tissue vitamin C in mice. J Nutr. 1987 Feb;117(2):291-7. doi: 10.1093/jn/117.2.291. PMID: 3559744.

(70) Levine M, Wang Y, Padayatty SJ, Morrow J. A new recommended dietary allowance of vitamin C for healthy young women. Proc Natl Acad Sci U S A. 2001 Aug 14;98(17):9842-6. doi: 10.1073/pnas.171318198. PMID: 11504949; PMCID: PMC55540.

(71) Anderson R, Theron A. Effects of ascorbate on leucocytes: Part III. In vitro and in vi-vo stimulation of abnormal neutrophil motility by ascorbate. S Afr Med J. 1979 Sep 8;56(11):429-33. PMID: 550365.

(72) Gregoraszczuk EL, Zajda K, Tekla J, Respekta N, Zdybał P, Such A. Vitamin C sup-plementation had no side effect in non-cancer, but had anticancer

properties in ovarian cancer cells. Int J Vitam Nutr Res. 2021 Jun;91(3-4):293-303. doi: 10.1024/0300-9831/a000634. Epub 2020 Feb 3. PMID: 32008465.

(73) Rivers JM. Safety of high-level vitamin C ingestion. Int J Vitam Nutr Res Suppl. 1989;30:95-102. PMID: 2507711.

(74) Suboticanec K, Folnegović-Smalc V, Turcin R, Mestrović B, Buzina R. Plasma levels and urinary vitamin C excretion in schizophrenic patients. Hum Nutr Clin Nutr. 1986 Nov;40(6):421-8. PMID: 3793523.

(75) Suboticanec K, Folnegović-Smalc V, Korbar M, Mestrović B, Buzina R. Vitamin C sta-tus in chronic schizophrenia. Biol Psychiatry. 1990 Dec 1;28(11):959-66. doi: 10.1016/0006-3223(90)90061-6. PMID: 2275953.

(76) Yue DK, McLennan S, McGill M, Fisher E, Heffernan S, Capogreco C, Turtle JR. Ab-normalities of ascorbic acid metabolism and diabetic control: differences between diabetic pa-tients and diabetic rats. Diabetes Res Clin Pract. 1990 Jul;9(3):239-44. doi: 10.1016/0168-8227(90)90051-t. PMID: 2226123.

(77) Preiser JC. Oxidative stress. JPEN J Parenter Enteral Nutr. 2012 Mar;36(2):147-54. doi: 10.1177/0148607111434963. Epub 2012 Feb 1. PMID: 22301329.

(78) Harrison FE, May JM. Vitamin C function in the brain: vital role of the ascorbate transporter SVCT2. Free Radic Biol Med. 2009;46(6):719-730. doi:10.1016/j.freeradbiomed.2008.12.018. Epub 2009 Jan 6. PMID: 19162177; PMCID: PMC2649700.

(79) Chan AC. Partners in defense, vitamin E and vitamin C. Can J Physiol Pharmacol. 1993 Sep;71(9):725-31. doi: 10.1139/y93-109. PMID: 8313238.

(80) Niki E. Interaction of ascorbate and alpha-tocopherol. Ann N Y Acad Sci. 1987;498:186-99. doi: 10.1111/j.1749-6632.1987.tb23761.x. PMID: 3304060.

(81) Ryan MJ, Dudash HJ, Docherty M, Geronilla KB, Baker BA, Haff GG, Cutlip RG, Alway SE. Vitamin E and C supplementation reduces oxidative stress, improves antioxidant enzymes and positive muscle work in chronically loaded muscles of aged rats. Exp Gerontol. 2010 Nov;45(11):882-95. doi:

10.1016/j.exger.2010.08.002. Epub 2010 Aug 10. PMID: 20705127; PMCID: PMC3104015.

(82) Amini L, Chekini R, Nateghi MR, Haghani H, Jamialahmadi T, Sathyapalan T, Saheb-kar A. The Effect of Combined Vitamin C and Vitamin E Supplementation on Oxidative Stress Markers in Women with Endometriosis: A Randomized, Triple-Blind Placebo-Controlled Clini-cal Trial. Pain Res Manag. 2021 May 26;2021:5529741. doi: 10.1155/2021/5529741. PMID: 34122682; PMCID: PMC8172324.

(83) Ciocoiu M, Badescu M, Paduraru I. Protecting antioxidative effects of vitamins E and C in experimental physical stress. J Physiol Biochem. 2007 Sep;63(3):187-94. doi: 10.1007/BF03165781. PMID: 18309774.

(84) Hillstrom RJ, Yacapin-Ammons AK, Lynch SM. Vitamin C inhibits lipid oxidation in human HDL. J Nutr. 2003 Oct;133(10):3047-51. doi: 10.1093/jn/133.10.3047. PMID: 14519782.

(85) Vojdani A, Bazargan M, Vojdani E, Wright J. New evidence for antioxidant properties of vitamin C. Cancer Detect Prev. 2000;24(6):508-23. Erratum in: Cancer Detect Prev 2001;25(2):222. PMID: 11198264.

(86) Putchala MC, Ramani P, Sherlin HJ, Premkumar P, Natesan A. Ascorbic acid and its pro-oxidant activity as a therapy for tumours of oral cavity -- a systematic review. Arch Oral Biol. 2013 Jun;58(6):563-74. doi: 10.1016/j.archoralbio.2013.01.016. Epub 2013 Mar 8. PMID: 23477602.

(87) Mühlhöfer A, Mrosek S, Schlegel B, Trommer W, Rozario F, Böhles H, Schremmer D, Zoller WG, Biesalski HK. High-dose intravenous vitamin C is not associated with an increase of pro-oxidative biomarkers. Eur J Clin Nutr. 2004 Aug;58(8):1151-8. doi: 10.1038/sj.ejcn.1601943. PMID: 15054428.

(88) Yanase F, Raman S, Naorungroj T, McCarthy A, Cree M, Schlapbach LJ, Bellomo R. Efficacy and Safety of Parenteral High-Dose Vitamin C Therapy in Pediatric Patients: A Scop-ing Review. Pediatr Crit Care Med. 2021 Jun 1;22(6):561-571. doi: 10.1097/PCC.0000000000002686. PMID: 33729732.

(89) A. Hacısevki , "AN OVERVIEW OF ASCORBIC ACID BIOCHEMISTRY", Journal of Faculty of Pharmacy of Ankara University, c. 38, sayı. 3, ss. 233-255, Eyl. 2009, doi:10.1501/Eczfak_0000000528

(90) Pullar JM, Carr AC, Bozonet SM, Vissers MCM. High Vitamin C Status Is Associated with Elevated Mood in Male Tertiary Students. Antioxidants (Basel). 2018;7(7):91. Published 2018 Jul 16. doi:10.3390/antiox7070091. PMID: 30012945; PMCID: PMC6071228.

(91) Carr AC, Shaw GM, Fowler AA, Natarajan R. Ascorbate-dependent vasopressor syn-thesis: a rationale for vitamin C administration in severe sepsis and septic shock?. Crit Care. 2015;19:418. Published 2015 Nov 27. doi:10.1186/s13054-015-1131-2.

(92) Yokoyama T, Date C, Kokubo Y, Yoshiike N, Matsumura Y, Tanaka H. Serum vita-min C concentration was inversely associated with subsequent 20-year incidence of stroke in a Japanese rural community. The Shibata study. Stroke. 2000 Oct;31(10):2287-94. doi: 10.1161/01.str.31.10.2287. PMID: 11022052.

(93) Zhang Q, Yan Q, Yang H, Wei W. Oxygen sensing and adaptability won the 2019 No-bel Prize in Physiology or medicine. Genes Dis. 2019 Oct 19;6(4):328-332. doi: 10.1016/j.gendis.2019.10.006. PMID: 31832511; PMCID: PMC6889041.

(94) Solak Y, Cetiner M, Siriopol D, Tarim K, Afsar B, Covic A, Kanbay M. Novel Masters of Erythropoiesis: Hypoxia Inducible Factors and Recent Advances in Anemia of Renal Dis-ease. Blood Purif. 2016;42(2):160-7. doi: 10.1159/000446273. Epub 2016 Jun 18. PMID: 27318465.

(95) Erler JT, Bennewith KL, Nicolau M, Dornhöfer N, Kong C, Le QT, Chi JT, Jeffrey SS, Giaccia AJ. Lysyl oxidase is essential for hypoxia-induced metastasis. Nature. 2006 Apr 27;440(7088):1222-6. doi: 10.1038/nature04695. Retraction in: Nature. 2020 Mar;579(7799):456. PMID: 16642001.

(96) Tian W, Wang Y, Xu Y, et al. The hypoxia-inducible factor renders cancer cells more sensitive to vitamin C-induced toxicity. J Biol Chem. 2014;289(6):3339-3351. doi:10.1074/jbc.M113.538157. Epub 2013 Dec 26. PMID: 24371136; PMCID: PMC3916538.

(97) Wilkes JG, O'Leary BR, Du J, et al. Pharmacologic ascorbate (P-AscH-) suppresses hypoxia-inducible Factor-1α (HIF-1α) in pancreatic adenocarcinoma. Clin Exp Metastasis. 2018;35(1-2):37-51. doi:10.1007/s10585-018-9876-z. Epub 2018 Feb 2. PMID: 29396728; PMCID: PMC5959274.

(98) Webb AL, Villamor E. Update: effects of antioxidant and non-antioxidant vitamin supplementation on immune function. Nutr Rev. 2007 May;65(5):181-217. doi: 10.1111/j.1753-4887.2007.tb00298.x. PMID: 17566547.

(99) Tajima S, Pinnell SR. Ascorbic acid preferentially enhances type I and III collagen gene transcription in human skin fibroblasts. J Dermatol Sci. 1996 Mar;11(3):250-3. doi: 10.1016/0923-1811(95)00640-0. PMID: 8785178.

(100) Ponec M, Weerheim A, Kempenaar J, Mulder A, Gooris GS, Bouwstra J, Mommaas AM. The formation of competent barrier lipids in reconstructed human epidermis requires the presence of vitamin C. J Invest Dermatol. 1997 Sep;109(3):348-55. doi: 10.1111/1523-1747.ep12336024. PMID: 9284103.

(101) Fisher BJ, Kraskauskas D, Martin EJ, Farkas D, Wegelin JA, Brophy D, Ward KR, Voelkel NF, Fowler AA 3rd, Natarajan R. Mechanisms of attenuation of abdominal sepsis induced acute lung injury by ascorbic acid. Am J Physiol Lung Cell Mol Physiol. 2012 Jul 1;303(1):L20-32. doi: 10.1152/ajplung.00300.2011. Epub 2012 Apr 20. PMID: 22523283.

(102) Washko PW, Wang Y, Levine M. Ascorbic acid recycling in human neutrophils. J Biol Chem. 1993 Jul 25;268(21):15531-5. PMID: 8340380.

(103) Goldschmidt MC, Masin WJ, Brown LR, Wyde PR. The effect of ascorbic acid deficiency on leukocyte phagocytosis and killing of actinomyces viscosus. Int J Vitam Nutr Res. 1988;58(3):326-34. PMID: 2461911.

(104) Rebora A, Dallegri F, Patrone F. Neutrophil dysfunction and repeated infec-tions: influence of levamisole and ascorbic acid. Br J Dermatol. 1980 Jan;102(1):49-56. doi: 10.1111/j.1365-2133.1980.tb05671.x. PMID: 7378281.

(105) Anderson R, Theron A. Effects of ascorbate on leucocytes: Part I. Effects of ascorbate on neutrophil motility and intracellular cyclic nucleotide levels in vitro. S Afr Med J. 1979 Sep 1;56(10):394-400. PMID: 233044.

(106) Vohra K, Khan AJ, Telang V, Rosenfeld W, Evans HE. Improvement of neu-trophil migration by systemic vitamin C in neonates. J Perinatol. 1990 Jun;10(2):134-6. PMID: 2358895.

(107) Anderson R. Assessment of oral ascorbate in three children with chronic granu-lomatous disease and defective neutrophil motility over a 2-year

period. Clin Exp Immunol. 1981 Jan;43(1):180-8. PMID: 6265123; PMCID: PMC1537134.

(108) Patrone F, Dallegri F. Vitamina C e sistema fagocitario: recenti acquisizioni e prospettive [Vitamin C and phagocytic system: present status and perspectives (author's transl)]. Acta Vitaminol Enzymol. 1979;1(1-6):5-10. Italian. PMID: 400272.

(109) Härter L, Mica L, Stocker R, Trentz O, Keel M. Mcl-1 correlates with reduced apoptosis in neutrophils from patients with sepsis. J Am Coll Surg. 2003 Dec;197(6):964-73. doi: 10.1016/j.jamcollsurg.2003.07.008. PMID: 14644285.

(110) Mikirova N, Riordan N, Casciari J. Modulation of Cytokines in Cancer Patients by Intravenous Ascorbate Therapy. Med Sci Monit. 2016 Jan 3;22:14-25. doi: 10.12659/msm.895368. PMID: 26724916; PMCID: PMC4756791.

(111) Czaikoski PG, Mota JM, Nascimento DC, Sônego F, Castanheira FV, Melo PH, Scortegagna GT, Silva RL, Barroso-Sousa R, Souto FO, Pazin-Filho A, Figueiredo F, Alves-Filho JC, Cunha FQ. Neutrophil Extracellular Traps Induce Organ Damage during Experimental and Clinical Sepsis. PLoS One. 2016 Feb 5;11(2):e0148142. doi: 10.1371/journal.pone.0148142. PMID: 26849138; PMCID: PMC4743982.

(112) Elks PM, van Eeden FJ, Dixon G, Wang X, Reyes-Aldasoro CC, Ingham PW, Whyte MK, Walmsley SR, Renshaw SA. Activation of hypoxia-inducible factor-1α (Hif-1α) delays inflammation resolution by reducing neutrophil apoptosis and reverse migration in a zebrafish inflammation model. Blood. 2011 Jul 21;118(3):712-22. doi: 10.1182/blood-2010-12-324186. Epub 2011 May 9. PMID: 21555741.

(113) McInturff AM, Cody MJ, Elliott EA, Glenn JW, Rowley JW, Rondina MT, Yost CC. Mammalian target of rapamycin regulates neutrophil extracellular trap formation via in-duction of hypoxia-inducible factor 1 α. Blood. 2012 Oct 11;120(15):3118-25. doi: 10.1182/blood-2012-01-405993. Epub 2012 Aug 23. PMID: 22919032; PMCID: PMC3471519.

(114) Mohammed BM, Fisher BJ, Kraskauskas D, Farkas D, Brophy DF, Fowler AA 3rd, Natarajan R. Vitamin C: a novel regulator of neutrophil

extracellular trap formation. Nutri-ents. 2013 Aug 9;5(8):3131-51. doi: 10.3390/nu5083131. PMID: 23939536; PMCID: PMC3775246.

(115) Tanaka M, Muto N, Gohda E, Yamamoto I. Enhancement by ascorbic acid 2-glucoside or repeated additions of ascorbate of mitogen-induced IgM and IgG productions by human peripheral blood lymphocytes. Jpn J Pharmacol. 1994 Dec;66(4):451-6. doi: 10.1254/jjp.66.451. PMID: 7723222.

(116) Manning J, Mitchell B, Appadurai DA, et al. Vitamin C promotes maturation of T-cells. Antioxid Redox Signal. 2013;19(17):2054-2067. doi:10.1089/ars.2012.4988. Epub 2013 Feb 5. PMID: 23249337; PMCID: PMC3869442.

(117) Gao YL, Lu B, Zhai JH, Liu YC, Qi HX, Yao Y, Chai YF, Shou ST. The Paren-teral Vitamin C Improves Sepsis and Sepsis-Induced Multiple Organ Dysfunction Syndrome via Preventing Cellular Immunosuppression. Mediators Inflamm. 2017;2017:4024672. doi: 10.1155/2017/4024672. Epub 2017 Jan 22. Retraction in: Mediators Inflamm. 2020 Sep 4;2020:8462563. PMID: 28210072; PMCID: PMC5292190.

(118) Kasahara H, Kondo T, Nakatsukasa H, Chikuma S, Ito M, Ando M, Kurebayashi Y, Sekiya T, Yamada T, Okamoto S, Yoshimura A. Generation of allo-antigen-specific induced Treg stabilized by vitamin C treatment and its application for prevention of acute graft versus host disease model. Int Immunol. 2017 Dec 18;29(10):457-469. doi: 10.1093/intimm/dxx060. PMID: 29126272.

(119) Young JI, Züchner S, Wang G. Regulation of the Epigenome by Vitamin C. An-nu Rev Nutr. 2015;35:545-64. doi: 10.1146/annurev-nutr-071714-034228. Epub 2015 May 6. PMID: 25974700; PMCID: PMC4506708.

(120) Nikolouli E, Hardtke-Wolenski M, Hapke M, Beckstette M, Geffers R, Floess S, Jaeckel E, Huehn J. Alloantigen-Induced Regulatory T Cells Generated in Presence of Vitamin C Display Enhanced Stability of Foxp3 Expression and Promote Skin Allograft Acceptance. Front Immunol. 2017 Jun 28;8:748. doi: 10.3389/fimmu.2017.00748. PMID: 28702031; PMCID: PMC5487376.

(121) Nieman DC, Peters EM, Henson DA, Nevines EI, Thompson MM. Influence of vitamin C supplementation on cytokine changes following an

ultramarathon. J Interferon Cy-tokine Res. 2000 Nov;20(11):1029-35. doi: 10.1089/10799900050198480. PMID: 11096461.

(122) Mohammad Gholizadeh, Said Abdul Ghafour Saeedy, Arash Abdi, Fatemeh Khademi, Keivan Lorian, Cain C.T. Clark, Kurosh Djafarian, Vitamin C reduces interleukin-6 plasma concentration: a systematic review and meta-analysis of randomized clinical trials, Clinical Nutrition Open Science,

volume 40 2021, Pages 1-14, ISSN 2667-2685, https://doi.org/10.1016/j.nutos.2021.09.003.

(123) Kim Y, Kim H, Bae S, Choi J, Lim SY, Lee N, Kong JM, Hwang YI, Kang JS, Lee WJ. Vitamin C Is an Essential Factor on the Anti-viral Immune Responses through the Pro-duction of Interferon-α/β at the Initial Stage of Influenza A Virus (H3N2) Infection. Immune Netw. 2013 Apr;13(2):70-4. doi: 10.4110/in.2013.13.2.70. Epub 2013 Apr 30. PMID: 23700397; PMCID: PMC3659258.

(124) Colunga Biancatelli RML, Berrill M, Marik PE. The antiviral properties of vita-min C. Expert Rev Anti Infect Ther. 2020 Feb;18(2):99-101. doi: 10.1080/14787210.2020.1706483. Epub 2019 Dec 23. PMID: 31852327.

(125) Mikirova N, Hunninghake R. Effect of high dose vitamin C on Epstein-Barr vi-ral infection. Med Sci Monit. 2014;20:725-732. Published 2014 May 3;20:725-32. doi: 10.12659/MSM.890423. PMID: 24793092; PMCID: PMC4015650.

(126) Mousavi S, Bereswill S, Heimesaat MM. Immunomodulatory and Antimicrobial Effects of Vitamin C. Eur J Microbiol Immunol (Bp). 2019 Aug 16;9(3):73-79. doi: 10.1556/1886.2019.00016. PMID: 31662885; PMCID: PMC6798581.

(127) Lynch SR, Cook JD. Interaction of vitamin C and iron. Ann N Y Acad Sci. 1980;355:32-44. doi: 10.1111/j.1749-6632.1980.tb21325.x. PMID: 6940487.

(128) Hallberg L, Brune M, Rossander L. The role of vitamin C in iron absorption. Int J Vitam Nutr Res Suppl. 1989;30:103-8. PMID: 2507689.

(129) Lane DJ, Richardson DR. The active role of vitamin C in mammalian iron me-tabolism: much more than just enhanced iron absorption! Free Radic Biol

Med. 2014 Oct;75:69-83. doi: 10.1016/j.freeradbiomed.2014.07.007. Epub 2014 Jul 15. PMID: 25048971.

(130) Li N, Zhao G, Wu W, Zhang M, Liu W, Chen Q, Wang X. The Efficacy and Safety of Vitamin C for Iron Supplementation in Adult Patients With Iron Deficiency Anemia: A Randomized Clinical Trial. JAMA Netw Open. 2020 Nov 2;3(11):e2023644. doi: 10.1001/jamanetworkopen.2020.23644. PMID: 33136134; PMCID: PMC7607440.

(131) Gerster H. High-dose vitamin C: a risk for persons with high iron stores? Int J Vitam Nutr Res. 1999 Mar;69(2):67-82. doi: 10.1024/0300-9831.69.2.67. PMID: 10218143.

(132) Brissot P, Deugnier Y, Le Treut A, Regnouard F, Simon M, Bourel M. Ascorbic acid status in idiopathic hemochromatosis. Digestion. 1978;17(6):479-87. doi: 10.1159/000198154. PMID: 710734.

(133) Ginter E. Cholesterol: vitamin C controls its transformation to bile acids. Sci-ence. 1973 Feb 16;179(4074):702-4. doi: 10.1126/science.179.4074.702. PMID: 4685043.

(134) Ginter E. Ascorbic acid in cholesterol and bile acid metabolism. Ann N Y Acad Sci. 1975 Sep 30;258:410-21. doi: 10.1111/j.1749-6632.1975.tb29299.x. PMID: 1060410.

(135) Jenkins SA. Vitamin C status, serum cholesterol levels and bile composition in the pregnant guinea-pig. Br J Nutr. 1980 Jan;43(1):95-100. doi: 10.1079/bjn19800068. PMID: 7370221.

(136) McRae MP. The efficacy of vitamin C supplementation on reducing total serum cholesterol in human subjects: a review and analysis of 51 experimental trials. J Chiropr Med. 2006 Spring;5(1):2-12. doi: 10.1016/S0899-3467(07)60127-X. PMID: 19674666; PMCID: PMC2647052.

(137) McRae MP. Vitamin C supplementation lowers serum low-density lipoprotein cholesterol and triglycerides: a meta-analysis of 13 randomized controlled trials. J Chiropr Med. 2008;7(2):48-58. doi:10.1016/j.jcme.2008.01.002. PMID: 19674720; PMCID: PMC2682928.

(138) Filis K, Anastassopoulou A, Sigala F, Theodorou D, Manouras A, Leandros E, Sigalas P, Hepp W, Bramis J. High-dose ascorbic acid decreases cholesterolemic factors of an atherogenic diet in guinea pigs. Int J Vitam Nutr Res. 2007 Mar;77(2):125-9. doi: 10.1024/0300-9831.77.2.125. PMID: 17896585.

(139) Juraschek SP, Miller ER 3rd, Gelber AC. Effect of oral vitamin C supplementa-tion on serum uric acid: a meta-analysis of randomized controlled trials. Arthritis Care Res (Hoboken). 2011 Sep;63(9):1295-306. doi: 10.1002/acr.20519. PMID: 21671418; PMCID: PMC3169708.

(140) Stein HB, Hasan A, Fox IH. Ascorbic acid-induced uricosuria. A consequency of megavitamin therapy. Ann Intern Med. 1976 Apr;84(4):385-8. doi: 10.7326/0003-4819-84-4-385. PMID: 1259282.

(141) Chade AR, Rodriguez-Porcel M, Herrmann J, Krier JD, Zhu X, Lerman A, Ler-man LO. Beneficial effects of antioxidant vitamins on the stenotic kidney. Hypertension. 2003 Oct;42(4):605-12. doi: 10.1161/01.HYP.0000089880.32275.7C. Epub 2003 Aug 18. PMID: 12925565.

(142) Brzezińska O, Styrzyński F, Makowska J, Walczak K. Role of Vitamin C in Prophylaxis and Treatment of Gout-A Literature Review. Nutrients. 2021 Feb 22;13(2):701. doi: 10.3390/nu13020701. PMID: 33671646; PMCID: PMC7926958.

(143) Moser MA, Chun OK. Vitamin C and Heart Health: A Review Based on Find-ings from Epidemiologic Studies. Int J Mol Sci. 2016 Aug 12;17(8):1328. doi: 10.3390/ijms17081328. PMID: 27529239; PMCID: PMC5000725.

(144) Polymeropoulos E, Bagos P, Papadimitriou M, Rizos I, Patsouris E, Toumpoulis I. Vitamin C for the Prevention of Postoperative Atrial Fibrillation after Cardiac Surgery: A Me-ta-Analysis. Adv Pharm Bull. 2016 Jun;6(2):243-50. doi: 10.15171/apb.2016.033. Epub 2016 Jun 30. PMID: 27478787; PMCID: PMC4961983.

(145) Papoulidis P, Ananiadou O, Chalvatzoulis E, Ampatzidou F, Koutsogiannidis C, Karaiskos T, Madesis A, Drossos G. The role of ascorbic acid in the prevention of atrial fibril-lation after elective on-pump myocardial revascularization surgery: a single-center experience--a pilot study. Interact

Cardiovasc Thorac Surg. 2011 Feb;12(2):121-4. doi: 10.1510/icvts.2010.240473. Epub 2010 Nov 23. PMID: 21098510.

(146) Trankle CR, Puckett L, Swift-Scanlan T, DeWilde C, Priday A, Sculthorpe R, El-lenbogen KA, Fowler A, Koneru JN. Vitamin C Intravenous Treatment In the Setting of Atrial Fibrillation Ablation: Results From the Randomized, Double-Blinded, Placebo-Controlled CIT-RIS-AF Pilot Study. J Am Heart Assoc. 2020 Feb 4;9(3): e014213. doi: 10.1161/JAHA.119.014213. Epub 2020 Jan 30. PMID: 32013700; PMCID: PMC7033876.

(147) Kamali A, Yavari S, Yazdi B, Rostami A. Prophylactic effect of Amiodarone and in combination with vitamin C in reducing atrial fibrillation after coronary artery bypass. Eur J Transl Myol. 2021 Sep 1;31(3). doi: 10.4081/ejtm.2021.8981. PMID: 34579514.

(148) Korantzopoulos P, Galaris D. The Protective Role of Vitamin C on Endothelial Dysfunction. Journal of Clinical and Basic Cardiology 2003; 6 (1-4), 3-6

(149) May, James M, and Fiona E Harrison. "Role of vitamin C in the function of the vascular endothelium." Antioxidants & redox signaling vol. 19,17 (2013): 2068-83. doi:10.1089/ars.2013.5205. Epub 2013 May 29. PMID: 23581713; PMCID: PMC3869438.

(150) Sun YP, Zhu BQ, Sievers RE, Norkus EP, Parmley WW, Deedwania PC. Effects of antioxidant vitamins C and E on atherosclerosis in lipid-fed rabbits. Cardiology. 1998 Mar;89(3):189-94. doi: 10.1159/000006786. PMID: 9570433.

(151) Agarwal M, Mehta PK, Dwyer JH, Dwyer KM, Shircore AM, Nordstrom CK, Sun P, Paul-Labrador M, Yang Y, Merz CN. Differing Relations to Early Atherosclerosis be-tween Vitamin C from Supplements vs. Food in the Los Angeles Atherosclerosis Study: A Pro-spective Cohort Study. Open Cardiovasc Med J. 2012;6:113-21. doi: 10.2174/1874192401206010113. Epub 2012 Sep 7. PMID: 23002405; PMCID: PMC3447163.

(152) Arun MZ, Üstünes L, Sevin G, Özer E. Effects of vitamin C treatment on collar-induced intimal thickening. Drug Des Devel Ther. 2015 Dec 15;9:6461-73. doi: 10.2147/DDDT.S97020. PMID: 26719672; PMCID: PMC4687616.

(153) Ivanov, Vadim et al. "Vitamin C inhibits the calcification process in human vascular smooth muscle cells." American journal of cardiovascular disease vol. 10,2 108-116. 15 Jun. 2020

(154) Rath M, Pauling L. Immunological evidence for the accumulation of lipopro-tein(a) in the atherosclerotic lesion of the hypoascorbemic guinea pig. Proc Natl Acad Sci U S A. 1990 Dec;87(23):9388-90. doi: 10.1073/pnas.87.23.9388. PMID: 2147514; PMCID: PMC55170.

(155) Wong, A. , Mohamed, A. and Niedzwiecki, A. (2016) Atherosclerosis and the Cholesterol Theory: A Reappraisal. World Journal of Cardiovascular Diseases, 6, 391-409. doi: 10.4236/wjcd.2016.611044.

(156) Juraschek SP, Guallar E, Appel LJ, Miller ER 3rd. Effects of vitamin C supple-mentation on blood pressure: a meta-analysis of randomized controlled trials. Am J Clin Nutr. 2012 May;95(5):1079-88. doi: 10.3945/ajcn.111.027995. Epub 2012 Apr 4. PMID: 22492364; PMCID: PMC3325833.

(157) Ran L, Zhao W, Tan X, et al. Association between Serum Vitamin C and the Blood Pressure: A Systematic Review and Meta-Analysis of Observational Studies. Cardiovasc Ther. 2020;2020:4940673. Published 2020 Apr 29. doi:10.1155/2020/4940673

(158) Nam CM, Oh KW, Lee KH, Jee SH, Cho SY, Shim WH, Suh I. Vitamin C intake and risk of ischemic heart disease in a population with a high prevalence of smoking. J Am Coll Nutr. 2003 Oct;22(5):372-8. doi: 10.1080/07315724.2003.10719320. PMID: 14559929.

(159) Schectman G, Byrd JC, Gruchow HW. The influence of smoking on vitamin C status in adults. Am J Public Health. 1989;79(2):158-162. doi:10.2105/ajph.79.2.158

(160) Spoelstra-de Man AME, Elbers PWG, Oudemans-van Straaten HM. Making sense of early high-dose intravenous vitamin C in ischemia/reperfusion injury. Crit Care. 2018 Mar 20;22(1):70. doi: 10.1186/s13054-018-1996-y. PMID: 29558975; PMCID: PMC5861638.

(161) Grooth HJ, Spoelstra-de Man AME, Oudemans-van Straaten HM. Early plasma Vitamin C concentration, organ dysfunction and ICU mortality. Intensive Care Med. 2014;40(Suppl 1):S199

(162) van Zanten AR, Sztark F, Kaisers UX, Zielmann S, Felbinger TW, Sablotzki AR, De Waele JJ, Timsit JF, Honing ML, Keh D, Vincent JL, Zazzo JF, Fijn HB, Petit L, Preiser JC, van Horssen PJ, Hofman Z. High-protein enteral nutrition enriched with immune-modulating nutrients vs standard high-protein enteral nutrition and nosocomial infections in the ICU: a randomized clinical trial. JAMA. 2014 Aug 6;312(5):514-24. doi: 10.1001/jama.2014.7698. PMID: 25096691.

(163) Tsai MS, Huang CH, Tsai CY, Chen HW, Lee HC, Cheng HJ, Hsu CY, Wang TD, Chang WT, Chen WJ. Ascorbic acid mitigates the myocardial injury after cardiac arrest and electrical shock. Intensive Care Med. 2011 Dec;37(12):2033-40. doi: 10.1007/s00134-011-2362-6. Epub 2011 Sep 28. PMID: 21953354.

(164) Nishinaka Y, Sugiyama S, Yokota M, Saito H, Ozawa T. The effects of a high dose of ascorbate on ischemia-reperfusion-induced mitochondrial dysfunction in canine hearts. Heart Vessels. 1992;7(1):18-23. doi: 10.1007/BF01745863. PMID: 1583008.

(165) Oudemans-van Straaten HM, Spoelstra-de Man AM, de Waard MC. Vitamin C revisited. Crit Care. 2014 Aug 6;18(4):460. doi: 10.1186/s13054-014-0460-x. PMID: 25185110; PMCID: PMC4423646.

(166) Rozemeijer S, de Grooth HJ, Elbers PWG, Girbes ARJ, den Uil CA, Dubois EA, Wils EJ, Rettig TCD, van Zanten ARH, Vink R, van den Bogaard B, Bosman RJ, Oudemans-van Straaten HM, de Man AME. Early high-dose vitamin C in post-cardiac arrest syndrome (VITaCCA): study protocol for a randomized, double-blind, multi-center, placebo-controlled trial. Trials. 2021 Aug 18;22(1):546. doi: 10.1186/s13063-021-05483-3. PMID: 34407846; PMCID: PMC8371424.

(167) Kamel AY, Dave NJ, Zhao VM, Griffith DP, Connor MJ Jr, Ziegler TR. Micro-nutrient Alterations During Continuous Renal Replacement Therapy in Critically Ill Adults: A Retrospective Study. Nutr Clin Pract. 2018 Jun;33(3):439-446. doi: 10.1177/0884533617716618. Epub 2017 Dec 18. PMID: 28727945.

(168) Shah FA, Pike F, Alvarez K, Angus D, Newman AB, Lopez O, Tate J, Kapur V, Wilsdon A, Krishnan JA, Hansel N, Au D, Avdalovic M, Fan VS, Barr RG, Yende S. Bidirec-tional relationship between cognitive function and

pneumonia. Am J Respir Crit Care Med. 2013 Sep 1;188(5):586-92. doi: 10.1164/rccm.201212-2154OC. PMID: 23848267; PMCID: PMC3827700.

(169) Artenstein AW, Higgins TL, Opal SM. Sepsis and scientific revolutions. Crit Care Med. 2013 Dec;41(12):2770-2. doi: 10.1097/CCM.0b013e31829eb98f. PMID: 23989175.

(170) Marik PE. Hydrocortisone, Ascorbic Acid and Thiamine (HAT Therapy) for the Treatment of Sepsis. Focus on Ascorbic Acid. Nutrients. 2018 Nov 14;10(11):1762. doi: 10.3390/nu10111762. PMID: 30441816; PMCID: PMC626597.

(171) Fowler AA 3rd, Syed AA, Knowlson S, et al. Phase I safety trial of intravenous ascorbic acid in patients with severe sepsis. J Transl Med. 2014;12:32. Published 2014 Jan 31. doi:10.1186/1479-5876-12-32

(172) Langley RJ, Tsalik EL, van Velkinburgh JC, et al. An integrated clinico-metabolomic model improves prediction of death in sepsis. Sci Transl Med. 2013;5(195):195ra95. doi:10.1126/scitranslmed.3005893

(173) Szakmany T, Hauser B, Radermacher P. N-acetylcysteine for sepsis and system-ic inflammatory response in adults. Cochrane Database Syst Rev. 2012 Sep 12;2012(9):CD006616. doi: 10.1002/14651858.CD006616.pub2. PMID: 22972094; PMCID: PMC6517277.

(174) Landry DW, Levin HR, Gallant EM, Ashton RC Jr, Seo S, D'Alessandro D, Oz MC, Oliver JA. Vasopressin deficiency contributes to the vasodilation of septic shock. Circula-tion. 1997 Mar 4;95(5):1122-5. doi: 10.1161/01.cir.95.5.1122. PMID: 9054839.

(175) Hooper MH, Carr A, Marik PE. The adrenal-vitamin C axis: from fish to guinea pigs and primates. Crit Care. 2019 Jan 28;23(1):29. doi: 10.1186/s13054-019-2332-x. PMID: 30691525; PMCID: PMC6348603.

(176) Marik PE, Khangoora V, Rivera R, Hooper MH, Catravas J. Hydrocortisone, Vitamin C, and Thiamine for the Treatment of Severe Sepsis and Septic Shock: A Retrospec-tive Before-After Study. Chest. 2017 Jun;151(6):1229-1238. doi: 10.1016/j.chest.2016.11.036. Epub 2016 Dec 6. PMID: 27940189.

(177) Kashiouris MG, L'Heureux M, Cable CA, Fisher BJ, Leichtle SW, Fowler AA. The Emerging Role of Vitamin C as a Treatment for Sepsis. Nutrients. 2020 Jan 22;12(2):292. doi: 10.3390/nu12020292. PMID: 31978969; PMCID: PMC7070236.

(178) Li J. Evidence is stronger than you think: a meta-analysis of vitamin C use in patients with sepsis. Crit Care. 2018;22(1):258. Published 2018 Oct 11. doi:10.1186/s13054-018-2191-x

(179) Rizzo JA, Rowan MP, Driscoll IR, Chung KK, Friedman BC. Vitamin C in Burn Resuscitation. Crit Care Clin. 2016 Oct;32(4):539-46. doi: 10.1016/j.ccc.2016.06.003. Epub 2016 Aug 2. PMID: 27600125.

(180) Matsuda T, Tanaka H, Williams S, Hanumadass M, Abcarian H, Reyes H. Re-duced fluid volume requirement for resuscitation of third-degree burns with high-dose vitamin C. J Burn Care Rehabil. 1991 Nov-Dec;12(6):525-32. doi: 10.1097/00004630-199111000-00007. PMID: 1779006.

(181) Tanaka H, Matsuda T, Miyagantani Y, Yukioka T, Matsuda H, Shimazaki S. Reduction of resuscitation fluid volumes in severely burned patients using ascorbic acid ad-ministration: a randomized, prospective study. Arch Surg. 2000 Mar;135(3):326-31. doi: 10.1001/archsurg.135.3.326. PMID: 10722036.

(182) Nakajima M, Kojiro M, Aso S, Matsui H, Fushimi K, Kaita Y, Goto H, Yamagu-chi Y, Yasunaga H. Effect of high-dose vitamin C therapy on severe burn patients: a nation-wide cohort study. Crit Care. 2019 Dec 12;23(1):407. doi: 10.1186/s13054-019-2693-1. PMID: 31831039; PMCID: PMC6909452.

(183) DE PASQUALINI CD. The effect of ascorbic acid on hemorrhagic shock in the guinea pig. Am J Physiol. 1946 Nov;147(3):598-601. doi: 10.1152/ajplegacy.1946.147.3.598. PMID: 21002954.

(184) Nabzdyk CS, Bittner EA. Vitamin C in the critically ill - indications and contro-versies. World J Crit Care Med. 2018 Oct 16;7(5):52-61. doi: 10.5492/wjccm.v7.i5.52. PMID: 30370227; PMCID: PMC6201324.

(185) Qi MZ, Yao Y, Xie RL, Sun SL, Sun WW, Wang JL, Chen Y, Zhao B, Chen EZ, Mao EQ. Intravenous Vitamin C attenuates hemorrhagic shock-related renal injury through the induction of SIRT1 in rats. Biochem Biophys Res

Commun. 2018 Jun 22;501(2):358-364. doi: 10.1016/j.bbrc.2018.04.111. PMID: 29673592.

(186) Travica N, Ried K, Hudson I, Scholey A, Pipingas A, Sali A. The effects of sur-gery on plasma/serum vitamin C concentrations: a systematic review and meta-analysis. Br J Nutr. 2022 Jan 28;127(2):233-247. doi: 10.1017/S0007114520004353. Epub 2020 Nov 4. PMID: 33143761.

(187) Chen S, Roffey DM, Dion CA, Arab A, Wai EK. Effect of Perioperative Vita-min C Supplementation on Postoperative Pain and the Incidence of Chronic Regional Pain Syndrome: A Systematic Review and Meta-Analysis. Clin J Pain. 2016 Feb;32(2):179-85. doi: 10.1097/AJP.0000000000000218. PMID: 25654537.

(188) Ayatollahi V, Dehghanpour Farashah S, Behdad S, Vaziribozorg S, Rabbani Anari M. Effect of intravenous vitamin C on postoperative pain in uvulopalatopharyngoplasty with tonsillectomy. Clin Otolaryngol. 2017 Feb;42(1):139-143. doi: 10.1111/coa.12684. Epub 2016 Jun 7. PMID: 27219124.

(189) Carr AC, McCall C. The role of vitamin C in the treatment of pain: new insights. J Transl Med. 2017 Apr 14;15(1):77. doi: 10.1186/s12967-017-1179-7. PMID: 28410599; PMCID: PMC5391567.

(190) Mochizucki D. Serotonin and noradrenaline reuptake inhibitors in animal mod-els of pain. Hum Psychopharmacol. 2004 Oct;19 Suppl 1:S15-9. doi: 10.1002/hup.620. PMID: 15378668.

(191) Evangelou A, Kalfakakou V, Georgakas P, Koutras V, Vezyraki P, Iliopoulou L, Vadalouka A. Ascorbic acid (vitamin C) effects on withdrawal syndrome of heroin abusers. In Vivo. 2000 Mar-Apr;14(2):363-6. PMID: 10836211.

(192) Wang D, Wang M, Zhang H, Zhu H, Zhang N, Liu J. Effect of Intravenous In-jection of Vitamin C on Postoperative Pulmonary Complications in Patients Undergoing Cardi-ac Surgery: A Double-Blind, Randomized Trial. Drug Des Devel Ther. 2020 Aug 11;14:3263-3270. doi: 10.2147/DDDT.S254150. PMID: 32848365; PMCID: PMC7431173.

(193) Deana R, Bharaj BS, Verjee ZH, Galzigna L. Changes relevant to catecholamine metabolism in liver and brain of ascorbic acid deficient guinea-pigs. Int J Vitam Nutr Res. 1975;45(2):175-82. PMID: 809379.

(194) Lee SH, Lumelsky N, Studer L, Auerbach JM, McKay RD. Efficient generation of midbrain and hindbrain neurons from mouse embryonic stem cells. Nat Biotechnol. 2000 Jun;18(6):675-9. doi: 10.1038/76536. PMID: 10835609.

(195) Huff TC, Sant DW, Camarena V, Van Booven D, Andrade NS, Mustafi S, Monje PV, Wang G. Vitamin C regulates Schwann cell myelination by promoting DNA de-methylation of pro-myelinating genes. J Neurochem. 2021 Jun;157(6):1759-1773. doi: 10.1111/jnc.15015. Epub 2020 Apr 14. PMID: 32219848; PMCID: PMC7530063.

(196) Moretti M, Fraga DB, Rodrigues ALS. Preventive and therapeutic potential of ascorbic acid in neurodegenerative diseases. CNS Neurosci Ther. 2017 Dec;23(12):921-929. doi: 10.1111/cns.12767. Epub 2017 Oct 4. PMID: 28980404; PMCID: PMC6492647.

(197) Kook SY, Lee KM, Kim Y, Cha MY, Kang S, Baik SH, Lee H, Park R, Mook-Jung I. High-dose of vitamin C supplementation reduces amyloid plaque burden and amelio-rates pathological changes in the brain of 5XFAD mice. Cell Death Dis. 2014 Feb 27;5(2):e1083. doi: 10.1038/cddis.2014.26. PMID: 24577081; PMCID: PMC3944243.

(198) Rivière S, Birlouez-Aragon I, Nourhashémi F, Vellas B. Low plasma vitamin C in Alzheimer patients despite an adequate diet. Int J Geriatr Psychiatry. 1998 Nov;13(11):749-54. doi: 10.1002/(sici)1099-1166(1998110)13:11<749::aid-gps860>3.0.co;2-t. PMID: 9850871.

(199) Fernandes JT, Tenreiro S, Gameiro A, Chu V, Outeiro TF, Conde JP. Modula-tion of alpha-synuclein toxicity in yeast using a novel microfluidic-based gradient generator. Lab Chip. 2014 Oct 21;14(20):3949-57. doi: 10.1039/c4lc00756e. PMID: 25167219.

(200) Recchia A, Debetto P, Negro A, Guidolin D, Skaper SD, Giusti P. Alpha-synuclein and Parkinson's disease. FASEB J. 2004 Apr;18(6):617-26. doi: 10.1096/fj.03-0338rev. PMID: 15054084.

(201) Férnandez-Calle P, Jiménez-Jiménez FJ, Molina JA, Cabrera-Valdivia F, Vázquez A, García Urra D, Bermejo F, Cruz Matallana M, Codoceo R. Serum levels of ascor-bic acid (vitamin C) in patients with Parkinson's disease. J Neurol

Sci. 1993 Aug;118(1):25-8. doi: 10.1016/0022-510x(93)90240-y. PMID: 8229047.

(202) Ide K, Yamada H, Umegaki K, Mizuno K, Kawakami N, Hagiwara Y, Matsu-moto M, Yoshida H, Kim K, Shiosaki E, Yokochi T, Harada K. Lymphocyte vitamin C levels as potential biomarker for progression of Parkinson's disease. Nutrition. 2015 Feb;31(2):406-8. doi: 10.1016/j.nut.2014.08.001. Epub 2014 Aug 23. PMID: 25592020.

(203) Fahn S. A pilot trial of high-dose alpha-tocopherol and ascorbate in early Park-inson's disease. Ann Neurol. 1992;32 Suppl:S128-32. doi: 10.1002/ana.410320722. PMID: 1510371.

(204) Nagayama H, Hamamoto M, Ueda M, Nito C, Yamaguchi H, Katayama Y. The effect of ascorbic acid on the pharmacokinetics of levodopa in elderly patients with Parkinson disease. Clin Neuropharmacol. 2004 Nov-Dec;27(6):270-3. doi: 10.1097/01.wnf.0000150865.21759.bc. PMID: 15613930.

(205) Eldridge CF, Bunge MB, Bunge RP, Wood PM. Differentiation of axon-related Schwann cells in vitro. I. Ascorbic acid regulates basal lamina assembly and myelin formation. J Cell Biol. 1987 Aug;105(2):1023-34. doi: 10.1083/jcb.105.2.1023. PMID: 3624305; PMCID: PMC2114758.

(206) Babri S, Mehrvash F, Mohaddes G, Hatami H, Mirzaie F. Effect of intrahippo-campal administration of vitamin C and progesterone on learning in a model of multiple sclero-sis in rats. Adv Pharm Bull. 2015 Mar;5(1):83-7. doi: 10.5681/apb.2015.011. Epub 2015 Mar 5. PMID: 25789223; PMCID: PMC4352227.

(207) Ambali SF, Idris SB, Onukak C, Shittu M, Ayo JO. Ameliorative effects of vit-amin C on short-term sensorimotor and cognitive changes induced by acute chlorpyrifos expo-sure in Wistar rats. Toxicol Ind Health. 2010 Oct;26(9):547-58. doi: 10.1177/0748233710373086. Epub 2010 Jun 16. PMID: 20554631.

(208) Besler HT, Comoğlu S, Okçu Z. Serum levels of antioxidant vitamins and lipid peroxidation in multiple sclerosis. Nutr Neurosci. 2002 Jun;5(3):215-20. doi: 10.1080/10284150290029205. PMID: 12041878.

(209) Ghadirian P, Jain M, Ducic S, Shatenstein B, Morisset R. Nutritional factors in the aetiology of multiple sclerosis: a case-control study in Montreal,

Canada. Int J Epidemiol. 1998 Oct;27(5):845-52. doi: 10.1093/ije/27.5.845. PMID: 9839742.

(210) Moretti M, Budni J, Ribeiro CM, Rieger DK, Leal RB, Rodrigues ALS. Sub-chronic administration of ascorbic acid elicits antidepressant-like effect and modulates cell survival signaling pathways in mice. J Nutr Biochem. 2016 Dec;38:50-56. doi: 10.1016/j.jnutbio.2016.09.004. Epub 2016 Sep 14. PMID: 27721116.

(211) Moretti M, Budni J, Ribeiro CM, Rodrigues AL. Involvement of different types of potassium channels in the antidepressant-like effect of ascorbic acid in the mouse tail sus-pension test. Eur J Pharmacol. 2012 Jul 15;687(1-3):21-7. doi: 10.1016/j.ejphar.2012.04.041. Epub 2012 May 2. PMID: 22575518.

(212) Zhao B, Fei J, Chen Y, Ying YL, Ma L, Song XQ, Wang L, Chen EZ, Mao EQ. Pharmacological preconditioning with vitamin C attenuates intestinal injury via the induction of heme oxygenase-1 after hemorrhagic shock in rats. PLoS One. 2014 Jun 13;9(6):e99134. doi: 10.1371/journal.pone.0099134. PMID: 24927128; PMCID: PMC4057195.

(213) Kocot J, Luchowska-Kocot D, Kiełczykowska M, Musik I, Kurzepa J. Does Vitamin C Influence Neurodegenerative Diseases and Psychiatric Disorders? Nutrients. 2017 Jun 27;9(7):659. doi: 10.3390/nu9070659. PMID: 28654017; PMCID: PMC5537779.

(214) Gariballa S. Poor vitamin C status is associated with increased depression symp-toms following acute illness in older people. Int J Vitam Nutr Res. 2014;84(1-2):12-7. doi: 10.1024/0300-9831/a000188. PMID: 25835231.

(215) Fritz H, Flower G, Weeks L, Cooley K, Callachan M, McGowan J, Skidmore B, Kirchner L, Seely D. Intravenous Vitamin C and Cancer: A Systematic Review. Integr Cancer Ther. 2014 Jul;13(4):280-300. doi: 10.1177/1534735414534463. Epub 2014 May 26. PMID: 24867961.

(216) Spector R. Dehydroascorbic acid for the treatment of acute ischemic stroke. Med Hypotheses. 2016 Apr;89:32-6. doi: 10.1016/j.mehy.2016.01.021. Epub 2016 Feb 6. PMID: 26968905.

(217) Chen GC, Lu DB, Pang Z, Liu QF. Vitamin C intake, circulating vitamin C and risk of stroke: a meta-analysis of prospective studies. J Am Heart

Assoc. 2013 Nov 27;2(6):e000329. doi: 10.1161/JAHA.113.000329. PMID: 24284213; PMCID: PMC3886767.

(218) Anthony HM, Schorah CJ. Severe hypovitaminosis C in lung-cancer patients: the utilization of vitamin C in surgical repair and lymphocyte-related host resistance. Br J Can-cer. 1982 Sep;46(3):354-67. doi: 10.1038/bjc.1982.211. PMID: 7126425; PMCID: PMC2011112.

(219) McCORMICK WJ. Cancer: the preconditioning factor in pathogenesis; a new etiologic approach. Arch Pediatr (N Y). 1954 Oct;71(10):313-22. PMID: 13208373.

(220) Cameron E, Pauling L. Supplemental ascorbate in the supportive treatment of cancer: Prolongation of survival times in terminal human cancer. Proc Natl Acad Sci U S A. 1976 Oct;73(10):3685-9. doi: 10.1073/pnas.73.10.3685. PMID: 1068480; PMCID: PMC431183.

(221) Cameron E, Pauling L. Supplemental ascorbate in the supportive treatment of cancer: reevaluation of prolongation of survival times in terminal human cancer. Proc Natl Acad Sci U S A. 1978 Sep;75(9):4538-42. doi: 10.1073/pnas.75.9.4538. PMID: 279931; PMCID: PMC336151.

(222) Creagan ET, Moertel CG, O'Fallon JR, Schutt AJ, O'Connell MJ, Rubin J, Frytak S. Failure of high-dose vitamin C (ascorbic acid) therapy to benefit patients with advanced cancer. A controlled trial. N Engl J Med. 1979 Sep 27;301(13):687-90. doi: 10.1056/NEJM197909273011303. PMID: 384241.

(223) Moertel CG, Fleming TR, Creagan ET, Rubin J, O'Connell MJ, Ames MM. High-dose vitamin C versus placebo in the treatment of patients with advanced cancer who have had no prior chemotherapy. A randomized double-blind comparison. N Engl J Med. 1985 Jan 17;312(3):137-41. doi: 10.1056/NEJM198501173120301. PMID: 3880867.

(224) Benade L, Howard T, Burk D. Synergistic killing of Ehrlich ascites carcinoma cells by ascorbate and 3-amino-1,2,4,-triazole. Oncology. 1969;23(1):33-43. doi: 10.1159/000224465. PMID: 5774953.

(225) Leung PY, Miyashita K, Young M, Tsao CS. Cytotoxic effect of ascorbate and its derivatives on cultured malignant and nonmalignant cell lines. Anticancer Res. 1993 Mar-Apr;13(2):475-80. PMID: 8517665.

(226) Chen Q, Espey MG, Sun AY, Pooput C, Kirk KL, Krishna MC, Khosh DB, Drisko J, Levine M. Pharmacologic doses of ascorbate act as a prooxidant and decrease growth of aggressive tumor xenografts in mice. Proc Natl Acad Sci U S A. 2008 Aug 12;105(32):11105-9. doi: 10.1073/pnas.0804226105. Epub 2008 Aug 4. PMID: 18678913; PMCID: PMC2516281.

(227) Liberti MV, Locasale JW. The Warburg Effect: How Does it Benefit Cancer Cells? Trends Biochem Sci. 2016 Mar;41(3):211-218. doi: 10.1016/j.tibs.2015.12.001. Epub 2016 Jan 5. Erratum in: Trends Biochem Sci. 2016 Mar;41(3):287. Erratum in: Trends Bio-chem Sci. 2016 Mar;41(3):287. PMID: 26778478; PMCID: PMC4783224.

(228) Yun J, Rago C, Cheong I, Pagliarini R, Angenendt P, Rajagopalan H, Schmidt K, Willson JK, Markowitz S, Zhou S, Diaz LA Jr, Velculescu VE, Lengauer C, Kinzler KW, Vo-gelstein B, Papadopoulos N. Glucose deprivation contributes to the development of KRAS pathway mutations in tumor cells. Science. 2009 Sep 18;325(5947):1555-9. doi: 10.1126/science.1174229. Epub 2009 Aug 6. PMID: 19661383; PMCID: PMC2820374.

(229) Yun J, Mullarky E, Lu C, Bosch KN, Kavalier A, Rivera K, Roper J, Chio II, Giannopoulou EG, Rago C, Muley A, Asara JM, Paik J, Elemento O, Chen Z, Pappin DJ, Dow LE, Papadopoulos N, Gross SS, Cantley LC. Vitamin C selectively kills KRAS and BRAF mu-tant colorectal cancer cells by targeting GAPDH. Science. 2015 Dec 11;350(6266):1391-6. doi: 10.1126/science.aaa5004. Epub 2015 Nov 5. PMID: 26541605; PMCID: PMC4778961.

(230) Rees DC, Kelsey H, Richards JD. Acute haemolysis induced by high dose ascorbic acid in glucose-6-phosphate dehydrogenase deficiency. BMJ. 1993 Mar 27;306(6881):841-2. doi: 10.1136/bmj.306.6881.841. PMID: 8490379; PMCID: PMC1677333.

(231) Mingay M, Chaturvedi A, Bilenky M, Cao Q, Jackson L, Hui T, Moksa M, Heravi-Moussavi A, Humphries RK, Heuser M, Hirst M. Vitamin C-induced epigenomic re-modelling in IDH1 mutant acute myeloid leukaemia. Leukemia. 2018 Jan;32(1):11-20. doi: 10.1038/leu.2017.171. Epub 2017 Jun 2. PMID: 28663574; PMCID: PMC5770587.

(232) Iamsawat S, Tian L, Daenthanasanmak A, Wu Y, Nguyen HD, Bastian D, Yu XZ. Vitamin C stabilizes CD8+ iTregs and enhances their therapeutic

potential in controlling murine GVHD and leukemia relapse. Blood Adv. 2019 Dec 23;3(24):4187-4201. doi: 10.1182/bloodadvances.2019000531. PMID: 31856270; PMCID: PMC6929397.

(233) Aguilera O, Muñoz-Sagastibelza M, Torrejón B, Borrero-Palacios A, Del Puerto-Nevado L, Martínez-Useros J, Rodriguez-Remirez M, Zazo S, García E, Fraga M, Rojo F, Gar-cía-Foncillas J. Vitamin C uncouples the Warburg metabolic switch in KRAS mutant colon cancer. Oncotarget. 2016 Jul 26;7(30):47954-47965. doi: 10.18632/oncotarget.10087. PMID: 27323830; PMCID: PMC5216991.

(234) Mamede AC, Pires AS, Abrantes AM, Tavares SD, Gonçalves AC, Casalta-Lopes JE, Sarmento-Ribeiro AB, Maia JM, Botelho MF. Cytotoxicity of ascorbic acid in a hu-man colorectal adenocarcinoma cell line (WiDr): in vitro and in vivo studies. Nutr Cancer. 2012;64(7):1049-57. doi: 10.1080/01635581.2012.713539. Epub 2012 Sep 13. PMID: 22974001.

(235) Nakanishi K, Hiramoto K, Sato EF, Ooi K. High-Dose Vitamin C Administration Inhibits the Invasion and Proliferation of Melanoma Cells in Mice Ovary. Biol Pharm Bull. 2021;44(1):75-81. doi: 10.1248/bpb.b20-00637. PMID: 33390553.

(236) Mustafi S, Sant DW, Liu ZJ, Wang G. Ascorbate induces apoptosis in melanoma cells by suppressing Clusterin expression. Sci Rep. 2017 Jun 16;7(1):3671. doi: 10.1038/s41598-017-03893-5. PMID: 28623268; PMCID: PMC5473908.

(237) Du J, Martin SM, Levine M, Wagner BA, Buettner GR, Wang SH, Taghiyev AF, Du C, Knudson CM, Cullen JJ. Mechanisms of ascorbate-induced cytotoxicity in pancreatic cancer. Clin Cancer Res. 2010 Jan 15;16(2):509-20. doi: 10.1158/1078-0432.CCR-09-1713. Epub 2010 Jan 12. PMID: 20068072; PMCID: PMC2807999.

(238) Wang G, Yin T, Wang Y. In vitro and in vivo assessment of high-dose vitamin C against murine tumors. Exp Ther Med. 2016 Nov;12(5):3058-3062. doi: 10.3892/etm.2016.3707. Epub 2016 Sep 16. PMID: 27882116; PMCID: PMC5103746.

(239) Pollard HB, Levine MA, Eidelman O, Pollard M. Pharmacological ascorbic acid suppresses syngeneic tumor growth and metastases in hormone-refractory prostate cancer. In Vivo. 2010 May-Jun;24(3):249-55. PMID: 20554995.

(240) Chen P, Yu J, Chalmers B, Drisko J, Yang J, Li B, Chen Q. Pharmacological ascorbate induces cytotoxicity in prostate cancer cells through ATP depletion and induction of autophagy. Anticancer Drugs. 2012 Apr;23(4):437-44. doi: 10.1097/CAD.0b013e32834fd01f. PMID: 22205155.

(241) Campbell EJ, Vissers MCM, Wohlrab C, Hicks KO, Strother RM, Bozonet SM, Robinson BA, Dachs GU. Pharmacokinetic and anti-cancer properties of high dose ascorbate in solid tumours of ascorbate-dependent mice. Free Radic Biol Med. 2016 Oct;99:451-462. doi: 10.1016/j.freeradbiomed.2016.08.027. Epub 2016 Aug 24. PMID: 27567539.

(242) Ma Y, Chapman J, Levine M, Polireddy K, Drisko J, Chen Q. High-dose paren-teral ascorbate enhanced chemosensitivity of ovarian cancer and reduced toxicity of chemo-therapy. Sci Transl Med. 2014 Feb 5;6(222):222ra18. doi: 10.1126/scitranslmed.3007154. PMID: 24500406.

(243) Böttger F, Vallés-Martí A, Cahn L, Jimenez CR. High-dose intravenous vitamin C, a promising multi-targeting agent in the treatment of cancer. J Exp Clin Cancer Res. 2021 Oct 30;40(1):343. doi: 10.1186/s13046-021-02134-y. PMID: 34717701; PMCID: PMC8557029.

(244) Boyera N, Galey I, Bernard BA. Effect of vitamin C and its derivatives on col-lagen synthesis and cross-linking by normal human fibroblasts. Int J Cosmet Sci. 1998 Jun;20(3):151-8. doi: 10.1046/j.1467-2494.1998.171747.x. PMID: 18505499.

(245) Polireddy K, Dong R, Reed G, Yu J, Chen P, Williamson S, Violet PC, Pessetto Z, Godwin AK, Fan F, Levine M, Drisko JA, Chen Q. High Dose Parenteral Ascorbate Inhibit-ed Pancreatic Cancer Growth and Metastasis: Mechanisms and a Phase I/IIa study. Sci Rep. 2017 Dec 7;7(1):17188. doi: 10.1038/s41598-017-17568-8. PMID: 29215048; PMCID: PMC5719364.

(246) Kuiper C, Dachs GU, Munn D, Currie MJ, Robinson BA, Pearson JF, Vissers MC. Increased Tumor Ascorbate is Associated with Extended Disease-

Free Survival and De-creased Hypoxia-Inducible Factor-1 Activation in Human Colorectal Cancer. Front Oncol. 2014 Feb 4;4:10. doi: 10.3389/fonc.2014.00010. PMID: 24551593; PMCID: PMC3912592.

(247) Klutstein M, Nejman D, Greenfield R, Cedar H. DNA Methylation in Cancer and Aging. Cancer Res. 2016 Jun 15;76(12):3446-50. doi: 10.1158/0008-5472.CAN-15-3278. Epub 2016 Jun 2. PMID: 27256564.

(248) Lee Chong T, Ahearn EL, Cimmino L. Reprogramming the Epigenome With Vitamin C. Front Cell Dev Biol. 2019 Jul 16;7:128. doi: 10.3389/fcell.2019.00128. PMID: 31380368; PMCID: PMC6646595.

(249) Agathocleous M, Meacham CE, Burgess RJ, Piskounova E, Zhao Z, Crane GM, Cowin BL, Bruner E, Murphy MM, Chen W, Spangrude GJ, Hu Z, DeBerardinis RJ, Morrison SJ. Ascorbate regulates haematopoietic stem cell function and leukaemogenesis. Nature. 2017 Sep 28;549(7673):476-481. doi: 10.1038/nature23876. Epub 2017 Aug 21. PMID: 28825709; PMCID: PMC5910063.

(250) Cimmino L, Dolgalev I, Wang Y, Yoshimi A, Martin GH, Wang J, Ng V, Xia B, Witkowski MT, Mitchell-Flack M, Grillo I, Bakogianni S, Ndiaye-Lobry D, Martín MT, Guil-lamot M, Banh RS, Xu M, Figueroa ME, Dickins RA, Abdel-Wahab O, Park CY, Tsirigos A, Neel BG, Aifantis I. Restoration of TET2 Function Blocks Aberrant Self-Renewal and Leuke-mia Progression. Cell. 2017 Sep 7;170(6):1079-1095.e20. doi: 10.1016/j.cell.2017.07.032. Epub 2017 Aug 17. PMID: 28823558; PMCID: PMC5755977.

(251) Ang A, Pullar JM, Currie MJ, Vissers MCM. Vitamin C and immune cell func-tion in inflammation and cancer. Biochem Soc Trans. 2018 Oct 19;46(5):1147-1159. doi: 10.1042/BST20180169. Epub 2018 Oct 8. PMID: 30301842; PMCID: PMC6195639.

(252) Magrì A, Germano G, Lorenzato A, Lamba S, Chilà R, Montone M, Amodio V, Ceruti T, Sassi F, Arena S, Abrignani S, D'Incalci M, Zucchetti M, Di Nicolantonio F, Bardelli A. High-dose vitamin C enhances cancer immunotherapy. Sci Transl Med. 2020 Feb 26;12(532):eaay8707. doi: 10.1126/scitranslmed.aay8707. PMID: 32102933.

(253) Yeom CH, Jung GC, Song KJ. Changes of terminal cancer patients' health-related quality of life after high dose vitamin C administration. J Korean Med Sci. 2007 Feb;22(1):7-11. doi: 10.3346/jkms.2007.22.1.7. PMID: 17297243; PMCID: PMC2693571.

(254) Tu H, Li H, Wang Y, Niyyati M, Wang Y, Leshin J, Levine M. Low Red Blood Cell Vitamin C Concentrations Induce Red Blood Cell Fragility: A Link to Diabetes Via Glu-cose, Glucose Transporters, and Dehydroascorbic Acid. EBioMedicine. 2015 Oct 3;2(11):1735-50. doi: 10.1016/j.ebiom.2015.09.049. PMID: 26870799; PMCID: PMC4740302.

(255) Dakhale GN, Chaudhari HV, Shrivastava M. Supplementation of vitamin C re-duces blood glucose and improves glycosylated hemoglobin in type 2 diabetes mellitus: a ran-domized, double-blind study. Adv Pharmacol Sci. 2011;2011:195271. doi: 10.1155/2011/195271. Epub 2011 Dec 28. PMID: 22242019; PMCID: PMC3254006.

(256) Bansal A, Hadimani CP. Low Plasma Ascorbate Levels in Type 2 Diabetic Pa-tients With Adequate Dietary Vitamin C. J Lab Physicians. 2021 Jun;13(2):139-143. doi: 10.1055/s-0041-1730751. Epub 2021 Jun 16. PMID: 34483559; PMCID: PMC8409123.

(257) Das UN. Vitamin C for Type 2 Diabetes Mellitus and Hypertension. Arch Med Res. 2019 Feb;50(2):11-14. doi: 10.1016/j.arcmed.2019.05.004. Epub 2019 May 23. PMID: 31349946.

(258) Zhang C, Williams MA, Frederick IO, King IB, Sorensen TK, Kestin MM, Da-show EE, Luthy DA. Vitamin C and the risk of gestational diabetes mellitus: a case-control study. J Reprod Med. 2004 Apr;49(4):257-66. PMID: 15134150.

(259) Liu C, Zhong C, Chen R, Zhou X, Wu J, Han J, Li X, Zhang Y, Gao Q, Xiao M, Hu X, Xiong G, Han W, Yang X, Hao L, Yang N. Higher dietary vitamin C intake is associated with a lower risk of gestational diabetes mellitus: A longitudinal cohort study. Clin Nutr. 2020 Jan;39(1):198-203. doi: 10.1016/j.clnu.2019.01.015. Epub 2019 Feb 2. PMID: 30773371.

(260) Reiss GR, Werness PG, Zollman PE, Brubaker RF. Ascorbic acid levels in the aqueous humor of nocturnal and diurnal mammals. Arch Ophthalmol. 1986

May;104(5):753-5. doi: 10.1001/archopht.1986.01050170143039. PMID: 3707416.

(261) Jacques PF, Taylor A, Hankinson SE, Willett WC, Mahnken B, Lee Y, Vaid K, Lahav M. Long-term vitamin C supplement use and prevalence of early age-related lens opaci-ties. Am J Clin Nutr. 1997 Oct;66(4):911-6. doi: 10.1093/ajcn/66.4.911. PMID: 9322567.

(262) Age-Related Eye Disease Study Research Group. A randomized, placebo-controlled, clinical trial of high-dose supplementation with vitamins C and E and beta carotene for age-related cataract and vision loss: AREDS report no. 9. Arch Ophthalmol. 2001 Oct;119(10):1439-52. doi: 10.1001/archopht.119.10.1439. Erratum in: Arch Ophthalmol. 2008 Sep;126(9):1251. PMID: 11594943; PMCID: PMC1472812.

(263) Wei L, Liang G, Cai C, Lv J. Association of vitamin C with the risk of age-related cataract: a meta-analysis. Acta Ophthalmol. 2016 May;94(3):e170-6. doi: 10.1111/aos.12688. Epub 2015 Mar 4. PMID: 25735187.

(264) Zanon-Moreno V, Ciancotti-Olivares L, Asencio J, Sanz P, Ortega-Azorin C, Pinazo-Duran MD, Corella D. Association between a SLC23A2 gene variation, plasma vitamin C levels, and risk of glaucoma in a Mediterranean population. Mol Vis. 2011;17:2997-3004. Epub 2011 Nov 17. PMID: 22171153; PMCID: PMC3236071.

(265) Hysi PG, Khawaja AP, Menni C, Tamraz B, Wareham N, Khaw KT, Foster PJ, Benet LZ, Spector TD, Hammond CJ. Ascorbic acid metabolites are involved in intraocular pressure control in the general population. Redox Biol. 2019 Jan;20:349-353. doi: 10.1016/j.redox.2018.10.004. Epub 2018 Oct 13. PMID: 30391827; PMCID: PMC6223183.

(266) Telang PS. Vitamin C in dermatology. Indian Dermatol Online J. 2013 Apr;4(2):143-6. doi: 10.4103/2229-5178.110593. PMID: 23741676; PMCID: PMC3673383.

(267) Sinclair PR, Gorman N, Shedlofsky SI, Honsinger CP, Sinclair JF, Karagas MR, Anderson KE. Ascorbic acid deficiency in porphyria cutanea tarda. J Lab Clin Med. 1997 Aug;130(2):197-201. doi: 10.1016/s0022-2143(97)90096-2. PMID: 9280147.

(268) Shin J, Kim YJ, Kwon O, Kim NI, Cho Y. Associations among plasma vitamin C, epidermal ceramide and clinical severity of atopic dermatitis. Nutr Res Pract. 2016 Aug;10(4):398-403. doi: 10.4162/nrp.2016.10.4.398. Epub 2016 Apr 29. PMID: 27478546; PMCID: PMC4958642.

(269) Wang K, Jiang H, Li W, Qiang M, Dong T, Li H. Role of Vitamin C in Skin Dis-eases. Front Physiol. 2018 Jul 4;9:819. doi: 10.3389/fphys.2018.00819. PMID: 30022952; PMCID: PMC6040229.

(270) Miles SL, Fischer AP, Joshi SJ, Niles RM. Ascorbic acid and ascorbate-2-phosphate decrease HIF activity and malignant properties of human melanoma cells. BMC Cancer. 2015 Nov 7;15:867. doi: 10.1186/s12885-015-1878-5. PMID: 26547841; PMCID: PMC4636772.

(271) Gustafson CB, Yang C, Dickson KM, Shao H, Van Booven D, Harbour JW, Liu ZJ, Wang G. Epigenetic reprogramming of melanoma cells by vitamin C treatment. Clin Epige-netics. 2015 Apr 29;7(1):51. doi: 10.1186/s13148-015-0087-z. PMID: 25977731; PMCID: PMC4430922.

(272) Marik PE, Long A. ARDS complicating pustular psoriasis: treatment with low-dose corticosteroids, vitamin C and thiamine. BMJ Case Rep. 2018 Feb 2;2018:bcr2017223475. doi: 10.1136/bcr-2017-223475. PMID: 29420246; PMCID: PMC5812384.

(273) Kitahata K, Matsuo K, Hara Y, Naganuma T, Oiso N, Kawada A, Nakayama T. Ascorbic acid derivative DDH-1 ameliorates psoriasis-like skin lesions in mice by suppressing inflammatory cytokine expression. J Pharmacol Sci. 2018 Dec;138(4):284-288. doi: 10.1016/j.jphs.2018.11.002. Epub 2018 Nov 20. PMID: 30503675.

(274) Li F, Yuan CW, Xu S, Zu T, Woappi Y, Lee CAA, Abarzua P, Wells M, Ramsey MR, Frank NY, Wu X, Mandinova A, Frank MH, Lian CG, Murphy GF. Loss of the Epigenetic Mark 5-hmC in Psoriasis: Implications for Epidermal Stem Cell Dysregulation. J Invest Derma-tol. 2020 Jun;140(6):1266-1275.e3. doi: 10.1016/j.jid.2019.10.016. Epub 2019 Dec 11. PMID: 31837302; PMCID: PMC7931370.

(275) Vollbracht C, Raithel M, Krick B, Kraft K, Hagel AF. Intravenous vitamin C in the treatment of allergies: an interim subgroup analysis of a long-

term observational study. J Int Med Res. 2018 Sep;46(9):3640-3655. doi: 10.1177/0300060518777044. Epub 2018 Jun 27. PMID: 29950123; PMCID: PMC6136002.

(276) Hagel AF, Layritz CM, Hagel WH, Hagel HJ, Hagel E, Dauth W, Kressel J, Reg-net T, Rosenberg A, Neurath MF, Molderings GJ, Raithel M. Intravenous infusion of ascorbic acid decreases serum histamine concentrations in patients with allergic and non-allergic diseas-es. Naunyn Schmiedebergs Arch Pharmacol. 2013 Sep;386(9):789-93. doi: 10.1007/s00210-013-0880-1. Epub 2013 May 11. PMID: 23666445.

(277) Johnston CS. The antihistamine action of ascorbic acid. Subcell Biochem. 1996;25:189-213. doi: 10.1007/978-1-4613-0325-1_10. PMID: 8821975.

(278) Clemetson CA. Histamine and ascorbic acid in human blood. J Nutr. 1980 Apr;110(4):662-8. doi: 10.1093/jn/110.4.662. PMID: 7365537.

(279) Pavlović S, Fraser R. Effects of different levels of vitamin C intake on the vit-amin C concentration in guinea pigs plasma and the effect of vitamin C intake on anaphylaxis. Med Interne. 1988 Jul-Sep;26(3):235-44. PMID: 3187363.

(280) Miura K, Matsuno H, Iwaoka Y, Ito H, Tai A. Antiallergic Activity of 6-Deoxy-2-O-methyl-6-(N-hexadecanoyl)amino-l-ascorbic Acid. Molecules. 2021 Aug 3;26(15):4684. doi: 10.3390/molecules26154684. PMID: 34361837; PMCID: PMC8348947.

(281) Aditi A, Graham DY. Vitamin C, gastritis, and gastric disease: a historical re-view and update. Dig Dis Sci. 2012 Oct;57(10):2504-15. doi: 10.1007/s10620-012-2203-7. Epub 2012 Apr 28. PMID: 22543844; PMCID: PMC3874117.

(282) Simon JA, Hudes ES, Perez-Perez GI. Relation of serum ascorbic acid to Heli-cobacter pylori serology in US adults: the Third National Health and Nutrition Examination Survey. J Am Coll Nutr. 2003 Aug;22(4):283-9. doi: 10.1080/07315724.2003.10719305. PMID: 12897042.

(283) Mowat C, McColl KE. Alterations in intragastric nitrite and vitamin C levels dur-ing acid inhibitory therapy. Best Pract Res Clin Gastroenterol. 2001 Jun;15(3):523-37. doi: 10.1053/bega.2000.0196. PMID: 11403544.

(284) Zojaji H, Talaie R, Mirsattari D, Haghazali M, Molaei M, Mohsenian N, De-rakhshan F, Zali MR. The efficacy of Helicobacter pylori eradication regimen with and without vitamin C supplementation. Dig Liver Dis. 2009 Sep;41(9):644-7. doi: 10.1016/j.dld.2008.09.008. Epub 2009 Jun 2. PMID: 19493713.

(285) Correa P, Fontham ET, Bravo JC, Bravo LE, Ruiz B, Zarama G, Realpe JL, Malcom GT, Li D, Johnson WD, Mera R. Chemoprevention of gastric dysplasia: randomized trial of antioxidant supplements and anti-helicobacter pylori therapy. J Natl Cancer Inst. 2000 Dec 6;92(23):1881-8. doi: 10.1093/jnci/92.23.1881. PMID: 11106679.

(286) Correa P. Human gastric carcinogenesis: a multistep and multifactorial process--First American Cancer Society Award Lecture on Cancer Epidemiology and Prevention. Cancer Res. 1992 Dec 15;52(24):6735-40. PMID: 1458460.

(287) Verdú EF, Armstrong D, Fraser R, Viani F, Idström JP, Cederberg C, Blum AL. Effect of Helicobacter pylori status on intragastric pH during treatment with omeprazole. Gut. 1995 Apr;36(4):539-43. doi: 10.1136/gut.36.4.539. PMID: 7737560; PMCID: PMC1382493.

(288) Scott P, Bruce C, Schofield D, Shiel N, Braganza JM, McCloy RF. Vitamin C status in patients with acute pancreatitis. Br J Surg. 1993 Jun;80(6):750-4. doi: 10.1002/bjs.1800800632. PMID: 8330166.

(289) Du WD, Yuan ZR, Sun J, Tang JX, Cheng AQ, Shen DM, Huang CJ, Song XH, Yu XF, Zheng SB. Therapeutic efficacy of high-dose vitamin C on acute pancreatitis and its potential mechanisms. World J Gastroenterol. 2003 Nov;9(11):2565-9. doi: 10.3748/wjg.v9.i11.2565. PMID: 14606098; PMCID: PMC4656542.

(290) Xu LL, Zhao B, Sun SL, Yu SF, Wang YM, Ji R, Yang ZT, Ma L, Yao Y, Chen Y, Sheng HQ, Chen EZ, Mao EQ. High-dose vitamin C alleviates pancreatic injury via the NRF2/NQO1/HO-1 pathway in a rat model of severe acute pancreatitis. Ann Transl Med. 2020 Jul;8(14):852. doi: 10.21037/atm-19-4552. PMID: 32793696; PMCID: PMC7396777.

(291) Su M, Liang X, Xu X, Wu X, Yang B. Hepatoprotective benefits of vitamin C against perfluorooctane sulfonate-induced liver damage in mice

through suppressing inflamma-tory reaction and ER stress. Environ Toxicol Pharmacol. 2019 Jan;65:60-65. doi: 10.1016/j.etap.2018.12.004. Epub 2018 Dec 5. PMID: 30551094.

(292) Yu SJ, Bae S, Kang JS, Yoon JH, Cho EJ, Lee JH, Kim YJ, Lee WJ, Kim CY, Lee HS. Hepatoprotective effect of vitamin C on lithocholic acid-induced cholestatic liver inju-ry in Gulo(-/-) mice. Eur J Pharmacol. 2015 Sep 5;762:247-55. doi: 10.1016/j.ejphar.2015.06.008. Epub 2015 Jun 6. PMID: 26057690.

(293) Liang T, Chen X, Su M, Chen H, Lu G, Liang K. Vitamin C exerts beneficial hepatoprotection against Concanavalin A-induced immunological hepatic injury in mice through inhibition of NF-κB signal pathway. Food Funct. 2014 Sep;5(9):2175-82. doi: 10.1039/c4fo00224e. PMID: 25030772.

(294) Mondal R, Biswas S, Chatterjee A, Mishra R, Mukhopadhyay A, Bhadra RK, Mukhopadhyay PK. Protection against arsenic-induced hematological and hepatic anomalies by supplementation of vitamin C and vitamin E in adult male rats. J Basic Clin Physiol Phar-macol. 2016 Nov 1;27(6):643-652. doi: 10.1515/jbcpp-2016-0020. PMID: 27464034.

(295) He Z, Li X, Yang H, Wu P, Wang S, Cao D, Guo X, Xu Z, Gao J, Zhang W, Luo X. Effects of Oral Vitamin C Supplementation on Liver Health and Associated Parameters in Patients With Non-Alcoholic Fatty Liver Disease: A Randomized Clinical Trial. Front Nutr. 2021 Sep 14;8:745609. doi: 10.3389/fnut.2021.745609. PMID: 34595203; PMCID: PMC8478121.

(296) Su M, Guo C, Liu M, Liang X, Yang B. Therapeutic targets of vitamin C on liver injury and associated biological mechanisms: A study of network pharmacology. Int Im-munopharmacol. 2019 Jan;66:383-387. doi: 10.1016/j.intimp.2018.11.048. Epub 2018 Dec 5. PMID: 30530052.

(297) Wang C, Lv H, Yang W, Li T, Fang T, Lv G, Han Q, Dong L, Jiang T, Jiang B, Yang G, Wang H. SVCT-2 determines the sensitivity to ascorbate-induced cell death in cholan-giocarcinoma cell lines and patient derived xenografts. Cancer Lett. 2017 Jul 10;398:1-11. doi: 10.1016/j.canlet.2017.03.039. Epub 2017 Apr 4. PMID: 28385602.

(298) Subramanian VS, Sabui S, Subramenium GA, Marchant JS, Said HM. Tumor necrosis factor alpha reduces intestinal vitamin C uptake: a role for NF-κB-mediated signaling. Am J Physiol Gastrointest Liver Physiol. 2018 Aug 1;315(2):G241-G248. doi: 10.1152/ajpgi.00071.2018. Epub 2018 Apr 6. PMID: 29631379; PMCID: PMC6139644.

(299) Xu J, Xu C, Chen X, Cai X, Yang S, Sheng Y, Wang T. Regulation of an antiox-idant blend on intestinal redox status and major microbiota in early weaned piglets. Nutrition. 2014 May;30(5):584-9. doi: 10.1016/j.nut.2013.10.018. Epub 2013 Oct 30. PMID: 24698350.

(300) Kondo K, Hiramoto K, Yamate Y, Goto K, Sekijima H, Ooi K. Ameliorative Ef-fect of High-Dose Vitamin C Administration on Dextran Sulfate Sodium-Induced Colitis Mouse Model. Biol Pharm Bull. 2019;42(6):954-959. doi: 10.1248/bpb.b18-00967. PMID: 31155592.

(301) Ali S, Hussain S, Khan R, Mumtaz S, Ashraf N, Andleeb S, Shakir HA, Tahir HM, Khan MKA, Ulhaq M. Renal toxicity of heavy metals (cadmium and mercury) and their amelioration with ascorbic acid in rabbits. Environ Sci Pollut Res Int. 2019 Feb;26(4):3909-3920. doi: 10.1007/s11356-018-3819-8. Epub 2018 Dec 13. PMID: 30547340.

(302) Lihm H, Kim H, Chang H, Yoon M, Lee K, Choi J. Vitamin C modulates lead excretion in rats. Anat Cell Biol. 2013 Dec;46(4):239-45. doi: 10.5115/acb.2013.46.4.239. Epub 2013 Dec 24. PMID: 24386596; PMCID: PMC3875841.

(303) Simon JA, Hudes ES. Relationship of ascorbic acid to blood lead levels. JAMA. 1999 Jun 23-30;281(24):2289-93. doi: 10.1001/jama.281.24.2289. PMID: 10386552.

(304) S. Gajawat, G. Sancheti and P. K. Goyal, "Vitamin C against Concomitant Ex-posure to Heavy Metal and Radiation: A Study on Variations in Hepatic Cellular Counts," Asian Journal of Experimental Sciences, Vol. 19, No. 2, 2005, pp. 53-58.

(305) Alexander MS, Wilkes JG, Schroeder SR, Buettner GR, Wagner BA, Du J, Gib-son-Corley K, O'Leary BR, Spitz DR, Buatti JM, Berg DJ, Bodeker KL, Vollstedt S, Brown HA, Allen BG, Cullen JJ. Pharmacologic Ascorbate

Reduces Radiation-Induced Normal Tissue Toxicity and Enhances Tumor Radiosensitization in Pancreatic Cancer. Cancer Res. 2018 Dec 15;78(24):6838-6851. doi: 10.1158/0008-5472.CAN-18-1680. Epub 2018 Sep 25. PMID: 30254147; PMCID: PMC6295907.

(306) Tetsuo Yamamoto and Manabu Kinoshita. Radioprotective Effect of Vitamin C as an Antioxidant. DOI: 10.5772/intechopen.68988.

(307) Semra Ozdemir, Yusuf Ziya Tan, Dilek Ulker Cakır, Kubilay Ukınc, Mehmet Aşık, d Fatmanur Çelik. Investigation of the effect of vitamin C on the oxidative stress parame-ters induced by i-131 treatment applied in patients with hyperthyroidism. Nuclear Medicine and Biomedical Imaging. DOI: 10.15761/NMBI.1000140.

(308) DOUGLASS CD, KAMP GH. The effect of orally administered rutin on the ad-renal ascorbic acid level in guinea pigs. J Nutr. 1959 Apr 10;67(4):531-6. doi: 10.1093/jn/67.4.531. PMID: 13642143.

(309) COTEREAU H, GABE M, et al. Influence of vitamin P (vitamin C2) upon the amount of ascorbic acid in the organs of the guinea pig. Nature. 1948 Apr 10;161(4093):557. doi: 10.1038/161557a0. PMID: 18915110.

(310) Carr AC, Vissers MC. Synthetic or food-derived vitamin C--are they equally bi-oavailable? Nutrients. 2013 Oct 28;5(11):4284-304. doi: 10.3390/nu5114284. PMID: 24169506; PMCID: PMC3847730.

(311) Carr AC, Bozonet SM, Vissers MC. A randomised cross-over pharmacokinetic bioavailability study of synthetic versus kiwifruit-derived vitamin C. Nutrients. 2013 Nov 11;5(11):4451-61. doi: 10.3390/nu5114451. PMID: 24284610; PMCID: PMC3847741.

(312) Davis JL, Paris HL, Beals JW, Binns SE, Giordano GR, Scalzo RL, Schweder MM, Blair E, Bell C. Liposomal-encapsulated Ascorbic Acid: Influence on Vitamin C Bioa-vailability and Capacity to Protect Against Ischemia-Reperfusion Injury. Nutr Metab Insights. 2016 Jun 20;9:25-30. doi: 10.4137/NMI.S39764. PMID: 27375360; PMCID: PMC4915787.

(313) Gopi S, Balakrishnan P. Evaluation and clinical comparison studies on liposo-mal and non-liposomal ascorbic acid (vitamin C) and their enhanced

bioavailability. J Lipo-some Res. 2021 Dec;31(4):356-364. doi: 10.1080/08982104.2020.1820521. Epub 2020 Oct 6. PMID: 32901526.

(314) Parhizkar E, Rashedinia M, Karimi M, Alipour S. Design and development of vitamin C-encapsulated proliposome with improved in-vitro and ex-vivo antioxidant efficacy. J Microencapsul. 2018 May;35(3):301-311. doi: 10.1080/02652048.2018.1477845. Epub 2018 Jun 6. PMID: 29781344.

(315) Elmore AR. Final report of the safety assessment of L-Ascorbic Acid, Calcium Ascorbate, Magnesium Ascorbate, Magnesium Ascorbyl Phosphate, Sodium Ascorbate, and Sodium Ascorbyl Phosphate as used in cosmetics. Int J Toxicol. 2005;24 Suppl 2:51-111. doi: 10.1080/10915810590953851. PMID: 16154915.

(316) Jiang K, Tang K, Liu H, Xu H, Ye Z, Chen Z. Ascorbic Acid Supplements and Kidney Stones Incidence Among Men and Women: A systematic review and meta-analysis. Urol J. 2019 May 5;16(2):115-120. doi: 10.22037/uj.v0i0.4275. PMID: 30178451.

(317) Gerster H. No contribution of ascorbic acid to renal calcium oxalate stones. Ann Nutr Metab. 1997;41(5):269-82. doi: 10.1159/000177954. PMID: 9429689.

(318) Thomas LD, Elinder CG, Tiselius HG, Wolk A, Akesson A. Ascorbic acid sup-plements and kidney stone incidence among men: a prospective study. JAMA Intern Med. 2013 Mar 11;173(5):386-8. doi: 10.1001/jamainternmed.2013.2296. PMID: 23381591.

(319) Prier M, Carr AC, Baillie N. No Reported Renal Stones with Intravenous Vita-min C Administration: A Prospective Case Series Study. Antioxidants (Basel). 2018 May 21;7(5):68. doi: 10.3390/antiox7050068. PMID: 29883396; PMCID: PMC5981254.

(320) Takahashi N, Morimoto S, Okigaki M, Seo M, Someya K, Morita T, Matsubara H, Sugiura T, Iwasaka T. Decreased plasma level of vitamin C in chronic kidney disease: com-parison between diabetic and non-diabetic patients. Nephrol Dial Transplant. 2011 Apr;26(4):1252-7. doi: 10.1093/ndt/gfq547. Epub 2010 Sep 3. PMID: 20817670.

(321) Chaghouri P, Maalouf N, Peters SL, Nowak PJ, Peczek K, Zasowska-Nowak A, Nowicki M. Two Faces of Vitamin C in Hemodialysis Patients: Relation to Oxidative Stress and Inflammation. Nutrients. 2021 Feb 27;13(3):791. doi: 10.3390/nu13030791. PMID: 33673687; PMCID: PMC7997461.

(322) Karahan S, Afsar B, Kanbay M. Ascorbic acid: a promising agent in chronic kidney disease? Clin Kidney J. 2018 Aug;11(4):530-531. doi: 10.1093/ckj/sfy044. Epub 2018 Jun 26. PMID: 30094017; PMCID: PMC6070088.

(323) Kun-Ying Zhang, Li Zuo. Vitamin C supplementation in patients on mainte-nance dialysis. World J Clin Urol. Nov 24, 2014; 3(3): 344-350. Published online Nov 24, 2014. doi: 10.5410/wjcu.v3.i3.344.

(324) Lee JK, Jung SH, Lee SE, Han JH, Jo E, Park HS, Heo KS, Kim D, Park JS, Myung CS. Alleviation of ascorbic acid-induced gastric high acidity by calcium ascorbate in vitro and in vivo. Korean J Physiol Pharmacol. 2018 Jan;22(1):35-42. doi: 10.4196/kjpp.2018.22.1.35. Epub 2017 Dec 22. PMID: 29302210; PMCID: PMC5746510.

(325) Marik PE. Is intravenous vitamin C contraindicated in patients with G6PD defi-ciency? Crit Care. 2019 Apr 3;23(1):109. doi: 10.1186/s13054-019-2397-6. PMID: 30944032; PMCID: PMC6448313.

(326) Rino PB, Scolnik D, Fustiñana A, Mitelpunkt A, Glatstein M. Ascorbic acid for the treatment of methemoglobinemia: the experience of a large tertiary care pediatric hospital. Am J Ther. 2014 Jul-Aug;21(4):240-3. doi: 10.1097/MJT.0000000000000028. PMID: 24914501.

(327) Gan R, Eintracht S, Hoffer LJ. Vitamin C deficiency in a university teaching hospital. J Am Coll Nutr. 2008 Jun;27(3):428-33. doi: 10.1080/07315724.2008.10719721. PMID: 18838532.

(328) Sharma Y, Miller M, Shahi R, Doyle A, Horwood C, Hakendorf P, Thompson C. Vitamin C deficiency in Australian hospitalised patients: an observational study. Intern Med J. 2019 Feb;49(2):189-196. doi: 10.1111/imj.14030. PMID: 29968401.

(329) Basu TK. Vitamin C-aspirin interactions. Int J Vitam Nutr Res Suppl. 1982;23:83-90. PMID: 6811490.

(330) Candelario-Jalil E, Akundi RS, Bhatia HS, Lieb K, Appel K, Muñoz E, Hüll M, Fiebich BL. Ascorbic acid enhances the inhibitory effect of aspirin on neuronal cyclooxygen-ase-2-mediated prostaglandin E2 production. J Neuroimmunol. 2006 May;174(1-2):39-51. doi: 10.1016/j.jneuroim.2006.01.003. Epub 2006 Mar 10. PMID: 16529823.

(331) Konturek PC, Kania J, Gessner U, Konturek SJ, Hahn EG, Konturek JW. Effect of vitamin C-releasing acetylsalicylic acid on gastric mucosal damage before and after Helico-bacter pylori eradication therapy. Eur J Pharmacol. 2004 Dec 15;506(2):169-77. doi: 10.1016/j.ejphar.2004.10.048. PMID: 15588738.

(332) Aşcı H, Saygın M, Yeşilot Ş, Topsakal Ş, Cankara FN, Özmen Ö, Savran M. Protective effects of aspirin and vitamin C against corn syrup consumption-induced cardiac damage through sirtuin-1 and HIF-1α pathway. Anatol J Cardiol. 2016 Sep;16(9):648-54. doi: 10.5152/AnatolJCardiol.2015.6418. Epub 2015 Sep 15. PMID: 26645266; PMCID: PMC5331347.

(333) Wang SM, Fan JH, Taylor PR, Lam TK, Dawsey SM, Qiao YL, Abnet CC. As-sociation of plasma vitamin C concentration to total and cause-specific mortality: a 16-year prospective study in China. J Epidemiol Community Health. 2018 Dec;72(12):1076-1082. doi: 10.1136/jech-2018-210809. Epub 2018 Aug 12. PMID: 30100578; PMCID: PMC7579680.

(334) Khaw KT, Bingham S, Welch A, Luben R, Wareham N, Oakes S, Day N. Rela-tion between plasma ascorbic acid and mortality in men and women in EPIC-Norfolk prospec-tive study: a prospective population study. European Prospective Investigation into Cancer and Nutrition. Lancet. 2001 Mar 3;357(9257):657-63. doi: 10.1016/s0140-6736(00)04128-3. PMID: 11247548.

(335) Tveden-Nyborg P. Vitamin C Deficiency in the Young Brain-Findings from Ex-perimental Animal Models. Nutrients. 2021 May 15;13(5):1685. doi: 10.3390/nu13051685. PMID: 34063417; PMCID: PMC8156420.

(336) Mosdøl A, Erens B, Brunner EJ. Estimated prevalence and predictors of vitamin C deficiency within UK's low-income population. J Public Health (Oxf). 2008 Dec;30(4):456-60. doi: 10.1093/pubmed/fdn076. Epub 2008 Sep 23. PMID: 18812436.

(337) D.S. Hickey, Ph.D.; H.J. Roberts, Ph.D.; R.F. Cathcart, M.D. Dynamic Flow: A New Model for Ascorbate. Journal of Orthomolecular Medicine Vol. 20, No. 4, 2005.

(338) Patterson T, Isales CM, Fulzele S. Low level of Vitamin C and dysregulation of Vitamin C transporter might be involved in the severity of COVID-19 Infection. Aging Dis. 2021 Feb 1;12(1):14-26. doi: 10.14336/AD.2020.0918. PMID: 33532123; PMCID: PMC7801272.

(339) Boretti A, Banik BK. Intravenous vitamin C for reduction of cytokines storm in acute respiratory distress syndrome. PharmaNutrition. 2020 Jun;12:100190. doi: 10.1016/j.phanu.2020.100190. Epub 2020 Apr 21. PMID: 32322486; PMCID: PMC7172861.

(340) Moretti M, Fraga DB, Rodrigues ALS. Ascorbic Acid to Manage Psychiatric Disorders. CNS Drugs. 2017 Jul;31(7):571-583. doi: 10.1007/s40263-017-0446-8. PMID: 28600627.

(341) Vetvicka V, Vetvickova J. Combination of glucan, resveratrol and vitamin C demonstrates strong anti-tumor potential. Anticancer Res. 2012 Jan;32(1):81-7. Erratum in: An-ticancer Res. 2012 Feb;32(2):713. PMID: 22213291.

(342) Saitoh Y, Umezaki T, Yonekura N, Nakawa A. Resveratrol potentiates intracel-lular ascorbic acid enrichment through dehydroascorbic acid transport and/or its intracellular reduction in HaCaT cells. Mol Cell Biochem. 2020 Apr;467(1-2):57-64. doi: 10.1007/s11010-020-03700-2. Epub 2020 Feb 21. PMID: 32080778.

(343) Chung JH, Kim S, Lee SJ, Chung JO, Oh YJ, Shim SM. Green tea formulations with vitamin C and xylitol on enhanced intestinal transport of green tea catechins. J Food Sci. 2013 May;78(5):C685-90. doi: 10.1111/1750-3841.12112. Epub 2013 Apr 1. PMID: 23551173.

(344) Karade PG, Jadhav NR. Colon targeted curcumin microspheres laden with ascorbic acid for bioavailability enhancement. J Microencapsul. 2018 Jun;35(4):372-380. doi: 10.1080/02652048.2018.1501111. PMID: 30010458.

(345) de Oliveira IJ, de Souza VV, Motta V, Da-Silva SL. Effects of Oral Vitamin C Supplementation on Anxiety in Students: A Double-Blind,

Randomized, Placebo-Controlled Trial. Pak J Biol Sci. 2015 Jan;18(1):11-8. doi: 10.3923/pjbs.2015.11.18. PMID: 26353411.

(346) Pascoe MC, Thompson DR, Jenkins ZM, Ski CF. Mindfulness mediates the physiological markers of stress: Systematic review and meta-analysis. J Psychiatr Res. 2017 Dec;95:156-178. doi: 10.1016/j.jpsychires.2017.08.004. Epub 2017 Aug 23. PMID: 28863392.

(347) Purkayastha SS, Sharma RP, Ilavazhagan G, Sridharan K, Ranganathan S, Selvamurthy W. Effect of vitamin C and E in modulating peripheral vascular response to local cold stimulus in man at high altitude. Jpn J Physiol. 1999 Apr;49(2):159-67. doi: 10.2170/jjphysiol.49.159. PMID: 10393350.

(348) Hu X, Yuan L, Wang H, Li C, Cai J, Hu Y, Ma C. Efficacy and safety of vitamin C for atrial fibrillation after cardiac surgery: A meta-analysis with trial sequential analysis of randomized controlled trials. Int J Surg. 2017 Jan;37:58-64. doi: 10.1016/j.ijsu.2016.12.009. Epub 2016 Dec 9. PMID: 27956113.

(349) Dombrowski Y, O'Hagan T, Dittmer M, Penalva R, Mayoral SR, Bankhead P, Fle-ville S, Eleftheriadis G, Zhao C, Naughton M, Hassan R, Moffat J, Falconer J, Boyd A, Hamil-ton P, Allen IV, Kissenpfennig A, Moynagh PN, Evergren E, Perbal B, Williams AC, Ingram RJ, Chan JR, Franklin RJM, Fitzgerald DC. Regulatory T cells promote myelin regeneration in the central nervous system. Nat Neurosci. 2017 May;20(5):674-680. doi: 10.1038/nn.4528. Epub 2017 Mar 13. PMID: 28288125; PMCID: PMC5409501.

(350) Ravindran RD, Vashist P, Gupta SK, Young IS, Maraini G, Camparini M, Jayanthi R, John N, Fitzpatrick KE, Chakravarthy U, Ravilla TD, Fletcher AE. Prevalence and risk fac-tors for vitamin C deficiency in north and south India: a two centre population based study in people aged 60 years and over. PLoS One. 2011;6(12):e28588. doi: 10.1371/journal.pone.0028588. Epub 2011 Dec 6. PMID: 22163038; PMCID: PMC3232233.

(351) Ried K, Travica N, Sali A. The acute effect of high-dose intravenous vitamin C and other nutrients on blood pressure: a cohort study. Blood Press Monit. 2016 Jun;21(3):160-7. doi: 10.1097/MBP.0000000000000178. PMID: 26910646; PMCID: PMC4864764.

(352) Na IS, Nguyen K, Potenzi B, Cheah M. Now you C me: a case of scurvy present-ing as depression and anaemia. BMJ Case Rep. 2020 Mar 4;13(3):e233645. doi: 10.1136/bcr-2019-233645. PMID: 32139451; PMCID: PMC7059414.

(353) Wilson R, Willis J, Gearry R, Skidmore P, Fleming E, Frampton C, Carr A. Inade-quate Vitamin C Status in Prediabetes and Type 2 Diabetes Mellitus: Associations with Gly-caemic Control, Obesity, and Smoking. Nutrients. 2017 Sep 9;9(9):997. doi: 10.3390/nu9090997. PMID: 28891932; PMCID: PMC5622757.

(354) Cho YW, Yoo WS, Kim SJ, Chung IY, Seo SW, Yoo JM. Efficacy of systemic vit-amin C supplementation in reducing corneal opacity resulting from infectious keratitis. Medi-cine (Baltimore). 2014 Nov;93(23):e125. doi: 10.1097/MD.0000000000000125. PMID: 25415664; PMCID: PMC4616340.

(355) Berger UV, Lu XC, Liu W, Tang Z, Slusher BS, Hediger MA. Effect of middle cerebral artery occlusion on mRNA expression for the sodium-coupled vitamin C transporter SVCT2 in rat brain. J Neurochem. 2003 Aug;86(4):896-906. doi: 10.1046/j.1471-4159.2003.01891.x. PMID: 12887688.

(356) Xu Y, Zheng X, Liang B, Gao J, Gu Z. Vitamins for Prevention of Contrast-induced Acute Kidney Injury: A Systematic Review and Trial Sequential Analysis. Am J Car-diovasc Drugs. 2018 Oct;18(5):373-386. doi: 10.1007/s40256-018-0274-3. PMID: 29633091.

(357) Brahma B, Forman RE, Stewart EE, Nicholson C, Rice ME. Ascorbate inhibits edema in brain slices. J Neurochem. 2000 Mar;74(3):1263-70. doi: 10.1046/j.1471-4159.2000.741263.x. PMID: 10693960.

(358) McNulty PH, Robertson BJ, Tulli MA, Hess J, Harach LA, Scott S, Sinoway LI. Effect of hyperoxia and vitamin C on coronary blood flow in patients with ischemic heart dis-ease. J Appl Physiol (1985). 2007 May;102(5):2040-5. doi: 10.1152/japplphysiol.00595.2006. Epub 2007 Feb 15. PMID: 17303710.

(359) Johnston CS, Martin LJ, Cai X. Antihistamine effect of supplemental ascorbic ac-id and neutrophil chemotaxis. J Am Coll Nutr. 1992 Apr;11(2):172-6. PMID: 1578094.

(360) He H , Qiao Y , Zhang Z , Wu Z , Liu D , Liao Z , Yin D , He M . Dual action of vitamin C in iron supplement therapeutics for iron deficiency anemia: prevention of liver dam-age induced by iron overload. Food Funct. 2018 Oct 17;9(10):5390-5401. doi: 10.1039/c7fo02057k. PMID: 30272083.

(361) Lefferts EC, Hibner BA, Lefferts WK, Lima NS, Baynard T, Haus JM, Lane-Cordova AD, Phillips SA, Fernhall B. Oral vitamin C restores endothelial function during acute inflammation in young and older adults. Physiol Rep. 2021 Nov;9(21):e15104. doi: 10.14814/phy2.15104. PMID: 34762777; PMCID: PMC8582295.

(362) Leichtle SW, Sarma AK, Strein M, Yajnik V, Rivet D, Sima A, Brophy GM. High-Dose Intravenous Ascorbic Acid: Ready for Prime Time in Traumatic Brain Injury? Neurocrit Care. 2020 Feb;32(1):333-339. doi: 10.1007/s12028-019-00829-x. PMID: 31440996.

(363) Vissers MC, Bozonet SM, Pearson JF, Braithwaite LJ. Dietary ascorbate intake affects steady state tissue concentrations in vitamin C-deficient mice: tissue deficiency after suboptimal intake and superior bioavailability from a food source (kiwifruit). Am J Clin Nutr. 2011 Feb;93(2):292-301. doi: 10.3945/ajcn.110.004853. Epub 2010 Dec 1. PMID: 21123463.

(364) Henmi H, Endo T, Kitajima Y, Manase K, Hata H, Kudo R. Effects of ascorbic acid supplementation on serum progesterone levels in patients with a luteal phase defect. Fertil Steril. 2003 Aug;80(2):459-61. doi: 10.1016/s0015-0282(03)00657-5. PMID: 12909517.

(365) Moon JM, Chun BJ. The efficacy of high doses of vitamin C in patients with paraquat poisoning. Hum Exp Toxicol. 2011 Aug;30(8):844-50. doi: 10.1177/0960327110385633. Epub 2010 Oct 4. PMID: 20921062.

(366) Aghajanian P, Hall S, Wongworawat MD, Mohan S. The Roles and Mechanisms of Actions of Vitamin C in Bone: New Developments. J Bone Miner Res. 2015 Nov;30(11):1945-55. doi: 10.1002/jbmr.2709. Epub 2015 Oct 7. PMID: 26358868; PMCID: PMC4833003.

(367) Carr AC, Cook J. Intravenous Vitamin C for Cancer Therapy - Identifying the Current Gaps in Our Knowledge. Front Physiol. 2018 Aug

23;9:1182. doi: 10.3389/fphys.2018.01182. PMID: 30190680; PMCID: PMC6115501.

(368) Ugwa EA, Iwasam EA, Nwali MI. Low Serum Vitamin C Status Among Pregnant Women Attending Antenatal Care at General Hospital Dawakin Kudu, Northwest Nigeria. Int J Prev Med. 2016 Feb 11;7:40. doi: 10.4103/2008-7802.176166. PMID: 27014432; PMCID: PMC4785790.

(369) Yuki K, Murat D, Kimura I, Ohtake Y, Tsubota K. Reduced-serum vitamin C and increased uric acid levels in normal-tension glaucoma. Graefes Arch Clin Exp Ophthalmol. 2010 Feb;248(2):243-8. doi: 10.1007/s00417-009-1183-6. Epub 2009 Sep 8. PMID: 19763599.

(370) Li T, Zeng J, Li DH, Yang GY, Wang K, Deng HF, Jiang H. Efficacy of intrave-nous vitamin C intervention for septic patients: A systematic review and meta-analysis based on randomized controlled trials. Am J Emerg Med. 2021 Dec;50:242-250. doi: 10.1016/j.ajem.2021.08.012. Epub 2021 Aug 12. PMID: 34416515.

(371) Otten AT, Bourgonje AR, Peters V, Alizadeh BZ, Dijkstra G, Harmsen HJM. Vit-amin C Supplementation in Healthy Individuals Leads to Shifts of Bacterial Populations in the Gut-A Pilot Study. Antioxidants (Basel). 2021 Aug 12;10(8):1278. doi: 10.3390/antiox10081278. PMID: 34439526; PMCID: PMC8389205.

(372) Wacker DA, Burton SL, Berger JP, Hegg AJ, Heisdorffer J, Wang Q, Medcraft EJ, Reilkoff RA. Evaluating Vitamin C in Septic Shock: A Randomized Controlled Trial of Vitamin C Monotherapy. Crit Care Med. 2022 May 1;50(5):e458-e467. doi: 10.1097/CCM.0000000000005427. Epub 2022 Jan 5. PMID: 34982738.

(373) Mortazavi SM, Rahimi S, Mosleh-Shirazi MA, Arjomandi M, Soleimani A, Koohi Hossein-Abadi O, Haghani M, Alavi M. A Comparative Study on the Life-Saving Radi-oprotective Effects of Vitamins A, E, C and Over-the-Counter Multivitamins. J Biomed Phys Eng. 2015 Jun 1;5(2):59-66. PMID: 26157731; PMCID: PMC4479387.

(374) Sinclair AJ, Taylor PB, Lunec J, Girling AJ, Barnett AH. Low plasma ascorbate levels in patients with type 2 diabetes mellitus consuming adequate

dietary vitamin C. Diabet Med. 1994 Nov;11(9):893-8. doi: 10.1111/j.1464-5491.1994.tb00375.x. PMID: 7705029.

(375) Chen K, Suh J, Carr AC, Morrow JD, Zeind J, Frei B. Vitamin C suppresses oxi-dative lipid damage in vivo, even in the presence of iron overload. Am J Physiol Endocrinol Metab. 2000 Dec;279(6):E1406-12. doi: 10.1152/ajpendo.2000.279.6.E1406. PMID: 11093930.

(376) Vetvicka V, Vetvickova J. Glucan–resveratrol–vitamin C combination offers protection against toxic agents. Toxins (Basel). 2012 Nov 9;4(11):1301-8. doi: 10.3390/toxins4111301. PMID: 23202317; PMCID: PMC3509709.

(377) Guo H, Ding J, Liu Q, Li Y, Liang J, Zhang Y. Vitamin C and Metabolic Syn-drome: A Meta-Analysis of Observational Studies. Front Nutr. 2021 Oct 8;8:728880. doi: 10.3389/fnut.2021.728880. PMID: 34692744; PMCID: PMC8531097.

(378) Carr AC, Maggini S. Vitamin C and Immune Function. Nutrients. 2017 Nov 3;9(11):1211. doi: 10.3390/nu9111211. PMID: 29099763; PMCID: PMC5707683.

(379) Zhang J, Ying X, Lu Q, Kallner A, Xiu RJ, Henriksson P, Björkhem I. A single high dose of vitamin C counteracts the acute negative effect on microcirculation induced by smoking a cigarette. Microvasc Res. 1999 Nov;58(3):305-11. doi: 10.1006/mvre.1999.2183. PMID: 10527771.

(380) Jia L, Jia Q, Shang Y, Dong X, Li L. Vitamin C intake and risk of renal cell car-cinoma: a meta-analysis. Sci Rep. 2015 Dec 8;5:17921. doi: 10.1038/srep17921. PMID: 26643589; PMCID: PMC4672306.

(381) Winterbourn CC. Protection by ascorbate against acetylphenylhydrazine-induced Heinz body formation in glucose-6-phosphate dehydrogenase deficient erythrocytes. Br J Haematol. 1979 Feb;41(2):245-22. doi: 10.1111/j.1365-2141.1979.tb05853.x. PMID: 427033.

(382) Jensen MP, Jacobs BM, Dobson R, Bandres-Ciga S, Blauwendraat C, Schrag A, Noyce AJ; International Parkinson's Disease Genomics Consortium (IPDGC). Lower Lympho-cyte Count is Associated With Increased Risk of Parkinson's Disease. Ann Neurol. 2021 Apr;89(4):803-812. doi:

10.1002/ana.26034. Epub 2021 Feb 22. PMID: 33527442; PMCID: PMC9012149.

(383) Travica N, Ried K, Hudson I, Scholey A, Pipingas A, Sali A. The effects of cardiovascular and orthopaedic surgery on vitamin concentrations: a narrative review of the lit-erature and mechanisms of action. Crit Rev Food Sci Nutr. 2021 Oct 7:1-31. doi: 10.1080/10408398.2021.1983762. Epub ahead of print. PMID: 34619992.

(384) Colpo E, de Bem AF, Pieniz S, Schettert SD, dos Santos RM, Farias IL, Bertoncello I, Moreira CM, Barbosa NV, Moretto MB, Rocha JB. A single high dose of ascor-bic acid and iron is not correlated with oxidative stress in healthy volunteers. Ann Nutr Metab. 2008;53(2):79-85. doi: 10.1159/000162257. Epub 2008 Oct 14. PMID: 18852484.

(385) Aschauer S, Gouya G, Klickovic U, Storka A, Weisshaar S, Vollbracht C, Krick B, Weiss G, Wolzt M. Effect of systemic high dose vitamin C therapy on forearm blood flow reactivity during endotoxemia in healthy human subjects. Vascul Pharmacol. 2014 Apr;61(1):25-9. doi: 10.1016/j.vph.2014.01.007. Epub 2014 Feb 8. PMID: 24512733.

(386) Lee JY, Choi HY, Yune TY. Fluoxetine and vitamin C synergistically inhibits blood-spinal cord barrier disruption and improves functional recovery after spinal cord injury. Neuropharmacology. 2016 Oct;109:78-87. doi: 10.1016/j.neuropharm.2016.05.018. Epub 2016 May 30. PMID: 27256500.

(387) Chen C, Yang Q, Ma X. Synergistic effect of ascorbic acid and taurine in the treatment of a spinal cord injury-induced model in rats. 3 Biotech. 2020 Feb;10(2):50. doi: 10.1007/s13205-019-2032-x. Epub 2020 Jan 16. PMID: 32002341; PMCID: PMC6965563.

(388) Liao JW, Song YM. [Preliminary study of the effects of high-dose Vitamin C on acute spinal cord injury in rats]. Sichuan Da Xue Xue Bao Yi Xue Ban. 2004 Nov;35(6):854-7. Chinese. PMID: 15573773.

(389) N. Mikirova, A. Rogers, J. Casciari, P. Taylor. Effect of high dose intravenous ascorbic acid on the level of inflammation in patients with rheumatoid arthritis. Riordan Clinic, Wichita, USA.

DOI: 10.4236/mri.2012.12004.

(390) Chaitanya NC, Badam R, Siva Prasad Reddy G, Alwala A, Srinivas P, Saawarn N, Chintada S, Akhila M, Bontala P, Inamdar P, Mannava H. ANALGESIC EFFECT OF IN-TRAVENOUS ASCORBIC ACID VERSUS ACELCOFENAC POST-TRANSALVEOLAR EX-TRACTION: A CASE-CONTROL STUDY. J Popul Ther Clin Pharmacol. 2019 Aug 19;26(2):e43-e52. doi: 10.15586/jptcp.v26i2.626. PMID: 31577085.

(391) Bernardo D, Martínez-Abad B, Vallejo-Diez S, Montalvillo E, Benito V, Anta B, Fernández-Salazar L, Blanco-Quirós A, Garrote JA, Arranz E. Ascorbate-dependent decrease of the mucosal immune inflammatory response to gliadin in coeliac disease patients. Allergol Immunopathol (Madr). 2012 Jan-Feb;40(1):3-8. doi: 10.1016/j.aller.2010.11.003. Epub 2011 Mar 21. PMID: 21420224.

(392) de Grooth HJ, Manubulu-Choo WP, Zandvliet AS, Spoelstra-de Man AME, Girbes AR, Swart EL, Oudemans-van Straaten HM. Vitamin C Pharmacokinetics in Critically Ill Patients: A Randomized Trial of Four IV Regimens. Chest. 2018 Jun;153(6):1368-1377. doi: 10.1016/j.chest.2018.02.025. Epub 2018 Mar 6. PMID: 29522710.

(393) Zhang N, Zhao W, Hu ZJ, Ge SM, Huo Y, Liu LX, Gao BL. Protective effects and mechanisms of high-dose vitamin C on sepsis-associated cognitive impairment in rats. Sci Rep. 2021 Jul 15;11(1):14511. doi: 10.1038/s41598-021-93861-x. Erratum in: Sci Rep. 2022 Jan 28;12(1):1874. PMID: 34267240; PMCID: PMC8282649.

(394) Jung SY, Lee MT, Baek MS, Kim WY. Vitamin C for ≥ 5 days is associated with decreased hospital mortality in sepsis subgroups: a nationwide cohort study. Crit Care. 2022 Jan 5;26(1):3. doi: 10.1186/s13054-021-03872-3. PMID: 34983595; PMCID: PMC8728994.

(395) Hess AL, Halalau A, Dokter JJ, Paydawy TS, Karabon P, Bastani A, Baker RE, Balla AK, Galens SA. High-dose intravenous vitamin C decreases rates of mechanical ventila-tion and cardiac arrest in severe COVID-19. Intern Emerg Med. 2022 Mar 29:1–10. doi: 10.1007/s11739-022-02954-6. Epub ahead of print. PMID: 35349005; PMCID: PMC8961256.

(396) Neale RJ, Lim H, Turner J, Freeman C, Kemm JR. The excretion of large vita-min C loads in young and elderly subjects: an ascorbic acid tolerance

test. Age Ageing. 1988 Jan;17(1):35-41. doi: 10.1093/ageing/17.1.35. PMID: 3364309.

(397) Doshida Y, Itabashi M, Takei T, Takino Y, Sato A, Yumura W, Maruyama N, Ishigami A. Reduced Plasma Ascorbate and Increased Proportion of Dehydroascorbic Acid Levels in Patients Undergoing Hemodialysis. Life (Basel). 2021 Sep 28;11(10):1023. doi: 10.3390/life11101023. PMID: 34685394; PMCID: PMC8538838.

(398) Cree BAC, Cutter G, Wolinsky JS, Freedman MS, Comi G, Giovannoni G, Hartung HP, Arnold D, Kuhle J, Block V, Munschauer FE, Sedel F, Lublin FD; SPI2 investiga-tive teams. Safety and efficacy of MD1003 (high-dose biotin) in patients with progressive mul-tiple sclerosis (SPI2): a randomised, double-blind, placebo-controlled, phase 3 trial. Lancet Neurol. 2020 Dec;19(12):988-997. doi: 10.1016/S1474-4422(20)30347-1. Epub 2020 Oct 23. PMID: 33222767.

(399) Chiu D, Vichinsky E, Ho SL, Liu T, Lubin BH. Vitamin C deficiency in patients with sickle cell anemia. Am J Pediatr Hematol Oncol. 1990 Fall;12(3):262-7. doi: 10.1097/00043426-199023000-00003. PMID: 2240472.

(400) Righi NC, Schuch FB, De Nardi AT, Pippi CM, de Almeida Righi G, Puntel GO, da Silva AMV, Signori LU. Effects of vitamin C on oxidative stress, inflammation, muscle soreness, and strength following acute exercise: meta-analyses of randomized clinical trials. Eur J Nutr. 2020 Oct;59(7):2827-2839. doi: 10.1007/s00394-020-02215-2. Epub 2020 Mar 11. PMID: 32162041.

(401) Mason SA, Baptista R, Della Gatta PA, Yousif A, Russell AP, Wadley GD. High-dose vitamin C supplementation increases skeletal muscle vitamin C concentration and SVCT2 transporter expression but does not alter redox status in healthy males. Free Radic Biol Med. 2014 Dec;77:130-8. doi: 10.1016/j.freeradbiomed.2014.09.013. Epub 2014 Sep 19. PMID: 25242204.

(402) Farahani-Jam S, Yaghmaei M, Vahdat Shariatpanahi Z. Effect of intravenous ascorbic acid administration on hemorrhage and wound complications in total abdominal hys-terectomy: A prospective randomized clinical trial. Clin Nutr ESPEN. 2022 Jun;49:74-78. doi: 10.1016/j.clnesp.2022.03.024. Epub 2022 Mar 26. PMID: 35623878.

(403) DePhillipo NN, Aman ZS, Kennedy MI, Begley JP, Moatshe G, LaPrade RF. Efficacy of Vitamin C Supplementation on Collagen Synthesis and Oxidative Stress After Musculoskeletal Injuries: A Systematic Review. Orthop J Sports Med. 2018 Oct 25;6(10):2325967118804544. doi: 10.1177/2325967118804544. PMID: 30386805; PMCID: PMC6204628.

(404) Campbell EJ, Vissers MC, Bozonet S, Dyer A, Robinson BA, Dachs GU. Re-storing physiological levels of ascorbate slows tumor growth and moderates HIF-1 pathway ac-tivity in Gulo(-/-) mice. Cancer Med. 2015 Feb;4(2):303-14. doi: 10.1002/cam4.349. Epub 2014 Oct 30. PMID: 25354695; PMCID: PMC4329013.

(405) Gao P, Zhang H, Dinavahi R, Li F, Xiang Y, Raman V, Bhujwalla ZM, Felsh-er DW, Cheng L, Pevsner J, Lee LA, Semenza GL, Dang CV. HIF-dependent antitumorigenic effect of antioxidants in vivo. Cancer Cell. 2007 Sep;12(3):230-8. doi: 10.1016/j.ccr.2007.08.004. PMID: 17785204; PMCID: PMC2084208.

(406) Jarisch R, Weyer D, Ehlert E, Koch CH, Pinkowski E, Jung P, Kähler W, Girgensohn R, Kowalski J, Weisser B, Koch A. Impact of oral vitamin C on histamine levels and seasickness. J Vestib Res. 2014;24(4):281-8. doi: 10.3233/VES-140509. PMID: 25095772.

(407) Wang Y, Liu XJ, Robitaille L, Eintracht S, MacNamara E, Hoffer LJ. Effects of vitamin C and vitamin D administration on mood and distress in acutely hospitalized pa-tients. Am J Clin Nutr. 2013 Sep;98(3):705-11. doi: 10.3945/ajcn.112.056366. Epub 2013 Jul 24. PMID: 23885048.

(408) Murata A, Morishige F, Yamaguchi H. Prolongation of survival times of termi-nal cancer patients by administration of large doses of ascorbate. Int J Vitam Nutr Res Suppl. 1982;23:103-13. PMID: 6811475.

(409) Chen J, He J, Ogden LG, Batuman V, Whelton PK. Relationship of serum an-tioxidant vitamins to serum creatinine in the US population. Am J Kidney Dis. 2002 Mar;39(3):460-8. doi: 10.1053/ajkd.2002.31389. PMID: 11877564.

(410) Taylor A, Jacques PF, Nowell T, Perrone G, Blumberg J, Handelman G, Jozwiak B, Nadler D. Vitamin C in human and guinea pig aqueous, lens and

plasma in relation to intake. Curr Eye Res. 1997 Sep;16(9):857-64. doi: 10.1076/ceyr.16.9.857.5039. PMID: 9288446.

(411) Ferrigno L, Aldigeri R, Rosmini F, Sperduto RD, Maraini G; Italian-American Cataract Study Group. Associations between plasma levels of vitamins and cataract in the Ital-ian-American Clinical Trial of Nutritional Supplements and Age-Related Cataract (CTNS): CTNS Report #2. Ophthalmic Epidemiol. 2005 Apr;12(2):71-80. doi: 10.1080/09286580590932815. PMID: 16019690.

(412) Kim SM, Lim SM, Yoo JA, Woo MJ, Cho KH. Consumption of high-dose vitamin C (1250 mg per day) enhances functional and structural properties of serum lipopro-tein to improve anti-oxidant, anti-atherosclerotic, and anti-aging effects via regulation of anti-inflammatory microRNA. Food Funct. 2015 Nov;6(11):3604-12. doi: 10.1039/c5fo00738k. Epub 2015 Sep 3. PMID: 26333284.

(413) Bendich A, Langseth L. The health effects of vitamin C supplementation: a re-view. J Am Coll Nutr. 1995 Apr;14(2):124-36. doi: 10.1080/07315724.1995.10718484. Erra-tum in: J Am Coll Nutr 1995 Aug;14(4):398. Erratum in: J Am Coll Nutr 1995 Jun;14(3):218. PMID: 7790686.

(414) He J, Mao E, Xu W, Zhao B, Jing F, Bian X, Chen E. [High dose vitamin C significantly reduces the nephrotoxicity of vancomycin in critically ill patients]. Zhonghua Wei Zhong Bing Ji Jiu Yi Xue. 2020 Apr;32(4):468-472. Chinese. doi: 10.3760/cma.j.cn121430-20200110-00083. PMID: 32527355.

(415) LAHIRI S, LLOYD BB. The effect of stress and corticotrophin on the con-centrations of vitamin C in blood and tissues of the rat. Biochem J. 1962 Sep;84(3):478-83. doi: 10.1042/bj0840478. PMID: 14461597; PMCID: PMC1243700.

(416) Heuser G, Vojdani A. Enhancement of natural killer cell activity and T and B cell function by buffered vitamin C in patients exposed to toxic chemicals: the role of protein kinase-C. Immunopharmacol Immunotoxicol. 1997 Aug;19(3):291-312. doi: 10.3109/08923979709046977. PMID: 9248859.

(417) Park JH, Kim SY, Kim DW, Lee WG, Rhee KH, Youn HS. Correlation be-tween Helicobacter pylori infection and vitamin C levels in whole blood, plasma, and gastric juice, and the pH of gastric juice in Korean children. J Pediatr

Gastroenterol Nutr. 2003 Jul;37(1):53-62. doi: 10.1097/00005176-200307000-00009. PMID: 12827006.

(418) Jenab M, Riboli E, Ferrari P, Sabate J, Slimani N, Norat T, Friesen M, Tjøn-neland A, Olsen A, Overvad K, Boutron-Ruault MC, Clavel-Chapelon F, Touvier M, Boeing H, Schulz M, Linseisen J, Nagel G, Trichopoulou A, Naska A, Oikonomou E, Krogh V, Panico S, Masala G, Sacerdote C, Tumino R, Peeters PH, Numans ME, Bueno-de-Mesquita HB, Büchner FL, Lund E, Pera G, Sanchez CN, Sánchez MJ, Arriola L, Barricarte A, Quirós JR, Hallmans G, Stenling R, Berglund G, Bingham S, Khaw KT, Key T, Allen N, Carneiro F, Mahlke U, Del Giudice G, Palli D, Kaaks R, Gonzalez CA. Plasma and dietary vitamin C levels and risk of gastric cancer in the European Prospective Investigation into Cancer and Nutrition (EPIC-EURGAST). Carcinogenesis. 2006 Nov;27(11):2250-7. doi: 10.1093/carcin/bgl096. Epub 2006 Jun 14. PMID: 16774936.

(419) Asmaa Ibrahim, Taha K. Alloush, Yousry Abo Elnaga, Mohamed Hamdy*, Mohamed M. Fouad. Serum Level of Vitamin C in a Sample of Egyptian Patients with Multiple Sclerosis. Neuroscience and Medicine > Vol.10 No.4, December 2019. DOI: 10.4236/nm.2019.104029.

(420) Jubiz W, Ramirez M. Effect of vitamin C on the absorption of levothyroxine in patients with hypothyroidism and gastritis. J Clin Endocrinol Metab. 2014 Jun;99(6):E1031-4. doi: 10.1210/jc.2013-4360. Epub 2014 Mar 6. PMID: 24601693.

(421) Sihver L, Mortazavi SMJ. Biological Protection in Deep Space Missions. J Bi-omed Phys Eng. 2021 Dec 1;11(6):663-674. doi: 10.31661/jbpe.v0i0.1193. PMID: 34904063; PMCID: PMC8649166.

(422) Sawicka-Glazer E, Czuczwar SJ. Vitamin C: a new auxiliary treatment of epi-lepsy? Pharmacol Rep. 2014 Aug;66(4):529-33. doi: 10.1016/j.pharep.2014.02.016. Epub 2014 Mar 11. PMID: 24948051.

(423) Panjwani U, Yadav DK, Kumar A, Singh SB, Selvamurthy W. Effect of vita-min C and E supplementation in modulating the peripheral nerve conduction following cold exposure in humans. Int J Biometeorol. 2003 Dec;48(2):103-7. doi: 10.1007/s00484-003-0183-1. Epub 2003 Jun 24. PMID: 12827484.

(424) Chen P, Reed G, Jiang J, Wang Y, Sunega J, Dong R, Ma Y, Esparham A, Ferrell R, Levine M, Drisko J, Chen Q. Pharmacokinetic Evaluation of Intravenous Vitamin C: A Classic Pharmacokinetic Study. Clin Pharmacokinet. 2022 Sep;61(9):1237-1249. doi: 10.1007/s40262-022-01142-1. Epub 2022 Jun 25. PMID: 35750958; PMCID: PMC9439974.

(425) Luo X, Ng C, He J, Yang M, Luo X, Herbert TP, Whitehead JP. Vitamin C protects against hypoxia, inflammation, and ER stress in primary human preadipocytes and ad-ipocytes. Mol Cell Endocrinol. 2022 Oct 1;556:111740. doi: 10.1016/j.mce.2022.111740. Epub 2022 Aug 4. PMID: 35932980.

(426) Oberley TD, Oberley LW. Antioxidant enzyme levels in cancer. Histol Histo-pathol. 1997 Apr;12(2):525-35. PMID: 9151141.

(427) Frei B, Stocker R, England L, Ames BN. Ascorbate: the most effective anti-oxidant in human blood plasma. Adv Exp Med Biol. 1990;264:155-63. doi: 10.1007/978-1-4684-5730-8_24. PMID: 2244489.

(428) Chen Q, Espey MG, Krishna MC, Mitchell JB, Corpe CP, Buettner GR, Shacter E, Levine M. Pharmacologic ascorbic acid concentrations selectively kill cancer cells: action as a pro-drug to deliver hydrogen peroxide to tissues. Proc Natl Acad Sci U S A. 2005 Sep 20;102(38):13604-9. doi: 10.1073/pnas.0506390102. Epub 2005 Sep 12. PMID: 16157892; PMCID: PMC1224653.

(429) Chen Q, Espey MG, Sun AY, Lee JH, Krishna MC, Shacter E, Choyke PL, Pooput C, Kirk KL, Buettner GR, Levine M. Ascorbate in pharmacologic concentrations selec-tively generates ascorbate radical and hydrogen peroxide in extracellular fluid in vivo. Proc Natl Acad Sci U S A. 2007 May 22;104(21):8749-54. doi: 10.1073/pnas.0702854104. Epub 2007 May 14. PMID: 17502596; PMCID: PMC1885574.

(430) Drisko JA, Serrano OK, Spruce LR, Chen Q, Levine M. Treatment of pancre-atic cancer with intravenous vitamin C: a case report. Anticancer Drugs. 2018 Apr;29(4):373-379. doi: 10.1097/CAD.0000000000000603. PMID: 29438178; PMCID: PMC5882293.

(431) Hah YS, Chung HJ, Sontakke SB, Chung IY, Ju S, Seo SW, Yoo JM, Kim SJ. Ascorbic acid concentrations in aqueous humor after systemic vitamin C

supplementation in patients with cataract: pilot study. BMC Ophthalmol. 2017 Jul 11;17(1):121. doi: 10.1186/s12886-017-0515-2. PMID: 28693452; PMCID: PMC5504646.

(432) Ahmad F, Liu P. (Ascorb)ing Pb Neurotoxicity in the Developing Brain. Anti-oxidants (Basel). 2020 Dec 21;9(12):1311. doi: 10.3390/antiox9121311. PMID: 33371438; PMCID: PMC7767447.

(433) Holford P, Carr AC, Zawari M, Vizcaychipi MP. Vitamin C Intervention for Critical COVID-19: A Pragmatic Review of the Current Level of Evidence. Life (Basel). 2021 Nov 1;11(11):1166. doi: 10.3390/life11111166. PMID: 34833042; PMCID: PMC8624950.

(434) Basaqr R, Skleres M, Jayswal R, Thomas DT. The effect of dietary nitrate and vitamin C on endothelial function, oxidative stress and blood lipids in untreated hypercho-lesterolemic subjects: A randomized double-blind crossover study. Clin Nutr. 2021 Apr;40(4):1851-1860. doi: 10.1016/j.clnu.2020.10.012. Epub 2020 Oct 14. PMID: 33115598.

(435) Di Tano M, Raucci F, Vernieri C, Caffa I, Buono R, Fanti M, Brandhorst S, Curigliano G, Nencioni A, de Braud F, Longo VD. Synergistic effect of fasting-mimicking diet and vitamin C against KRAS mutated cancers. Nat Commun. 2020 May 11;11(1):2332. doi: 10.1038/s41467-020-16243-3. PMID: 32393788; PMCID: PMC7214421.

(436) Samadikhah J, Golzari SE, Sabermarouf B, Karimzadeh I, Tizro P, Moham-mad Khanli H, Ghabili K. Efficacy of Combination Therapy of Statin and Vitamin C in Com-parison with Statin in the Prevention of Post-CABG Atrial Fibrillation. Adv Pharm Bull. 2014;4(1):97-100. doi: 10.5681/apb.2014.015. Epub 2013 Dec 23. PMID: 24409416; PMCID: PMC3885376.

(437) Zeman M, Vecka M, Perlík F, Hromádka R, Staňková B, Tvrzická E, Žák A. Niacin in the Treatment of Hyperlipidemias in Light of New Clinical Trials: Has Niacin Lost its Place? Med Sci Monit. 2015 Jul 25;21:2156-62. doi: 10.12659/MSM.893619. PMID: 26210594; PMCID: PMC4523006.

(438) Jackson TS, Xu A, Vita JA, Keaney JF Jr. Ascorbate prevents the interac-tion of superoxide and nitric oxide only at very high physiological

concentrations. Circ Res. 1998 Nov 2;83(9):916-22. doi: 10.1161/01.res.83.9.916. PMID: 9797340.

(439) Lauer AC, Groth N, Haag SF, Darvin ME, Lademann J, Meinke MC. Dose-dependent vitamin C uptake and radical scavenging activity in human skin measured with in vivo electron paramagnetic resonance spectroscopy. Skin Pharmacol Physiol. 2013;26(3):147-54. doi: 10.1159/000350833. Epub 2013 May 24. PMID: 23689595.

(440) Sherman DL, Keaney JF Jr, Biegelsen ES, Duffy SJ, Coffman JD, Vita JA. Pharmacological concentrations of ascorbic acid are required for the beneficial effect on endo-thelial vasomotor function in hypertension. Hypertension. 2000 Apr;35(4):936-41. doi: 10.1161/01.hyp.35.4.936. PMID: 10775565.

(441) Hong SY, Hwang KY, Lee EY, Eun SW, Cho SR, Han CS, Park YH, Chang SK. Effect of vitamin C on plasma total antioxidant status in patients with paraquat intoxica-tion. Toxicol Lett. 2002 Jan 5;126(1):51-9. doi: 10.1016/s0378-4274(01)00431-3. PMID: 11738270.

(442) Tessier DM, Khalil A, Trottier L, Fülöp T. Effects of vitamin C supplemen-tation on antioxidants and lipid peroxidation markers in elderly subjects with type 2 diabetes. Arch Gerontol Geriatr. 2009 Jan-Feb;48(1):67-72. doi: 10.1016/j.archger.2007.10.005. Epub 2008 Feb 20. PMID: 18077012.

(443) Wayner DD, Burton GW, Ingold KU. The antioxidant efficiency of vita-min C is concentration-dependent. Biochim Biophys Acta. 1986 Oct 29;884(1):119-23. doi: 10.1016/0304-4165(86)90234-5. PMID: 3768406.

(444) Nakano K, Suzuki S. Stress-induced change in tissue levels of ascorbic acid and histamine in rats. J Nutr. 1984 Sep;114(9):1602-8. doi: 10.1093/jn/114.9.1602. PMID: 6206215.

(445) Suzuki S, Nakano K. Decrease in urinary excretion of ascorbic acid and his-tamine in rats after repeated immobilization stress. J Nutr. 1984 Feb;114(2):441-6. doi: 10.1093/jn/114.2.441. PMID: 6694003.

(446) Gillani SW, Sulaiman SAS, Abdul MIM, Baig MR. Combined effect of met-formin with ascorbic acid versus acetyl salicylic acid on diabetes-related cardiovascular com-plication; a 12-month single blind multicenter randomized

control trial. Cardiovasc Diabetol. 2017 Aug 14;16(1):103. doi: 10.1186/s12933-017-0584-9. PMID: 28807030; PMCID: PMC5556597.

(447) Jarosz M, Dzieniszewski J, Dabrowska-Ufniarz E, Wartanowicz M, Ziem-lanski S, Reed PI. Effects of high dose vitamin C treatment on Helicobacter pylori infection and total vitamin C concentration in gastric juice. Eur J Cancer Prev. 1998 Dec;7(6):449-54. doi: 10.1097/00008469-199812000-00004. PMID: 9926292.

(448) Zabet MH, Mohammadi M, Ramezani M, Khalili H. Effect of high-dose Ascorbic acid on vasopressor's requirement in septic shock. J Res Pharm Pract. 2016 Apr-Jun;5(2):94-100. doi: 10.4103/2279-042X.179569. PMID: 27162802; PMCID: PMC4843590.

(449) Fowler AA 3rd, Truwit JD, Hite RD, Morris PE, DeWilde C, Priday A, Fisher B, Thacker LR 2nd, Natarajan R, Brophy DF, Sculthorpe R, Nanchal R, Syed A, Sturgill J, Martin GS, Sevransky J, Kashiouris M, Hamman S, Egan KF, Hastings A, Spencer W, Tench S, Mehkri O, Bindas J, Duggal A, Graf J, Zellner S, Yanny L, McPolin C, Hollrith T, Kramer D, Ojielo C, Damm T, Cassity E, Wieliczko A, Halquist M. Effect of Vitamin C Infusion on Organ Failure and Biomarkers of Inflammation and Vascular Injury in Patients With Sepsis and Severe Acute Respiratory Failure: The CITRIS-ALI Randomized Clinical Trial. JAMA. 2019 Oct 1;322(13):1261-1270. doi: 10.1001/jama.2019.11825. Erratum in: JAMA. 2020 Jan 28;323(4):379. PMID: 31573637; PMCID: PMC6777268.

(450) Borrelli E, Roux-Lombard P, Grau GE, Girardin E, Ricou B, Dayer J, Suter PM. Plasma concentrations of cytokines, their soluble receptors, and antioxidant vitamins can predict the development of multiple organ failure in patients at risk. Crit Care Med. 1996 Mar;24(3):392-7. doi: 10.1097/00003246-199603000-00006. PMID: 8625625.

(451) Seno T, Inoue N, Matsui K, Ejiri J, Hirata K, Kawashima S, Yokoyama M. Functional expression of sodium-dependent vitamin C transporter 2 in human endothelial cells. J Vasc Res. 2004 Jul-Aug;41(4):345-51. doi: 10.1159/000080525. Epub 2004 Aug 15. PMID: 15340249.

(452) Harling L, Rasoli S, Vecht JA, Ashrafian H, Kourliouros A, Athanasiou T. Do antioxidant vitamins have an anti-arrhythmic effect following cardiac surgery? A meta-analysis of randomised controlled trials. Heart. 2011

Oct;97(20):1636-42. doi: 10.1136/heartjnl-2011-300245. Epub 2011 Aug 23. PMID: 21865202.

(453) Marcial-Vega V, Idxian Gonzalez-Terron G, Levy TE. Intravenous ascorbic acid and hydrogen peroxide in the management of patients with chikungunya. Bol Asoc Med P R. 2015 Jan-Mar;107(1):20-4. PMID: 26035980.

(454) Shi R, Li ZH, Chen D, Wu QC, Zhou XL, Tie HT. Sole and combined vita-min C supplementation can prevent postoperative atrial fibrillation after cardiac surgery: A sys-tematic review and meta-analysis of randomized controlled trials. Clin Cardiol. 2018 Jun;41(6):871-878. doi: 10.1002/clc.22951. Epub 2018 May 15. PMID: 29603289; PMCID: PMC6489881.

(455) Peters C, Kouakanou L, Kabelitz D. A comparative view on vitamin C ef-fects on αβ- versus γδ T-cell activation and differentiation. J Leukoc Biol. 2020 Jun;107(6):1009-1022. doi: 10.1002/JLB.1MR1219-245R. Epub 2020 Feb 7. PMID: 32034803.

(456) Baba Y, Kuroiwa A, Uitti RJ, Wszolek ZK, Yamada T. Alterations of T-lymphocyte populations in Parkinson disease. Parkinsonism Relat Disord. 2005 Dec;11(8):493-8. doi: 10.1016/j.parkreldis.2005.07.005. Epub 2005 Sep 9. PMID: 16154792.

(457) Cárcamo JM, Pedraza A, Bórquez-Ojeda O, Golde DW. Vitamin C sup-presses TNF alpha-induced NF kappa B activation by inhibiting I kappa B alpha phosphoryla-tion. Biochemistry. 2002 Oct 29;41(43):12995-3002. doi: 10.1021/bi0263210. PMID: 12390026.

(458) Rouleau L, Antony AN, Bisetto S, Newberg A, Doria C, Levine M, Monti DA, Hoek JB. Synergistic effects of ascorbate and sorafenib in hepatocellular carcinoma: New insights into ascorbate cytotoxicity. Free Radic Biol Med. 2016 Jun;95:308-322. doi: 10.1016/j.freeradbiomed.2016.03.031. Epub 2016 Mar 30. PMID: 27036367; PMCID: PMC4867251.

(459) Babar M, Abdel-Latif MM, Ravi N, Murphy A, Byrne PJ, Kelleher D, Reynolds JV. Pilot translational study of dietary vitamin C supplementation in Barrett's esoph-agus. Dis Esophagus. 2010 Apr;23(3):271-6. doi: 10.1111/j.1442-2050.2009.01027.x. Epub 2009 Nov 23. PMID: 19930402.

(460) Ellulu MS, Rahmat A, Patimah I, Khaza'ai H, Abed Y. Effect of vitamin C on inflammation and metabolic markers in hypertensive and/or diabetic obese adults: a ran-domized controlled trial. Drug Des Devel Ther. 2015 Jul 1;9:3405-12. doi: 10.2147/DDDT.S83144. PMID: 26170625; PMCID: PMC4492638.

(461) Li Y, Feng L, Zhang X, Huang L, Song J, Chen G, Zhang Y, Zhang C, Li W, Feng Z. Intraoperative Vitamin C Reduces the Dosage of Propofol in Patients Undergoing Total Knee Replacement. J Pain Res. 2021 Jul 19;14:2201-2208. doi: 10.2147/JPR.S319172. PMID: 34321919; PMCID: PMC8302814.

(462) Patel V, Fisher M, Voelker M, Gessner U. Gastrointestinal effects of the addition of ascorbic acid to aspirin. Pain Pract. 2012 Jul;12(6):476-84. doi: 10.1111/j.1533-2500.2011.00517.x. Epub 2011 Dec 7. PMID: 22151399.

(463) McAlindon ME, Muller AF, Filipowicz B, Hawkey CJ. Effect of allopuri-nol, sulphasalazine, and vitamin C on aspirin induced gastroduodenal injury in human volun-teers. Gut. 1996 Apr;38(4):518-24. doi: 10.1136/gut.38.4.518. PMID: 8707080; PMCID: PMC1383107.

(464) Dammann HG, Saleki M, Torz M, Schulz HU, Krupp S, Schürer M, Timm J, Gessner U. Effects of buffered and plain acetylsalicylic acid formulations with and without ascorbic acid on gastric mucosa in healthy subjects. Aliment Pharmacol Ther. 2004 Feb 1;19(3):367-74. doi: 10.1111/j.1365-2036.2004.01742.x. PMID: 14984384.

(465) Teixeira A, Carrié AS, Généreau T, Herson S, Cherin P. Vitamin C deficiency in elderly hospitalized patients. Am J Med. 2001 Oct 15;111(6):502. doi: 10.1016/s0002-9343(01)00893-2. PMID: 11690581.

(466) Paolini R, Bernardini G, Molfetta R, Santoni A. NK cells and interferons. Cytokine Growth Factor Rev. 2015 Apr;26(2):113-20. doi: 10.1016/j.cytogfr.2014.11.003. Epub 2014 Nov 13. PMID: 25443799.

(467) Pipino F, Molfetta L. The Cathcart elliptical orthocentric endoprosthesis. A long-term clinical and radiographic study. Ital J Orthop Traumatol. 1989 Mar;15(1):5-14. PMID: 2661497.

(468) Miyaue N, Kubo M, Nagai M. Ascorbic acid can alleviate the degradation of levodopa and carbidopa induced by magnesium oxide. Brain

Behav. 2022 Jul;12(7):e2672. doi: 10.1002/brb3.2672. Epub 2022 Jun 17. PMID: 35712877; PMCID: PMC9304850.

(469) De Nuccio F, Cianciulli A, Porro C, Kashyrina M, Ruggiero M, Calvello R, Miraglia A, Nicolardi G, Lofrumento DD, Panaro MA. Inflammatory Response Modulation by Vitamin C in an MPTP Mouse Model of Parkinson's Disease. Biology (Basel). 2021 Nov 9;10(11):1155. doi: 10.3390/biology10111155. PMID: 34827148; PMCID: PMC8614932.

(470) Nikolova G, Karamalakova Y, Gadjeva V. Reducing oxidative toxicity of L-dopa in combination with two different antioxidants: an essential oil isolated from Rosa Damascena Mill., and vitamin C. Toxicol Rep. 2019 Mar 22;6:267-271. doi: 10.1016/j.toxrep.2019.03.006. PMID: 30984563; PMCID: PMC6444129.

(471) Sharshar T, Carlier R, Blanchard A, Feydy A, Gray F, Paillard M, Raphael JC, Gajdos P, Annane D. Depletion of neurohypophyseal content of vasopressin in septic shock. Crit Care Med. 2002 Mar;30(3):497-500. doi: 10.1097/00003246-200203000-00001. PMID: 11990905.

(472) Dionne CE, Laurin D, Desrosiers T, Abdous B, Le Sage N, Frenette J, Mondor M, Pelletier S. Serum vitamin C and spinal pain: a nationwide study. Pain. 2016 Nov;157(11):2527-2535. doi: 10.1097/j.pain.0000000000000671. PMID: 27434504.

(473) Jang AY, Han SH, Sohn IS, Oh PC, Koh KK. Lipoprotein(a) and Cardio-vascular Diseases - Revisited. Circ J. 2020 May 25;84(6):867-874. doi: 10.1253/circj.CJ-20-0051. Epub 2020 Apr 24. PMID: 32336721.

(474) Gao L, Chong E, Pendharkar S, Phillips A, Ke L, Li W, Windsor JA. The Challenges and Effects of Ascorbic Acid Treatment of Acute Pancreatitis: A Systematic Re-view and Meta-Analysis of Preclinical and Clinical Studies. Front Nutr. 2021 Oct 26;8:734558. doi: 10.3389/fnut.2021.734558. PMID: 34765629; PMCID: PMC8576576.

(475) Siriwardena AK, Mason JM, Balachandra S, Bagul A, Galloway S, Formela L, Hardman JG, Jamdar S. Randomised, double blind, placebo controlled trial of intravenous antioxidant (n-acetylcysteine, selenium, vitamin C) therapy in severe acute pancreatitis. Gut. 2007 Oct;56(10):1439-44. doi:

10.1136/gut.2006.115873. Epub 2007 Mar 13. PMID: 17356040; PMCID: PMC2000286.

(476) Mahwash Siddiqi, MD, Francesca Bryan, M.D, Faran Bokhari, MD, MBA, 535 Vitamin C in the Management of Burn Patients: A Review of Benefits and Risks, Journal of Burn Care & Research, Volume 42, Issue Supplement_1, April 2021, Pages S115–S116.

(477) Chen H, Karne RJ, Hall G, Campia U, Panza JA, Cannon RO 3rd, Wang Y, Katz A, Levine M, Quon MJ. High-dose oral vitamin C partially replenishes vitamin C levels in patients with Type 2 diabetes and low vitamin C levels but does not improve endothelial dys-function or insulin resistance. Am J Physiol Heart Circ Physiol. 2006 Jan;290(1):H137-45. doi: 10.1152/ajpheart.00768.2005. Epub 2005 Aug 26. PMID: 16126809.

(478) Ashor AW, Werner AD, Lara J, Willis ND, Mathers JC, Siervo M. Effects of vitamin C supplementation on glycaemic control: a systematic review and meta-analysis of randomised controlled trials. Eur J Clin Nutr. 2017 Dec;71(12):1371-1380. doi: 10.1038/ejcn.2017.24. Epub 2017 Mar 15. PMID: 28294172.

(479) Kim GN, Yoo WS, Park MH, Chung JK, Han YS, Chung IY, Seo SW, Yoo JM, Kim SJ. Clinical Features of Herpes Simplex Keratitis in a Korean Tertiary Referral Center: Efficacy of Oral Antiviral and Ascorbic Acid on Recurrence. Korean J Ophthalmol. 2018 Oct;32(5):353-360. doi: 10.3341/kjo.2017.0131. PMID: 30311457; PMCID: PMC6182212.

(480) Woodward M, Tunstall-Pedoe H, McColl K. Helicobacter pylori infection reduces systemic availability of dietary vitamin C. Eur J Gastroenterol Hepatol. 2001 Mar;13(3):233-7. doi: 10.1097/00042737-200103000-00003. PMID: 11293441.

(481) Yoshinaga M, Ohtani A, Harada N, Fukuda Y, Nawata H. Vitamin C inhibits corpus gastritis in Helicobacter pylori-infected patients during acid-suppressive therapy. J Gastroenterol Hepatol. 2001 Nov;16(11):1206-10. doi: 10.1046/j.1440-1746.2001.02626.x. PMID: 11903736.

(482) Kamiji MM, Oliveira RB. Efeito da administração de vitamina C sobre a colonização do estômago por Helicobacter pylori [Effect of vitamin C

administration on gastric colonization by Helicobacter pylori]. Arq Gastroenterol. 2005 Jul-Sep;42(3):167-72. Portu-guese. doi: 10.1590/s0004-28032005000300008. Epub 2005 Sep 22. PMID: 16200253.

(483) Mirvish SS, Wallcave L, Eagen M, Shubik P. Ascorbate-nitrite reaction: possible means of blocking the formation of carcinogenic N-nitroso compounds. Science. 1972 Jul 7;177(4043):65-8. doi: 10.1126/science.177.4043.65. PMID: 5041776.

(484) CRESCENZO VM, CAYER D. Plasma vitamin C levels in patients with peptic ulcer; response to oral load test of ascorbic acid. Gastroenterology. 1947 Jun;8(6):754-61. PMID: 20251629.

(485) Zullo A, Rinaldi V, Hassan C, Diana F, Winn S, Castagna G, Attili AF. Ascorbic acid and intestinal metaplasia in the stomach: a prospective, randomized study. Ali-ment Pharmacol Ther. 2000 Oct;14(10):1303-9. doi: 10.1046/j.1365-2036.2000.00841.x. PMID: 11012475.

(486) Hoang BV, Lee J, Choi IJ, Kim YW, Ryu KW, Kim J. Effect of dietary vitamin C on gastric cancer risk in the Korean population. World J Gastroenterol. 2016 Jul 21;22(27):6257-67. doi: 10.3748/wjg.v22.i27.6257. PMID: 27468215; PMCID: PMC4945984.

(487) Zhang C, Williams MA, Sorensen TK, King IB, Kestin MM, Thompson ML, Leisenring WM, Dashow EE, Luthy DA. Maternal plasma ascorbic Acid (vitamin C) and risk of gestational diabetes mellitus. Epidemiology. 2004 Sep;15(5):597-604. doi: 10.1097/01.ede.0000134864.90563.fa. PMID: 15308960.

(488) Osaikhuwuomwan JA, Okpere EE, Okonkwo CA, Ande AB, Idogun ES. Plasma vitamin C levels and risk of preterm prelabour rupture of membranes. Arch Gynecol Obstet. 2011 Sep;284(3):593-7. doi: 10.1007/s00404-010-1741-5. Epub 2010 Nov 3. PMID: 21046131.

(489) Ilhan N, Celik E, Kumbak B. Maternal plasma levels of interleukin-6, C-reactive protein, vitamins C, E and A, 8-isoprostane and oxidative status in women with pre-term premature rupture of membranes. J Matern Fetal Neonatal Med. 2015 Feb;28(3):316-9. doi: 10.3109/14767058.2014.916674. Epub 2014 May 22. PMID: 24749795.

(490) Sharma R, Mehta S. Ascorbic Acid concentration and preterm premature rupture of membranes. J Obstet Gynaecol India. 2014 Dec;64(6):417-20. doi: 10.1007/s13224-014-0570-z. Epub 2014 May 18. PMID: 25489145; PMCID: PMC4257913.

(491) Domith I, Socodato R, Portugal CC, Munis AF, Duarte-Silva AT, Paes-de-Carvalho R. Vitamin C modulates glutamate transport and NMDA receptor function in the retina. J Neurochem. 2018 Feb;144(4):408-420. doi: 10.1111/jnc.14260. Epub 2017 Dec 14. PMID: 29164598.

(492) Majewska MD, Bell JA. Ascorbic acid protects neurons from injury induced by glutamate and NMDA. Neuroreport. 1990 Nov-Dec;1(3-4):194-6. doi: 10.1097/00001756-199011000-00004. PMID: 1983355.

(493) Sandstrom MI, Rebec GV. Extracellular ascorbate modulates glutamate dynamics: role of behavioral activation. BMC Neurosci. 2007 May 16;8:32. doi: 10.1186/1471-2202-8-32. PMID: 17506898; PMCID: PMC1884166.

(494) Zeng X, Dong X, Xiao Q, Yao J. Vitamin C Inhibits Ubiquitination of Glutamate Transporter 1 (GLT-1) in Astrocytes by Downregulating HECTD1. ACS Chem Neu-rosci. 2022 Mar 2;13(5):676-687. doi: 10.1021/acschemneuro.1c00845. Epub 2022 Feb 11. PMID: 35148069.

(495) Rice ME, Forman RE, Chen BT, Avshalumov MV, Cragg SJ, Drew KL. Brain antioxidant regulation in mammals and anoxia-tolerant reptiles: balanced for neuropro-tection and neuromodulation. Comp Biochem Physiol C Toxicol Pharmacol. 2002 Dec;133(4):515-25. doi: 10.1016/s1532-0456(02)00116-3. PMID: 12458180.

(496) Carr A, Frei B. Does vitamin C act as a pro-oxidant under physiological conditions? FASEB J. 1999 Jun;13(9):1007-24. doi: 10.1096/fasebj.13.9.1007. PMID: 10336883.

(497) A.Bikker, J.Wielders, R.van Loo, M.Loubert. Ascorbic acid deficiency impairs wound healing in surgical patients: Four case reports. International Journal of Surgery Open.

Volume 2, 2016, Pages 15-18. doi.org/10.1016/j.ijso.2016.02.009.

(498) Sadeghpour A, Alizadehasl A, Kyavar M, Sadeghi T, Moludi J, Gholizadeh F, Totonchi Z, Ghadrdoost B. Impact of vitamin C supplementation on post-cardiac surgery ICU and hospital length of stay. Anesth Pain Med. 2015 Feb 19;5(1):e25337. doi: 10.5812/aapm.25337. PMID: 25789244; PMCID: PMC4350190.

(499) Ballmer PE, Reinhart WH, Jordan P, Bühler E, Moser UK, Gey KF. De-pletion of plasma vitamin C but not of vitamin E in response to cardiac operations. J Thorac Cardiovasc Surg. 1994 Aug;108(2):311-20. Erratum in: J Thorac Cardiovasc Surg 1995 Oct;110(4 Pt 1):1072. PMID: 8041179.

(500) Wannamethee SG, Bruckdorfer KR, Shaper AG, Papacosta O, Lennon L, Whincup PH. Plasma vitamin C, but not vitamin E, is associated with reduced risk of heart failure in older men. Circ Heart Fail. 2013 Jul;6(4):647-54. doi: 10.1161/CIRCHEARTFAILURE.112.000281. Epub 2013 May 31. PMID: 23729199.

(501) Pfister R, Sharp SJ, Luben R, Wareham NJ, Khaw KT. Plasma vitamin C predicts incident heart failure in men and women in European Prospective Investigation into Cancer and Nutrition-Norfolk prospective study. Am Heart J. 2011 Aug;162(2):246-53. doi: 10.1016/j.ahj.2011.05.007. Epub 2011 Jul 7. PMID: 21835284.

(502) Hemilä H, Chalker E, de Man AME. Vitamin C May Improve Left Ventricular Ejection Fraction: A Meta-Analysis. Front Cardiovasc Med. 2022 Feb 25;9:789729. doi: 10.3389/fcvm.2022.789729. PMID: 35282368; PMCID: PMC8913583.

(503) Hemilä H, Chalker E. Bias against Vitamin C in Mainstream Medicine: Examples from Trials of Vitamin C for Infections. Life (Basel). 2022 Jan 3;12(1):62. doi: 10.3390/life12010062. PMID: 35054455; PMCID: PMC8779885.

(504) Mason SA, Keske MA, Wadley GD. Effects of Vitamin C Supplementation on Glycemic Control and Cardiovascular Risk Factors in People With Type 2 Diabetes: A GRADE-Assessed Systematic Review and Meta-analysis of Randomized Controlled Trials. Diabetes Care. 2021 Feb;44(2):618-630. doi: 10.2337/dc20-1893. PMID: 33472962.

(505) Xie ZQ, Li HX, Tan WL, Yang L, Ma XW, Li WX, Wang QB, Shang CZ, Chen YJ. Association of Serum Vitamin C With NAFLD and MAFLD Among Adults in the United States. Front Nutr. 2022 Feb 4;8:795391. doi: 10.3389/fnut.2021.795391. PMID: 35187020; PMCID: PMC8854786.

(506) Qian Y, Wang L, Qiang X, Weng H, Jiang J, Che X, Li Q, Wang Z. Choroidal and retinal thickness in patients with vitamin C deficiency using swept-source opti-cal coherence tomography. BMC Ophthalmol. 2022 Jul 18;22(1):311. doi: 10.1186/s12886-022-02530-8. PMID: 35850684; PMCID: PMC9290199.

(507) Ottone T, Faraoni I, Fucci G, Divona M, Travaglini S, De Bellis E, Marchesi F, Angelini DF, Palmieri R, Gurnari C, Giansanti M, Nardozza AM, Montesano F, Fabiani E, Lindfors Rossi EL, Cerretti R, Cicconi L, De Bardi M, Catanoso ML, Battistini L, Massoud R, Venditti A, Voso MT. Vitamin C Deficiency in Patients With Acute Myeloid Leu-kemia. Front Oncol. 2022 Jun 27;12:890344. doi: 10.3389/fonc.2022.890344. PMID: 35832559; PMCID: PMC9271703.

(508) Johnston CS, Cox SK. Plasma-Saturating intakes of vitamin C confer maximal antioxidant protection to plasma. J Am Coll Nutr. 2001 Dec;20(6):623-7. doi: 10.1080/07315724.2001.10719159. PMID: 11771678.

(509) Ceriello A, Novials A, Ortega E, Canivell S, La Sala L, Pujadas G, Buc-ciarelli L, Rondinelli M, Genovese S. Vitamin C further improves the protective effect of glu-cagon-like peptide-1 on acute hypoglycemia-induced oxidative stress, inflammation, and endo-thelial dysfunction in type 1 diabetes. Diabetes Care. 2013 Dec;36(12):4104-8. doi: 10.2337/dc13-0750. Epub 2013 Oct 15. Erratum in: Diabetes Care. 2014 Jul;37(7):2063. PMID: 24130351; PMCID: PMC3836129.

(510) Sargeant LA, Wareham NJ, Bingham S, Day NE, Luben RN, Oakes S, Welch A, Khaw KT. Vitamin C and hyperglycemia in the European Prospective Investigation into Cancer--Norfolk (EPIC-Norfolk) study: a population-based study. Diabetes Care. 2000 Jun;23(6):726-32. doi: 10.2337/diacare.23.6.726. PMID: 10840986.

(511) Irawati Y, Kusnoputranto H, Achmadi UF, Safrudin A, Sitorus A, Risandi R, Wangsamuda S, Setia Asih PB, Syafruddin D. Blood lead levels and lead toxicity in children aged 1-5 years of Cinangka Village, Bogor Regency.

PLoS One. 2022 Feb 23;17(2):e0264209. doi: 10.1371/journal.pone.0264209. PMID: 35196330; PMCID: PMC8865693.

(512) Hauptman M, Niles JK, Gudin J, Kaufman HW. Individual- and Community-Level Factors Associated With Detectable and Elevated Blood Lead Levels in US Children: Results From a National Clinical Laboratory. JAMA Pediatr. 2021 Dec 1;175(12):1252-1260. doi: 10.1001/jamapediatrics.2021.3518. PMID: 34570188; PMCID: PMC8477303.

(513) Tian N, Thrasher KD, Gundy PD, Hughson MD, Manning RD Jr. Antioxidant treatment prevents renal damage and dysfunction and reduces arterial pressure in salt-sensitive hypertension. Hypertension. 2005 May;45(5):934-9. doi: 10.1161/01.HYP.0000160404.08866.5a. Epub 2005 Apr 18. PMID: 15837840.

(514) Hunt JR, Mullen LM, Lykken GI, Gallagher SK, Nielsen FH. Ascorbic acid: effect on ongoing iron absorption and status in iron-depleted young women. Am J Clin Nutr. 1990 Apr;51(4):649-55. doi: 10.1093/ajcn/51.4.649. PMID: 2321571.

(515) Dakhale GN, Khanzode SD, Khanzode SS, Saoji A. Supplementation of vitamin C with atypical antipsychotics reduces oxidative stress and improves the outcome of schizophrenia. Psychopharmacology (Berl). 2005 Nov;182(4):494-8. doi: 10.1007/s00213-005-0117-1. Epub 2005 Oct 19. PMID: 16133138.

(516) Levine M, Conry-Cantilena C, Wang Y, Welch RW, Washko PW, Dhariwal KR, Park JB, Lazarev A, Graumlich JF, King J, Cantilena LR. Vitamin C pharmaco-kinetics in healthy volunteers: evidence for a recommended dietary allowance. Proc Natl Acad Sci U S A. 1996 Apr 16;93(8):3704-9. doi: 10.1073/pnas.93.8.3704. PMID: 8623000; PMCID: PMC39676.

(517) Minor T, Niessen F, Klauke H, Isselhard W. No evidence for a protective effect of ascorbic acid on free radical generation and liver injury after hemorrhagic shock in rats. Shock. 1996 Apr;5(4):280-3. doi: 10.1097/00024382-199604000-00008. PMID: 8721388.

(518) Lagowska-Lenard M, Stelmasiak Z, Bartosik-Psujek H. Influence of vitamin C on markers of oxidative stress in the earliest period of ischemic stroke.

Pharmacol Rep. 2010 Jul-Aug;62(4):751-6. doi: 10.1016/s1734-1140(10)70334-0. PMID: 20885017.

(519) Mittermayer F, Pleiner J, Schaller G, Zorn S, Namiranian K, Kapiotis S, Bartel G, Wolfrum M, Brügel M, Thiery J, Macallister RJ, Wolzt M. Tetrahydrobiopterin cor-rects Escherichia coli endotoxin-induced endothelial dysfunction. Am J Physiol Heart Circ Physiol. 2005 Oct;289(4):H1752-7. doi: 10.1152/ajpheart.00057.2005. Epub 2005 Jun 17. PMID: 15964928.

(520) Marcé-Grau A, Martí-Sánchez L, Baide-Mairena H, Ortigoza-Escobar JD, Pérez-Dueñas B. Genetic defects of thiamine transport and metabolism: A review of clini-cal phenotypes, genetics, and functional studies. J Inherit Metab Dis. 2019 Jul;42(4):581-597. doi: 10.1002/jimd.12125. Epub 2019 Jun 24. PMID: 31095747.

(521) Ghomian N, Hafizi L, Takhti Z. The role of vitamin C in prevention of preterm premature rupture of membranes. Iran Red Crescent Med J. 2013 Feb;15(2):113-6. doi: 10.5812/ircmj.5138. Epub 2013 Feb 5. PMID: 23682322; PMCID: PMC3652497.

(522) Wong SK, Chin KY, Ima-Nirwana S. Vitamin C: A Review on its Role in the Management of Metabolic Syndrome. Int J Med Sci. 2020 Jun 27;17(11):1625-1638. doi: 10.7150/ijms.47103. PMID: 32669965; PMCID: PMC7359392.

(523) Virno M, Bucci MG, Pecori-Giraldi J, Cantore G. Intravenous glycer-ol-vitamin C (sodium salt) as osmotic agents to reduce intraocular pressure. Am J Ophthalmol. 1966 Nov;62(5):824-33. doi: 10.1016/0002-9394(66)91905-2. PMID: 5928830.

(524) Fung TC, Vuong HE, Luna CDG, Pronovost GN, Aleksandrova AA, Riley NG, Vavilina A, McGinn J, Rendon T, Forrest LR, Hsiao EY. Intestinal serotonin and fluoxetine exposure modulate bacterial colonization in the gut. Nat Microbiol. 2019 Dec;4(12):2064-2073. doi: 10.1038/s41564-019-0540-4. Epub 2019 Sep 2. PMID: 31477894; PMCID: PMC6879823.

(525) Fan H, Kou J, Han D, Li P, Zhang D, Wu Q, He Q. Association between vitamin C intake and the risk of pancreatic cancer: a meta-analysis of

observational studies. Sci Rep. 2015 Sep 11;5:13973. doi: 10.1038/srep13973. PMID: 26360104; PMCID: PMC4566085.

(526) Polidori MC, Mecocci P, Frei B. Plasma vitamin C levels are de-creased and correlated with brain damage in patients with intracranial hemorrhage or head trauma. Stroke. 2001 Apr;32(4):898-902. doi: 10.1161/01.str.32.4.898. PMID: 11283389.

(527) Heller R, Unbehaun A, Schellenberg B, Mayer B, Werner-Felmayer G, Werner ER. L-ascorbic acid potentiates endothelial nitric oxide synthesis via a chemical sta-bilization of tetrahydrobiopterin. J Biol Chem. 2001 Jan 5;276(1):40-7. doi: 10.1074/jbc.M004392200. PMID: 11022034.

(528) Frei B, England L, Ames BN. Ascorbate is an outstanding antioxidant in human blood plasma. Proc Natl Acad Sci U S A. 1989 Aug;86(16):6377-81. doi: 10.1073/pnas.86.16.6377. PMID: 2762330; PMCID: PMC297842.

(529) Mastrangelo D, Pelosi E, Castelli G, Lo-Coco F, Testa U. Mechanisms of anti-cancer effects of ascorbate: Cytotoxic activity and epigenetic modulation. Blood Cells Mol Dis. 2018 Mar;69:57-64. doi: 10.1016/j.bcmd.2017.09.005. Epub 2017 Sep 21. PMID: 28954710.

(530) Lo-Coco F, Avvisati G, Vignetti M, Thiede C, Orlando SM, Iacobelli S, Ferrara F, Fazi P, Cicconi L, Di Bona E, Specchia G, Sica S, Divona M, Levis A, Fiedler W, Cerqui E, Breccia M, Fioritoni G, Salih HR, Cazzola M, Melillo L, Carella AM, Brandts CH, Morra E, von Lilienfeld-Toal M, Hertenstein B, Wattad M, Lübbert M, Hänel M, Schmitz N, Link H, Kropp MG, Rambaldi A, La Nasa G, Luppi M, Ciceri F, Finizio O, Venditti A, Fab-biano F, Döhner K, Sauer M, Ganser A, Amadori S, Mandelli F, Döhner H, Ehninger G, Schlenk RF, Platzbecker U; Gruppo Italiano Malattie Ematologiche dell'Adulto; German-Austrian Acute Myeloid Leukemia Study Group; Study Alliance Leukemia. Retinoic acid and arsenic trioxide for acute promyelocytic leukemia. N Engl J Med. 2013 Jul 11;369(2):111-21. doi: 10.1056/NEJMoa1300874. PMID: 23841729.

(531) Noguera NI, Pelosi E, Angelini DF, Piredda ML, Guerrera G, Piras E, Battistini L, Massai L, Berardi A, Catalano G, Cicconi L, Castelli G, D'Angiò A, Pasquini L, Graziani G, Fioritoni G, Voso MT, Mastrangelo D, Testa U, Lo-Coco F. High-dose ascorbate and arsenic trioxide selectively kill acute myeloid

leukemia and acute promyelocytic leukemia blasts in vitro. Oncotarget. 2017 May 16;8(20):32550-32565. doi: 10.18632/oncotarget.15925. PMID: 28427227; PMCID: PMC5464808.

(532) Miller PG, Ebert BL. Leukaemia: Vitamin C regulates stem cells and cancer. Nature. 2017 Sep 28;549(7673):462-464. doi: 10.1038/nature23548. Epub 2017 Sep 6. PMID: 28869971.

(533) Amr M, El-Mogy A, Shams T, Vieira K, Lakhan SE. Efficacy of vitamin C as an adjunct to fluoxetine therapy in pediatric major depressive disorder: a random-ized, double-blind, placebo-controlled pilot study. Nutr J. 2013 Mar 9;12:31. doi: 10.1186/1475-2891-12-31. PMID: 23510529; PMCID: PMC3599706.

(534) Gokce N, Keaney JF Jr, Frei B, Holbrook M, Olesiak M, Zachariah BJ, Leeuwenburgh C, Heinecke JW, Vita JA. Long-term ascorbic acid administration reverses endothelial vasomotor dysfunction in patients with coronary artery disease. Circulation. 1999 Jun 29;99(25):3234-40. doi: 10.1161/01.cir.99.25.3234. PMID: 10385496.

(535) Long CL, Maull KI, Krishnan RS, Laws HL, Geiger JW, Borghesi L, Franks W, Lawson TC, Sauberlich HE. Ascorbic acid dynamics in the seriously ill and in-jured. J Surg Res. 2003 Feb;109(2):144-8. doi: 10.1016/s0022-4804(02)00083-5. PMID: 12643856.

(536) Mills KT, Stefanescu A, He J. The global epidemiology of hyper-tension. Nat Rev Nephrol. 2020 Apr;16(4):223-237. doi: 10.1038/s41581-019-0244-2. Epub 2020 Feb 5. PMID: 32024986; PMCID: PMC7998524.

(537) Carr AC, Bozonet SM, Pullar JM, Simcock JW, Vissers MC. Human skeletal muscle ascorbate is highly responsive to changes in vitamin C intake and plasma concentrations. Am J Clin Nutr. 2013 Apr;97(4):800-7. doi: 10.3945/ajcn.112.053207. Epub 2013 Feb 27. PMID: 23446899; PMCID: PMC3607654.

(538) Bunton-Stasyshyn RK, Saccon RA, Fratta P, Fisher EM. SOD1 Function and Its Implications for Amyotrophic Lateral Sclerosis Pathology: New and Renascent Themes. Neuroscientist. 2015 Oct;21(5):519-29. doi: 10.1177/1073858414561795. Epub 2014 Dec 9. PMID: 25492944.

(539) Ngo B, Van Riper JM, Cantley LC, Yun J. Targeting cancer vulnerabilities with high-dose vitamin C. Nat Rev Cancer. 2019 May;19(5):271-282. doi: 10.1038/s41568-019-0135-7. PMID: 30967651; PMCID: PMC6526932.

(540) Levy T.E. MedFox Publishing; Henderson, NV, USA: 2012. Primal Panacea. 350 p.

(541) Song X, Qu H, Yang Z, Rong J, Cai W, Zhou H. Efficacy and Safety of L-Carnitine Treatment for Chronic Heart Failure: A Meta-Analysis of Randomized Con-trolled Trials. Biomed Res Int. 2017;2017:6274854. doi: 10.1155/2017/6274854. Epub 2017 Apr 13. PMID: 28497060; PMCID: PMC5406747.

(542) Gao X, Curhan G, Forman JP, Ascherio A, Choi HK. Vitamin C in-take and serum uric acid concentration in men. J Rheumatol. 2008 Sep;35(9):1853-8. Epub 2008 May 1. PMID: 18464304; PMCID: PMC2853937.

(543) Miller ER 3rd, Pastor-Barriuso R, Dalal D, Riemersma RA, Appel LJ, Guallar E. Meta-analysis: high-dosage vitamin E supplementation may increase all-cause mortality. Ann Intern Med. 2005 Jan 4;142(1):37-46. doi: 10.7326/0003-4819-142-1-200501040-00110. Epub 2004 Nov 10. PMID: 15537682.

(544) Joachim C, Macni J, Drame M, Pomier A, Escarmant P, Veronique-Baudin J, Vinh-Hung V. Overall survival of colorectal cancer by stage at diagnosis: Data from the Martinique Cancer Registry. Medicine (Baltimore). 2019 Aug;98(35):e16941. doi: 10.1097/MD.0000000000016941. PMID: 31464932; PMCID: PMC6736397.

(545) Wilson CW. Ascorbic acid function and metabolism during colds. Ann N Y Acad Sci. 1975 Sep 30;258:529-39. doi: 10.1111/j.1749-6632.1975.tb29312.x. PMID: 1106304.

(546) Hung KC, Lin YT, Chen KH, Wang LK, Chen JY, Chang YJ, Wu SC, Chiang MH, Sun CK. The Effect of Perioperative Vitamin C on Postoperative Analgesic Consumption: A Meta-Analysis of Randomized Controlled Trials. Nutrients. 2020 Oct 12;12(10):3109. doi: 10.3390/nu12103109. PMID: 33053814; PMCID: PMC7600013.

(547) Dingchao H, Zhiduan Q, Liye H, Xiaodong F. The protective ef-fects of high-dose ascorbic acid on myocardium against reperfusion injury during and

after cardiopulmonary bypass. Thorac Cardiovasc Surg. 1994 Oct;42(5):276-8. doi: 10.1055/s-2007-1016504. PMID: 7863489.

(548) Gardner R, Liu X, Wang Y, Cole A, Heydrick S, Donnino MW, Moskowitz A. Vitamin C levels amongst initial survivors of out of hospital cardiac arrest. Re-suscitation. 2020 Nov;156:190-193. doi: 10.1016/j.resuscitation.2020.09.005. Epub 2020 Sep 16. PMID: 32946985; PMCID: PMC7934834.

(549) Sil S, Ghosh T, Gupta P, Ghosh R, Kabir SN, Roy A. Dual Role of Vitamin C on the Neuroinflammation Mediated Neurodegeneration and Memory Impairments in Colchicine Induced Rat Model of Alzheimer Disease. J Mol Neurosci. 2016 Dec;60(4):421-435. doi: 10.1007/s12031-016-0817-5. Epub 2016 Sep 24. PMID: 27665568.

(550) Rice ME, Russo-Menna I. Differential compartmentalization of brain ascorbate and glutathione between neurons and glia. Neuroscience. 1998 Feb;82(4):1213-23. doi: 10.1016/s0306-4522(97)00347-3. PMID: 9466441.

(551) Rice ME, Lee EJ, Choy Y. High levels of ascorbic acid, not glu-tathione, in the CNS of anoxia-tolerant reptiles contrasted with levels in anoxia-intolerant spe-cies. J Neurochem. 1995 Apr;64(4):1790-9. doi: 10.1046/j.1471-4159.1995.64041790.x. PMID: 7891107.

(552) Basili S, Tanzilli G, Mangieri E, Raparelli V, Di Santo S, Pignatelli P, Violi F. Intravenous ascorbic acid infusion improves myocardial perfusion grade during elec-tive percutaneous coronary intervention: relationship with oxidative stress markers. JACC Car-diovasc Interv. 2010 Feb;3(2):221-9. doi: 10.1016/j.jcin.2009.10.025. PMID: 20170881.

(553) Chen P, Stone J, Sullivan G, Drisko JA, Chen Q. Anti-cancer effect of pharmacologic ascorbate and its interaction with supplementary parenteral glutathione in preclinical cancer models. Free Radic Biol Med. 2011 Aug 1;51(3):681-7. doi: 10.1016/j.freeradbiomed.2011.05.031. Epub 2011 May 30. PMID: 21672627.

(554) Sun H, Saeedi P, Karuranga S, Pinkepank M, Ogurtsova K, Duncan BB, Stein C, Basit A, Chan JCN, Mbanya JC, Pavkov ME, Ramachandaran A, Wild SH, James S, Herman WH, Zhang P, Bommer C, Kuo S, Boyko EJ,

Magliano DJ. IDF Diabetes Atlas: Global, regional and country-level diabetes prevalence estimates for 2021 and projections for 2045. Diabetes Res Clin Pract. 2022 Jan;183:109119. doi: 10.1016/j.diabres.2021.109119. Epub 2021 Dec 6. Erratum in: Diabetes Res Clin Pract. 2023 Oct;204:110945. PMID: 34879977.

(555) Kiondo P, Welishe G, Wandabwa J, Wamuyu-Maina G, Bimenya GS, Okong P. Plasma vitamin C concentration in pregnant women with pre-eclampsia in Mu-lago hospital, Kampala, Uganda. Afr Health Sci. 2011 Dec;11(4):566-72. PMID: 22649436; PMCID: PMC3362966.

(556) Madruga de Oliveira A, Rondó PH, Mastroeni SS, Oliveira JM. Plasma concentrations of ascorbic acid in parturients from a hospital in Southeast Brazil. Clin Nutr. 2008 Apr;27(2):228-32. doi: 10.1016/j.clnu.2007.11.006. Epub 2008 Jan 30. PMID: 18234398.

(557) Marik PE, Hooper MH. Doctor-your septic patients have scurvy! Crit Care. 2018 Jan 29;22(1):23. doi: 10.1186/s13054-018-1950-z. PMID: 29378661; PMCID: PMC5789732.

(558) Korantzopoulos P, Kolettis TM, Kountouris E, Dimitroula V, Ka-ranikis P, Pappa E, Siogas K, Goudevenos JA. Oral vitamin C administration reduces early re-currence rates after electrical cardioversion of persistent atrial fibrillation and attenuates asso-ciated inflammation. Int J Cardiol. 2005 Jul 10;102(2):321-6. doi: 10.1016/j.ijcard.2004.12.041. PMID: 15982504.

(559) Wójciak P, Remlinger-Molenda A, Rybakowski J. Rola oksytocyny i wazopresyny w czynności ośrodkowego układu nerwowego i w zaburzeniach psychicznych [The role of oxytocin and vasopressin in central nervous system activity and mental disorders]. Psychiatr Pol. 2012 Nov-Dec;46(6):1043-52. Polish. PMID: 23479945.

(560) Vecchio M, Chiaramonte R, Testa G, Pavone V. Clinical Effects of L-Carnitine Supplementation on Physical Performance in Healthy Subjects, the Key to Suc-cess in Rehabilitation: A Systematic Review and Meta-Analysis from the Rehabilitation Point of View. J Funct Morphol Kinesiol. 2021 Nov 4;6(4):93. doi: 10.3390/jfmk6040093. PMID: 34842765; PMCID: PMC8628984.

(561) Almassi GH, Schowalter T, Nicolosi AC, Aggarwal A, Moritz TE, Henderson WG, Tarazi R, Shroyer AL, Sethi GK, Grover FL, Hammermeister

KE. Atrial fibril-lation after cardiac surgery: a major morbid event? Ann Surg. 1997 Oct;226(4):501-11; discus-sion 511-3. doi: 10.1097/00000658-199710000-00011. PMID: 9351718; PMCID: PMC1191069.

(562) Hemilä H, Suonsyrjä T. Vitamin C for preventing atrial fibrilla-tion in high risk patients: a systematic review and meta-analysis. BMC Cardiovasc Disord. 2017 Feb 1;17(1):49. doi: 10.1186/s12872-017-0478-5. PMID: 28143406; PMCID: PMC5286679.

(563) Antonic M, Lipovec R, Gregorcic F, Juric P, Kosir G. Periop-erative ascorbic acid supplementation does not reduce the incidence of postoperative atrial fi-brillation in on-pump coronary artery bypass graft patients. J Cardiol. 2017 Jan;69(1):98-102. doi: 10.1016/j.jjcc.2016.01.010. Epub 2016 Feb 23. PMID: 26917198.

(564) Scott C, Lateef SS, Hong CG, Dey AK, Manyak GA, Patel NH, Zhou W, Sorokin AV, Abdelrahman K, Uceda D, Teklu M, Wu C, Parel PM, Sandfort V, Chen MY, Mallek M, Ahlman M, Bluemke D, Mehta NN. Inflammation, coronary plaque progression, and statin use: A secondary analysis of the Risk Stratification with Image Guidance of HMG CoA Reductase Inhibitor Therapy (RIGHT) study. Clin Cardiol. 2022 Jun;45(6):622-628. doi: 10.1002/clc.23808. Epub 2022 Apr 2. PMID: 35366378; PMCID: PMC9175258.

(565) Kuzkaya N, Weissmann N, Harrison DG, Dikalov S. Interactions of peroxynitrite, tetrahydrobiopterin, ascorbic acid, and thiols: implications for uncoupling endo-thelial nitric-oxide synthase. J Biol Chem. 2003 Jun 20;278(25):22546-54. doi: 10.1074/jbc.M302227200. Epub 2003 Apr 10. PMID: 12692136.

(566) Clavo B, Santana-Rodríguez N, Llontop P, Gutiérrez D, Suárez G, López L, Rovira G, Martínez-Sánchez G, González E, Jorge IJ, Perera C, Blanco J, Rodríguez-Esparragón F. Ozone Therapy as Adjuvant for Cancer Treatment: Is Further Research Warrant-ed? Evid Based Complement Alternat Med. 2018 Sep 9;2018:7931849. doi: 10.1155/2018/7931849. PMID: 30271455; PMCID: PMC6151231.

(567) Hattori M, Yamazaki M, Ohashi W, Tanaka S, Hattori K, Todoroki K, Fujimori T, Ohtsu H, Matsuda N, Hattori Y. Critical role of endogenous histamine in promoting end-organ tissue injury in sepsis. Intensive Care Med Exp. 2016

Dec;4(1):36. doi: 10.1186/s40635-016-0109-y. Epub 2016 Nov 8. PMID: 27822777; PMCID: PMC5099302.

(568) Sasidharan Nair V, Song MH, Oh KI. Vitamin C Facilitates Demethylation of the Foxp3 Enhancer in a Tet-Dependent Manner. J Immunol. 2016 Mar 1;196(5):2119-31. doi: 10.4049/jimmunol.1502352. Epub 2016 Jan 29. PMID: 26826239.

(569) Uciechowski P, Dempke WCM. Interleukin-6: A Masterplayer in the Cytokine Network. Oncology. 2020;98(3):131-137. doi: 10.1159/000505099. Epub 2020 Jan 20. PMID: 31958792.

(570) Essien EU. Plasma levels of retinol, ascorbic acid and alpha-tocopherol in sickle cell anaemia. Cent Afr J Med. 1995 Feb;41(2):48-50. PMID: 7788666.

(571) Feduska ET, Thoma BN, Torjman MC, Goldhammer JE. Acute Amiodarone Pulmonary Toxicity. J Cardiothorac Vasc Anesth. 2021 May;35(5):1485-1494. doi: 10.1053/j.jvca.2020.10.060. Epub 2020 Nov 5. PMID: 33262034.

(572) Nielsen TK, Højgaard M, Andersen JT, Jørgensen NR, Zerahn B, Kristensen B, Henriksen T, Lykkesfeldt J, Mikines KJ, Poulsen HE. Weekly ascorbic acid infu-sion in castration-resistant prostate cancer patients: a single-arm phase II trial. Transl Androl Urol. 2017 Jun;6(3):517-528. doi: 10.21037/tau.2017.04.42. PMID: 28725594; PMCID: PMC5503969.

(573) Ren X, Santhosh SM, Coppo L, Ogata FT, Lu J, Holmgren A. The combination of ascorbate and menadione causes cancer cell death by oxidative stress and rep-licative stress. Free Radic Biol Med. 2019 Apr;134:350-358. doi: 10.1016/j.freeradbiomed.2019.01.037. Epub 2019 Jan 28. PMID: 30703479.

(574) Viviano KR, Lavergne SN, Goodman L, Vanderwielen B, Grundahl L, Padilla M, Trepanier LA. Glutathione, cysteine, and ascorbate concentrations in clinically ill dogs and cats. J Vet Intern Med. 2009 Mar-Apr;23(2):250-7. doi: 10.1111/j.1939-1676.2008.0238.x. Epub 2008 Dec 16. PMID: 19143933.

(575) Lo BC, Chen GY, Núñez G, Caruso R. Gut microbiota and systemic immunity in health and disease. Int Immunol. 2021 Mar 31;33(4):197-209. doi: 10.1093/intimm/dxaa079. PMID: 33367688; PMCID: PMC8011437.

(576) Dumitrescu L, Popescu-Olaru I, Cozma L, Tulbă D, Hinescu ME, Ceafalan LC, Gherghiceanu M, Popescu BO. Oxidative Stress and the Microbiota-Gut-Brain Axis. Oxid Med Cell Longev. 2018 Dec 9;2018:2406594. doi: 10.1155/2018/2406594. PMID: 30622664; PMCID: PMC6304899.

(577) Abouzid M, Główka F, Kagan L, Karaźniewicz-Łada M. Vitamin D Metabolism Gene Polymorphisms and Their Associated Disorders: A Literature Re-view. Curr Drug Metab. 2022;23(8):630-651. doi: 10.2174/1389200223666220627104139. PMID: 35761493.

(578) Kanbay M, Afsar B, Siriopol D, Unal HU, Karaman M, Sa-glam M, Eyileten T, Gezer M, Verim S, Oguz Y, Vural A, Ortiz A, Johnson RJ, Covic A, Yil-maz MI. Relevance of uric acid and asymmetric dimethylarginine for modeling cardiovascular risk prediction in chronic kidney disease patients. Int Urol Nephrol. 2016 Jul;48(7):1129-36. doi: 10.1007/s11255-016-1271-6. Epub 2016 Mar 23. PMID: 27007614.

(579) Gillis K, Stevens KK, Bell E, Patel RK, Jardine AG, Mor-ris STW, Schneider MP, Delles C, Mark PB. Ascorbic acid lowers central blood pressure and asymmetric dimethylarginine in chronic kidney disease. Clin Kidney J. 2018 Aug;11(4):532-539. doi: 10.1093/ckj/sfx158. Epub 2018 Feb 6. PMID: 30094018; PMCID: PMC6070083.

(580) Guide book for intravenous Vitamin C for cancer treatment (Kadokawa SSC, 2009) (in Japanese)

(581) Guide Book for Chelation Therapy, (JCIT, 2008) (in Japanese)

(582) Adolfo Panfili Medicina Ortomolecolare. Una tera-pia a misura d'uomo; Tecniche Nuove (Agosto 1995)

(583) Wen C, Li Y, Hu Q, Liu H, Xu X, Lü M. IV Vitamin C in Sep-sis: A Latest Systematic Review and Meta-Analysis. Int J Clin Pract. 2023 Jan 24;2023:6733465. doi: 10.1155/2023/6733465. PMID: 36743822; PMCID: PMC9889164.

(584) Alissa A, Alrashed MA, Alshaya AI, Al Sulaiman K, Alharbi S. Reevaluating vitamin C in sep-sis and septic shock: a potential benefit in severe cases? Front Med (Lausanne). 2024 Oct 29;11:1476242. doi: 10.3389/fmed.2024.1476242. PMID: 39540046; PMCID: PMC11558524.

(585) Bodeker KL, Smith BJ, Berg DJ, Chandrasekharan C, Sha-rif S, Fei N, Vollstedt S, Brown H, Chandler M, Lorack A, McMichael S, Wulfekuhle J, Wagner BA, Buettner GR, Allen BG, Caster JM, Dion B, Kamgar M, Buatti JM, Cullen JJ. A ran-domized trial of pharmacological ascorbate, gemcitabine, and nab-paclitaxel for metastatic pancreatic cancer. Redox Biol. 2024 Nov;77:103375. doi: 10.1016/j.redox.2024.103375. Epub 2024 Oct 2. PMID: 39369582; PMCID: PMC11491967.

(586) Wang F, He MM, Xiao J, Zhang YQ, Yuan XL, Fang WJ, Zhang Y, Wang W, Hu XH, Ma ZG, Yao YC, Zhuang ZX, Zhou FX, Ying JE, Yuan Y, Zou QF, Guo ZQ, Wu XY, Jin Y, Mai ZJ, Wang ZQ, Qiu H, Guo Y, Shi SM, Chen SZ, Luo HY, Zhang DS, Wang FH, Li YH, Xu RH. A Randomized, Open-Label, Multicenter, Phase 3 Study of High-Dose Vitamin C Plus FOLFOX ± Bevacizumab versus FOLFOX ± Bevacizumab in Unresectable Untreated Metastatic Colorectal Cancer (VITALITY Study). Clin Cancer Res. 2022 Oct 3;28(19):4232-4239. doi: 10.1158/1078-0432.CCR-22-0655. PMID: 35929990; PMCID: PMC9527503.

(587) Wang S, Lai F, Zhao L, Zhou J, Kong D, Yu H, Ding Y. As-sociation between vitamin C in serum and trouble sleeping based on NHANES 2017-2018. Sci Rep. 2024 Apr 27;14(1):9727. doi: 10.1038/s41598-024-56703-0. PMID: 38678062; PMCID: PMC11055852.

(588) Wang C, Zhao J, Zhou Q, Li J. Serum vitamin C levels and their correlation with chronic kidney disease in adults: a nationwide study. Ren Fail. 2024 Dec;46(1):2298079. doi: 10.1080/0886022X.2023.2298079. Epub 2024 Jan 8. PMID: 38186336; PMCID: PMC10776057.

(589) Bayu P, Wibisono JJ. Vitamin C and E antioxidant supple-mentation may significantly reduce pain symptoms in endometriosis: A systematic review and meta-analysis of randomized controlled trials. PLoS One. 2024 May 31;19(5):e0301867. doi: 10.1371/journal.pone.0301867. PMID: 38820340; PMCID: PMC11142610.

(590) Ranjbar Moghaddam M, Nasiri-Formi E, Merajikhah A. Efficacy of vitamin C supplementation in preventing and treating complex regional pain syndrome type I (CRPS-I) in Orthopedic patients: A systematic review and meta-

analysis. Int J Orthop Trauma Nurs. 2024 Nov;55:101140. doi: 10.1016/j.ijotn.2024.101140. Epub 2024 Oct 18. PMID: 39447383.

(591) Athanasiou A, Charalambous M, Anastasiou T, Aggeli K, Soteri-ades ES. Preoperative and postoperative administration of vitamin C in cardiac surgery patients - settings, dosages, duration, and clinical outcomes: a narrative review. Ann Med Surg (Lond). 2024 Apr 29;86(6):3591-3607. doi: 10.1097/MS9.0000000000002112. PMID: 38846824; PMCID: PMC11152825.

(592) Sun L, Zhao JH, Fan WY, Feng B, Liu WW, Chen RQ, Ban C, Dang AG, Wang M, Luo KT, Zhou GY, Yu FF, Ba Y. Therapeutic effects of high-dose vitamin C supplementation in patients with COVID-19: a meta-analysis. Nutr Rev. 2024 Aug 1;82(8):1056-1068. doi: 10.1093/nutrit/nuad105. PMID: 37682265.

(593) Kow CS, Hasan SS, Ramachandram DS. The effect of vitamin C on the risk of mortality in patients with COVID-19: a systematic review and meta-analysis of randomized controlled trials. Inflammopharmacology. 2023 Dec;31(6):3357-3362. doi: 10.1007/s10787-023-01200-5. Epub 2023 Apr 18. PMID: 37071316; PMCID: PMC10111321.

(594) Zhou L, Liu J, Zhou M. A comprehensive meta-analysis on the association between vitamin C intake and gestational diabetes mellitus: Insights and novel perspectives. Medicine (Baltimore). 2023 Aug 11;102(32):e34740. doi: 10.1097/MD.0000000000034740. PMID: 37565861; PMCID: PMC10419659.

(595) Lu CP, Dijk SW, Pandit A, Kranenburg L, Luik AI, Hu-nink MGM. The effect of mindfulness-based interventions on reducing stress in future health professionals: A systematic review and meta-analysis of randomized controlled trials. Appl Psychol Health Well Being. 2024 May;16(2):765-792. doi: 10.1111/aphw.12472. Epub 2023 Aug 1. PMID: 37527644.

(596) Golder JE, Bauer JD, Barker LA, Lemoh CN, Gibson SJ, Da-vidson ZE. Prevalence, risk factors, and clinical outcomes of vitamin C deficiency in adult hospitalized patients in high-income countries: a scoping review. Nutr Rev. 2024 Nov 1;82(11):1605-1621. doi: 10.1093/nutrit/nuad157. PMID: 38219216; PMCID: PMC11465154.

(597) Abu-Zaid A, Alrashidi H, Almouh A, Abualsaud ZM, Saleh AM, Aldawsari SB, Alajmi MM, Alomar O. Ascorbic Acid for Prevention of Intraoperative Blood Loss and Related Complications During Myomectomy: A Systematic Review and Meta-Analysis of Randomized Controlled Trials. Cureus. 2022 Nov 16;14(11):e31571. doi: 10.7759/cureus.31571. PMID: 36540502; PMCID: PMC9756975.

(598) Dai Y, Zhou J, Shi C. Inflammasome: structure, biological functions, and therapeutic targets. MedComm (2020). 2023 Oct 9;4(5):e391. doi: 10.1002/mco2.391. PMID: 37817895; PMCID: PMC10560975.

John Woodall. The Surgeons' Mate; London: Dawsons of Pall Mall, 1978

James Lind. A Treatise of the Scurvy, in Three Parts: Containing An Inquiry Into The Nature, Causes, And Cure, Of That Disease; Cambridge University Press (27 dicembre 2022)

Irwin Stone. The Healing Factor: Vitamin C Against Disease; New York: Grosset & Dunlap, 1972

Linus Pauling. Vitamin C and the Common Cold; W.H.Freeman & Co Ltd, 1970

Linus Pauling. How to Live Longer and Feel Better; New York: W. H. Freeman, 1986

Abram Hoffer e Linus Pauling. Vitamin C and Cancer: Discovery, Recovery, Controversy; Quarry Press, 2000

Norman Cousins. Anatomy of an Illness as Perceived by the Patient; W. W. Norton & Company

Made in United States
Orlando, FL
04 November 2026

90200182R00249